循证医学基础（双语）

Essentials for Evidence-based Medicine（Bilingual）

主　编　　　　　　陈世耀　　　　刘天舒
Chief Editor　　　Chen Shiyao　　Liu Tianshu

副主编　　　　　　吴尚洁
Vice Chief Editor　Wu Shangjie

人民卫生出版社
·北京·

图书在版编目（CIP）数据

循证医学基础：汉英对照 / 陈世耀，刘天舒主编
. —北京：人民卫生出版社，2022.11
ISBN 978-7-117-33817-2

Ⅰ. ①循… Ⅱ. ①陈… ②刘… Ⅲ. ①循证医学－高
等学校－教材－汉、英 Ⅳ. ①R499

中国版本图书馆 CIP 数据核字（2022）第 195724 号

人卫智网	www.ipmph.com	医学教育、学术、考试、健康， 购书智慧智能综合服务平台
人卫官网	www.pmph.com	人卫官方资讯发布平台

循证医学基础（双语）
Xunzheng Yixue Jichu（Shuangyu）

主　　编：陈世耀　刘天舒
出版发行：人民卫生出版社（中继线 010-59780011）
地　　址：北京市朝阳区潘家园南里 19 号
邮　　编：100021
E - mail：pmph @ pmph.com
购书热线：010-59787592　010-59787584　010-65264830
印　　刷：三河市国英印务有限公司
经　　销：新华书店
开　　本：787×1092　1/16　印张：26
字　　数：649 千字
版　　次：2022 年 11 月第 1 版
印　　次：2022 年 11 月第 1 次印刷
标准书号：ISBN 978-7-117-33817-2
定　　价：86.00 元

打击盗版举报电话：010-59787491　E-mail：WQ @ pmph.com
质量问题联系电话：010-59787234　E-mail：zhiliang @ pmph.com
数字融合服务电话：4001118166　E-mail：zengzhi @ pmph.com

编　委

（以姓氏笔画为序）

马莉莉　　　　　复旦大学附属中山医院
Ma Lili　　　　Zhongshan Hospital of Fudan University
让蔚清　　　　　南华大学公共卫生学院
Rang Weiqing　School of Public Health of University of South China
吕敏之　　　　　复旦大学循证医学中心
Lü Minzhi　　　Center for Evidence-based Medicine of Fudan University
刘广芝　　　　　河南省人民医院
Liu Guangzhi　Henan Provincial People's Hospital
刘天舒　　　　　复旦大学附属中山医院
Liu Tianshu　　Zhongshan Hospital of Fudan University
刘学东　　　　　空军军医大学西京医院
Liu Xuedong　Xijing Hospital of Air Force Medical University
刘晓清　　　　　北京协和医院
Liu Xiaoqing　Peking Union Medical College Hospital
许良智　　　　　四川大学华西第二医院
Xu Liangzhi　West China Second University Hospital of Sichuan University
孙良丹　　　　　安徽医科大学第一附属医院
Sun Liangdan　The First Affiliated Hospital of Anhui Medical University
李亚斐　　　　　陆军军医大学
Li Yafei　　　Army Medical University
李春波　　　　　上海市精神卫生中心
Li Chunbo　　Shanghai Mental Health Center
吴尚洁　　　　　中南大学湘雅二医院
Wu Shangjie　The Second Xiangya Hospital of Central South University
陈世耀　　　　　复旦大学附属中山医院
Chen Shiyao　Zhongshan Hospital of Fudan University
赵亚双　　　　　哈尔滨医科大学
Zhao Yashuang　Harbin Medical University
袁源智　　　　　复旦大学附属中山医院

全国高等学校循证医学类教材编写委员会

（全国高等医药教材建设研究会·人民卫生出版社）

顾　　问：王吉耀（复旦大学）　唐金陵（香港中文大学）

主任委员：詹思延（北京大学）

副主任委员

　　　　　杨克虎（兰州大学）

　　　　　陈世耀（复旦大学）

　　　　　刘建平（北京中医药大学）

　　　　　刘　鸣（四川大学华西医院）

常务委员（以姓氏笔画为序）

　　　　　王小钦　复旦大学附属华山医院

　　　　　王聪霞　西安交通大学医学部

　　　　　文　进　四川大学华西医院

　　　　　方向华　首都医科大学宣武医院

　　　　　田金徽　兰州大学循证医学中心

　　　　　刘天舒　复旦大学附属中山医院

　　　　　孙　凤　北京大学公共卫生学院

　　　　　吴大嵘　广州中医药大学

　　　　　吴尚洁　中南大学湘雅二医院

　　　　　邸阜生　天津市第三中心医院

　　　　　陈英耀　复旦大学公共卫生学院

　　　　　陈耀龙　兰州大学循证医学中心

　　　　　胡　虹　重庆医科大学

　　　　　姜林娣　复旦大学附属中山医院

　　　　　费宇彤　北京中医药大学

　　　　　徐佩茹　新疆医科大学第一附属医院

　　　　　商洪才　北京中医药大学东直门医院

　　　　　彭晓霞　首都医科大学附属北京儿童医院

秘　　书：孙　凤　北京大学公共卫生学院

全国高等学校循证医学类教材目录

1. 循证医学基础（双语）

2. 循证医学证据检索与评估

3. 系统综述与Meta分析

4. 循证临床实践及案例分析

5. 循证医疗卫生决策与管理

6. 循证医学与临床研究

7. 循证临床实践指南的制定与实施

8. 循证中医药

9. 循证医学回顾、现状和展望（双语）

前　言

　　循证医学是一种理念，强调临床医师在临床实践过程中，依据最新、最佳证据，结合实践经验、患者的意愿和价值观做出科学合理的决策。循证医学体现在处理患者的临床实践过程中，从提出临床问题开始，通过文献检索、文献评价、收集证据、评价证据，在充分评估实践条件和患者状态的基础上，进行证据的临床应用和患者的跟踪随访，完成循证实践的全过程。循证医学的核心是证据评价。最新、最佳证据的评价依据包括科学性、结果效应值以及是否适合患者三个维度。

　　在医学科技和人工智能辅助临床决策飞速发展的今天，遵循循证医学理念，充分考虑患者的意愿，联合科学研究中的最新、最佳证据为患者做出诊疗决策，是推动临床医学进步的关键。精准医学的本质是个体化的循证实践。根据每个患者的特点，权衡获益风险比，批判性地应用研究结果和指南，也是精准医学发展的方向。

　　《循证医学基础》旨在为医学生和临床医生提供一本简明扼要的循证医学教材，引导其形成批判性的文献阅读思维和个体化循证临床决策思维。

　　全书系统阐述了循证医学理念：第一层，按照证据收集、证据评价、证据应用的思路，提出临床问题并且转化为科学问题；第二层，从病因问题、诊断评价、治疗选择、预后评估、预防与筛查、不良反应等原始研究设计出发，通过案例进行了证据评价示范；第三层，同时介绍系统综述、临床指南、经济学分析与决策分析等二次研究证据的评价与应用。希望读者通过学习、掌握循证医学基本方法，更好地开展临床实践、服务患者。同时，我们希望循证医学回归初心。临床医师通过使用最新的证据以及制定的规范指南，确保循证实践，考虑并尊重患者的价值观，协助卫生政策的制定与发展，推动循证医学的发展和临床医学的进步。

　　全书采用中英文双语对照，作为国内临床医学双语教学（MBBS）的循证医学课程教材。书末配有两套模拟试卷，也是教学内容的核心，有利于对基本概念的深入理解。全书章节经过多轮专家互审与修改，力图简洁清晰。感谢复旦大学外国语言文学学院蔡和兵老师对英文进行了逐字逐句的修改，感谢复旦大学循证医学中心张宁萍、复旦大学附属华山医院曾于珍对部分章节提出了修改意见。

　　本书的出版得到 2020 年上海高校本科重点教改项目——"用循证医学理念推进医学生临床实践教学体系建设"的支持，本书涉及的概念在教改课程中进行了尝试，并通过学生反馈进行了反复修改。

　　由于水平限制，时间仓促，难免有不尽完善之处，恳请广大读者不吝赐教。

陈世耀

2022 年 10 月

Preface

Evidence-based medicine is a concept that emphasizes clinicians make scientific and reasonable decisions based on the latest and best evidence, along with practical experience and patients' wishes and values in the process of clinical practice. Evidence-based medicine is embodied in the clinical practice of treating patients. It starts from asking clinical questions, collecting evidence to evaluating evidence through literature search and literature evaluation; then applies evidence and follows up to complete the whole process of evidence-based practice on the basis of fully evaluating clinical conditions and patient status. The core of evidence-based medicine is evidence evaluation. The basis for evaluating the latest and best evidence includes three dimensions: scientificity, effect of results, and suitability for patients.

With rapid development of clinical decision-making assisted by medical technology and artificial intelligence, the key to advancing clinical medicine is the combination of following the concept of evidence-based medicine, taking full consideration of patients' wishes and utilizing the latest and best evidence in scientific researches to make diagnosis and treatment decisions. The essence of precision medicine is individualized evidence-based practice. Weighing the benefit-risk ratio and critically applying research results and guidelines according to the characteristics of each patient are also the advancing direction of precision medicine.

Essentials for Evidence-based Medicine aims to provide medical students and clinicians with a concise textbook of evidence-based medicine, guiding the formation of critical thinking for literature reading and individualized evidence-based clinical decision-making.

The whole book systematically expounds the concept of evidence-based medicine as follows: first, asking clinical questions and transforming them into scientific questions according to the ideas of evidence collection, evaluation and application; second, demonstrating evidence evaluation through cases on the basis of original research designs involving etiological problems, diagnostic evaluation, treatment selection, prognostic evaluation, prevention, screening and adverse reactions; third, introducing the evaluation and application of secondary research evidence such as systematic reviews, clinical guidelines, economic analysis and decision analysis. We expect to better carry out clinical practice and serve patients through learning and mastering the basic methods of evidence-based medicine. At the same time, we hope that evidence-based medicine returns to its original intention. With clinical evidence-based practice of utilizing the latest evidence and standardizing the formulation of guidelines, clinicians who consider and respect patients' wishes and values can assist in the formulation of health policies, contribute to the development of evidence-based medicine and promote the progression of clinical medicine.

The whole book is bilingual in Chinese and English which can be used as a teaching material for domestic MBBS evidence-based medicine courses. There are two quizzes which are also the core of the teaching content, and are conducive to in-depth understanding of basic concepts. All chapters have undergone multiple rounds of mutual review and revision by experts, intended to be concise and clear. I would like to appreciate Mr. Cai Hebing from the College of Foreign Languages and Literature, Fudan University for making word-for-word revision of the context. Thanks to Zhang Ningping from Evidence-Based Medicine Center, Fudan University and Zeng Yuzhen from Huashan Hospital, Fudan University for proposing amendments to some chapters.

This book is supported by the 2020 Key Education Reform Project for Undergraduates in Shanghai Universities — promoting the construction of the teaching system of medical students' clinical practice with the concept of evidence-based medicine. The concepts have been tested in the teaching reform course and have been repeatedly revised through feedback from students.

Since it is inevitable that there are many imperfections due to limited knowledge and time constraints, I sincerely ask readers for advice and communication.

Chen Shiyao
October 2022

目　录

Contents

第一章

循证医学概论

学习目标

1. **掌握** 循证医学基本理念、循证医学实践过程、临床决策个体化的意义和影响因素。
2. **熟悉** 个体化权衡证据应用的利弊。
3. **了解** 利用相关工具进行个体化实践的方法。

第一节 循证医学的基本理念

循证医学（evidence-based medicine）即遵循证据的临床医学，是临床流行病学理论和方法学在临床医疗实践中的具体应用。其核心思想是：在充分考虑患者意愿的条件下，医务人员严谨地、规范地、全面地运用在科学研究中得到的最新、最佳的证据（evidence）来诊治患者。循证医学这一概念最早由萨克特（Sackett）和他的同事提出，属于一种医学新理念，是将最佳证据、医师的临床经验、患者的价值观三者结合起来，对患者开展最有利的临床决策。1991 年，循证医学创始人之一戈登·盖亚特（Gordon Guyatt）博士首次提出"evidence-based medicine"，Cochrane 系统评价和 Cochrane 协作网随之诞生，随着专家共识和临床实践指南的普遍推荐，遵循循证医学理念进行临床决策不断增多，并逐渐成为规范。随着现代医疗的发展，信息增加、技术创新，临床医师面临着诸多挑战，如何选择适宜的诊断方法？如何为患者提供最安全、经济和有效的治疗方法？如何对患者进行最精确的预后估计？概括地说，就是如何获取临床研究结果并在科学评价之后循证实践，更好地服务患者，是循证医学的核心任务。

循证医学旨在整合多个证据综合形成解决临床问题的策略，通过对发病危险因素的分析，认识疾病的发生发展；通过对疾病的早期诊断的分析，提高诊断的准确性；通过对疾病的治疗方法的分析，选择合理有效的治疗方案；通过对疾病预后的分析，改善患者预后和生存质量；通过对临床用药的分析，促进卫生管理和科学决策。

2006 年，戈登·盖亚特（Gordon Guyatt）提出循证医学发展的五个方向，今天仍然有指导意义。

1. 把握最新的循证医学资源 在信息化的时代，临床医生面临的挑战是如何在最短的时间内为每个患者制订最佳的诊疗方案。最佳循证实践资源如同洋葱，一层一层包裹着。有些病例，医师只需要根据指南中的推荐意见进行诊疗，有些病例却需要医师深入一层去判断推荐意见的强弱程度,当推荐意见强度很低时,医师还需要了解更深一层信息,查看相关证据并对证据进行系统评价。同时,尽管有指南推荐,有 UpToDate、Clinical Evidence 等整合的电子资源推荐,通过简单地点击鼠标即可看到里面一层的信息,但新的证据不断出现并替代原有信息,临床医学更需要把握前沿,人工智能(AI)可能是一种解决途径,但仍需要个体化应用到患者。

2. 规范循证指南的制定　循证实践致力于颠覆临床医生历来习惯依靠专家指导意见的观念,赋予了临床医师在理解和应用证据时前所未有的自主性。循证实践指南需要专家按照规范制定。指南的制定过程包括:明确的临床问题、系统的文献检索与评价、证据的等级评定与指南条目的推荐意见。按照 GRADE 标准制定指南已成为共识,指南制定还需要结合地方政策与人群特征,指南评价通常采用临床指南研究与评估系统Ⅱ(AGREE Ⅱ)进行质量评价。

3. 确保循证实施　尽管循证指南促进临床诊疗进入新时代,然而,指南本身并不能确保临床诊疗规范。如何让临床医师在临床实践中使用高质量的证据成为每个国家都应该关注的问题,也是循证医学实际应用时面临的问题。

4. 确保临床决策符合患者价值观且乐于接受　循证医学的第三个要素是充分考虑患者的价值观和意愿。面临同样的医学问题,不同的患者可能有不同的决策,与其宗教信仰、生活环境、生活方式息息相关。

5. 卫生政策中引入循证原则　循证原理用于卫生政策研究中,结合卫生技术评估和成本 - 效益分析,协助卫生政策的制定和发展。

第二节　证据与证据评价

证据包括基础研究证据、临床研究证据、群体研究证据。临床实践中,循证医学更加关注来自临床、以患者为研究对象的临床研究证据。

按照临床研究的类型,证据包括原始研究报告,比如病例报告、病例对照研究、队列研究、随机对照临床试验等,还包括二次研究证据,比如系统综述(systemic review)与荟萃分析(meta-analysis)、临床指南、基于数据库的临床研究等。临床医师的实践经验也是一种循证医学证据,单纯的临床实践经验证据级别很弱,但结合文献结果与临床实践经验结合往往比文献本身的证据级别更高。

证据可以通过文献检索获得,有一系列文献检索的策略协助临床医师快速获取需要的证据,但数量庞大,评价需要更多时间和能力。简便的办法是直接寻找最新的临床实践指南、指南之后发表的系统综述、系统综述之后发表的原始研究,这一策略不仅省略了对指南与系统综述纳入的大量文献的评价,更可以获得最新的临床研究结果。

无论原始研究或者二次研究获得的证据应用于循证临床实践都需要进行评价。证据的评价标准有发表标准和应用标准,临床实践更关注应用标准:比如诊断试验评价,更关注研究中是否同时接受了金标准与待评价的诊断试验,并是否进行了盲法比较;比如干预研究,更关注研究中是否设置对照,有无随机分组与随机化隐藏,结果测量是否采用盲法或者重复测量;比如预后研究,更关注比较生存分析的两组队列是否有相同的起点,结局设置是否合理并通过客观的标准手段测量,是否失访,是否混杂因素影响预后等。

证据级别或者强弱的划分依据临床研究类型,以及样本量和人群代表性等多种因素。

临床决策中通常不仅依据一项研究结果所提供的证据，而是依据多种途径（基础研究、临床与人群研究）、多种研究类型（病例对照、队列研究、随机对照临床试验、基于真实数据进行的研究、meta 分析研究等）组成的证据体。

第三节 循证实践过程

循证临床实践强调：无论是诊断、治疗还是预防，都需要遵循证据，将经过评估、适合患者的最新、最佳证据推荐给患者。

循证实践过程通常包括以下五个步骤。

1. 提出一个需要回答的临床问题，并将其转化为科学问题，这是成功回答临床争议问题最关键的一步。比如，一位 40 岁男性患者，通过胃镜和病理诊断其患有早期胃癌，超声胃镜显示胃癌位于黏膜层，如何治疗是一般的问题，特殊问题是：对这例患者，采用内镜黏膜剥离术治疗还是腹腔镜手术切除治疗？转化为科学问题就是：内镜黏膜剥离术治疗能否替代腹腔镜手术切除治疗？

2. 寻找有效的证据：通过检索医学文献数据库，获得最佳的证据。简单的办法是查阅相关的指南推荐，进一步评价指南推荐条目后面的证据与证据级别，指南更新比较慢，可以检索指南纳入的证据时间点之后发表的最新文献结果并通过评价进行引用。

3. 批判性地评价证据的有效性和科学性。不仅原始研究需要评价，指南也需要评价。尽管不同的研究设计类型有不同的评价标准，但证据评价都需要考虑科学性、证据效应值以及适用人群的范围。

4. 比较文献中的人群特征与当前需要处理的患者特征，结合临床医生的个人临床经验、所在地区或者单位的医疗条件，做出临床处理决策。在应用证据时，需要结合评价判断偏倚，以及偏倚对结果效应值大小的影响，提出合理的决策预期。

5. 评估处理结果，包括短期或者长期结果，如果失败或者没有获得期望的结果，重新考虑临床问题并进行再次循证实践过程。

循证实践过程首先需要提出临床问题。阅读综述可以了解一般临床问题的处理进展，循证实践需要将临床上患者面临的矛盾转化为具体可以回答的科学问题，也就是将一般的临床问题转化为特定的科学问题的过程。这个过程遵循 PICO 原则。

（1）P：环境、患者和 / 或疾病状况（population, patient and/or problem）。首先，确定好需要你解决问题的患者的特征，也是证据的研究人群和目标应用人群。

（2）I：治疗干预（intervention）或者暴露（exposure）。思考要采取的措施，对于治疗方法，可以是一种药物或者一项干预措施；对于诊断方法，可以是一项检查或筛查项目；对于病因分析，可以是一种暴露因素。对干预措施或暴露特点了解越充分，判断越全面。

（3）C：对照（comparison）。与不施行这项措施比较，如果不施行这项措施结果会怎样？措施不同，结果不同。

（4）O：临床的结局（outcome）。明确所关注的临床结局。结局可以是直接的，比如止血；也可以是最终的，比如生存与死亡；还可以是中间结果或者替代终点，比如血清学指标、影像显示的疾病程度变化等。对于严重的疾病，关注的重点是生存与死亡；对于慢性疾病，关注的重点是它的并发症。

提出临床问题时，正确判断问题的类型有助于更好地找到答案。包括对症状和体征的解释、病因、诊断、治疗、预后、生命质量、成本-效果等问题。

使用任何证据前，必须对证据进行严格的评价。最佳证据应具有真实性、重要性和适用性三大特征。将证据用于解决患者问题时，必须将获得的证据与患者充分沟通后，了解并尊重患者的意愿，在患者理解和同意的基础上实施。临床实践应当考虑患者及其家庭、社会的实际状况、医疗服务提供者、医疗费用支付者的能力。对于需要长期治疗或观察的疾病，不但要考虑近期的成本-效果、成本-效用情况，还要考虑中长期的疾病治疗负担和预后情况，此时，医师应该提供足够的各方面证据信息，与患者进行良好的沟通，共同做出最佳的临床决策。

循证医学提倡将临床医生个人的临床实践经验与最佳的临床证据结合起来，为患者的诊治做出最优决策，这是一个医生必须具备的基本条件。忽视临床实践经验的医生即使得到了最好的证据也有可能用错，因为最好的临床证据在用于每一个具体患者时，必须因人而异，结合具体患者的临床特征与状态进行取舍。如果缺乏最好、最新的外部证据，临床医生可能应用已经过时的旧方法，无法给患者带来最优决策，甚至造成损害。当下，循证医学倡导有根据地对患者进行医疗服务，将医学研究最新、最佳结果用于临床实践的做法已被广大医务人员和患者所接受，在医学生和年轻医师中传承循证医学理念成为必然。

第四节　循证医学与精准医学

循证实践是从一般到个体的决策过程，将普遍理论应用于个体时，需要考量的因素包括生物学、病理生理学、社会心理因素及经济因素等。循证临床实践是遵循证据的实践，证据来源于临床医学实践和各种研究，代表的是群体。从理论到实践，是从总体到样本、从普遍到个体的过程，是一个推广应用的过程。要正确完成这个从证据到个体实施的过程，首先需要有真实的证据，还需要将证据正确地应用于个体，否则不但不能给患者提供最合适的诊疗方案，甚至还会给患者带来伤害，与循证医学的原则背道而驰。在循证医学实践中，一个误区是只关注证据，不关注证据的科学性和真实性；另一个误区是，只要有科学性和真实性的证据，就不顾一切地推荐或应用于所有患者，而忽视证据的可适用性以及相关的因素对于实践的影响，特别是患者的具体情况和价值观。因此，在循证医学实践中，如何结合每个患者的个体特征、需求和价值观，并正确推理、个体化应用，是至关重要的。

个体化处理是临床医生针对患者具体疾病采取最适合该患者的诊疗过程，是医生将自己的临床经验、现有的研究证据和患者疾病本身的病理生理状况的结合，再结合患者的意愿做出临床决策的过程。循证医学重视临床经验，反对仅依靠经验而忽略最新的可靠证据。随机对照临床研究证据由于其严格的入选标准和理想的治疗环境令其研究结果在运用到实际情况时受到质疑。如何将证据和临床经验结合在个体化处理中尤其重要。研究结果用于患者能否取得预期结果是临床医生最关注的问题。

生物学特征和社会经济学状态影响个体治疗的疗效，包括生物学特征、性别、伴发疾病、种族、年龄和疾病的病理特点。临床医师将随机对照临床研究的结果用于个体时，应充分考虑以上几个因素。

个体化处理需要考虑干预措施实施的获益、风险与依从性。

1. 能否把该方案用于某一患者　当患者的生物学特征不适用于该治疗方案时，医生应该根据其所处的社会环境改变综合考虑治疗的有效性和安全性，同时考虑患者对治疗方案的依从性。通常临床研究纳入的患者依从性远远高于日常诊疗中的患者。例如对于高血压的控制，依从性不同的患者获得的治疗有效性完全不同。还需要考虑临床医师胜任该治疗方案的能力，尤其在包括外科手术、介入治疗等在内的有创操作与手术的措施。治疗方案的选择还应该依据医生所在的医院的医疗条件和自身的能力，如果医院不具备该最优治疗条件或者医师不具备进行该操作的资质，应该选择二线治疗方案，以患者的安全为首要考虑因素。

2. 患者获益是否大于风险　医生能否对门诊患者很好地进行管理也是选择治疗方案应该考虑的因素。接受抗凝治疗的患者应该门诊随访 INR 值，然而，一些患者由于经济的原因或路途遥远等原因不能按时随访，会增加出血的风险。此时，作为医生，应该谨慎考虑是否对患者进行抗凝治疗以及抗凝治疗的具体方案。

3. 考虑分层与亚组　提供分层或者亚组分析证据是治疗决策个体化的前提。比如，一项临床研究对血清胆固醇升高的人群是否需要降血脂治疗进行了随机对照临床研究，纳入了 30～70 岁血清胆固醇升高的患者，研究结果显示，使用他汀类药物降血脂可以显著降低其心血管死亡事件发生的风险。此时，门诊来了一名 32 岁的女性患者，体检发现血清胆固醇升高，血压 110/70mmHg，没有家族糖尿病与心脏病病史，接诊医生是否要给她进行降血脂的药物治疗呢？随后，又进来一名 69 岁的男性患者，40 年吸烟史，血清胆固醇轻微升高，血压 140/85mmHg，他的母亲因为心脏病 20 年前去世，此时，接诊医生又该怎么做？很明显，这两名患者分别属于心血管死亡事件发生的低风险组和高风险组。如果仅凭一个随机对照试验的结论对他们进行相同的降血脂治疗，对那名年轻女性的作用可能仅仅是将原来 2% 的风险降为 1%，而对后面这名老年男性则是将心血管事件的风险从 40% 降到了 10%。对于前者，更推荐通过饮食、运动等健康生活方式的指导达到降血脂治疗效果，而后者除了健康生活方式指导之外，药物治疗更加迫切。

4. 结合患者的价值观和意愿考虑　充分考虑患者的价值观，尊重患者的选择是临床决策的决定因素。情况完全相同的两名患者在充分了解自己的疾病和治疗现状后，可能做出完全不同的决策。例如，服用阿司匹林可以预防脑栓塞但是却增加消化道出血的风险，大部分医生选择不使用阿司匹林，而大部分患者却选择继续服用阿司匹林，因为他们无法接受脑栓塞对自己生活质量的影响。

利用循证医学工具评估特定的疾病或状态，实施个体化循证决策是一个发展方向。UpToDate 等许多医学网站甚至手机应用程序均有针对各个疾病状态开发的评分工具，提供了各类疾病风险模型预测的个体化治疗依据。这些评分模型是根据已发表的最新循证医学证据，不断更新和修改的，可以通过输入患者个体化的资料，得到这一患者的风险评分，指导临床医师进行临床决策，制订诊疗方案，给临床工作带来了极大的便利。

以终末期肝病模型（model for end-stage liver disease，MELD）为例，2000 年马林乔克（Malinchoc）等为了预测经颈静脉肝内门腔内支架分流术（TIPSS）术后患者的生存时间和预后，提出了这一评估模型。其危险度评分如下：R=0.957×ln（血清肌酐浓度）+0.378× ln（血清胆红素浓度）+1.120×ln（INR）+0.643×（肝硬化的原因：酒精性、胆汁淤积性为 0，其余为1），比如一个丙肝肝硬化患者，血清肌酐 1.9mg/dl，血清胆红素 4.2mg/dl，INR1.2，则其风险评分计算如下：R =0.957×ln1.9+0.378×ln4.2+1.120×ln1.2+0.643×1=2.003。卡马斯（Kamath）为了方便应用，将上述公式计算所得分值乘以 10，结果四舍五入为最接近的整数，即风险评分为 20。随后，他对此进行回顾前瞻性研究，证明 MELD 模型可普遍用于预测进展期肝病患者的预后。根据患者的各项指标可预测慢性肝病患者的预后，帮助医生评估病情，决定治疗手段和治疗时间。更新的研究发现，血清钠是早期预测肝肾综合征的独立预测因子，同时也反映了肝硬化的门静脉高压并发症的影响，并提出了改良的 MELD 评分系统，MELDNa 模型，即 MESO，MESO=MELD/SNa×10。随着临床研究证据增多，不断对现有评分系统进行修改与完善，这是循证决策个体化的基础，更是循证医学的前进方向。

精准医学最早在肿瘤研究中提出，针对肿瘤分子分型与特点开发靶向药物治疗。精准医学是循证医学个体化理念在肿瘤领域针对分子分型进行决策的具体应用。当前，在肿瘤分子诊断与靶向药物开发、评价以及临床应用中，同样需要遵循循证医学理念：一是针对肿瘤患者的处理仍然需要强调一般生物学特征与社会经济学特征；二是强调肿瘤患者的分子靶标同样需要循证医学证据，尤其是大样本、多中心、针对不同肿瘤、不同肿瘤患者状态的随机对照临床研究。每一个肿瘤分子标志物，可以理解为疾病的一种临床病理状态。

第五节　走出循证医学误区

循证医学是一种理念，强调临床决策依据最佳证据、临床医生的经验、患者的意愿与价值观。无论是病例报告、队列研究或者随机对照临床试验，或者 meta 分析、指南等，都是证据。开展原始研究、meta 分析等二次研究，制定指南，利用数据库发表论文等，都是为循证医学提供证据，但其不是循证医学的本质。

循证医学强调证据，更强调证据评价。循证医学理念贯穿在临床实践的全过程中，从提出临床问题到转换为科学问题，到文献检索、证据评价、应用证据解决临床问题与后效评价，五步骤体现了循证实践的全过程，科学评价证据与个体化处理患者是循证医学临床实践的精髓，患者的结局是检验循证实践过程的最终标准。

误区一：大量低质量 meta 分析、网状 meta 分析成为循证医学证据，被错误推荐。meta 分析是一种二次研究方法，选题针对临床有争议的问题，如报道阳性或者阴性结果不一，为了评估不同研究的结果效应。meta 分析结果可以扩大样本量，增加人群代表性，可以在 Cochrane 网络注册，接受方法学指导。过程管理包括组建 meta 分析团队、系统检索与评价、按照写作与发表标准发表，尤其重要的是，meta 分析的科学解读与应用。

meta 分析质量是当前面临的一个问题，尤其是原始研究来源的质量。过度利用和解读 meta 分析结果是另一个问题。

首先，meta 分析需要一个团队，至少包括临床专家、方法专家、具体实施文献检索与评价的 2 名研究者。临床专家负责：选题、文献纳入的患者标准、文献结果的选择、研究结果的解释；方法专家负责：文献检索策略、文献评价标准、数据合成、结果呈现。其次，系统文献检索和科学文献质量评价是重点。方法学正确与否直接影响结果，高质量的文献是高质量的 meta 分析的基础。第三，采用规范的标准格式发表 meta 分析结果。如果不适合数据整合，尤其是低质量原始研究数据，应该选择系统综述而不是 meta 分析。避免低质量 meta 分析结果被错误利用。

误区二：指南依赖。尤其是与产品等利用相关的指南推荐。一是指南在制定时收到利益相关方的支持，制定过程出现问题；二是指南推荐被商家利用或者错误解读。指南是专家组系统制定的文件，帮助临床医生和患者根据特定的临床情况做出恰当决策的指导意见。

指南能规范医务人员的诊疗行为、提高医疗服务质量、节约医疗费用、提示未来临床研究的方向。

指南制定的过程包括：确定指南拟解决问题的重要性及制定指南的必要性和适应范围；成立专门小组，确立制定指南的规范程序；全面收集资料，系统分析，对证据分级；依据对证据的客观评价结果，提出推荐意见和推荐强度；组织小组以外的专家对指南评审、修改；发布指南，定期更新。

指南同样需要质量评价，指南有明显的地域性和时效性。指南评价包括科学性或严谨性、有效性或安全性、经济性、可用性或可行性、利益冲突等条目。指南应该可以通过AGREE Ⅱ标准评价。

实践循证医学指南同时需要突破自我，不断出现的新的证据为指南更新提供了基础，不断出现的新的临床问题也是开展临床研究的动力。

第六节 循证医学在中国的发展与挑战

我国从20世纪80年代引进了临床流行病学，在卫生部和世界银行资助下派出了一批临床医师到美国、加拿大、澳大利亚临床流行病中心学习，并成为国际临床流行病学网（INCLEN）成员单位。此批医师回国后，先后自1986年起在各院校本科生和研究生中开设了临床流行病学课程。原上海医科大学和华西医科大学分别获批成为我国的临床流行病学地区与资源培训中心（R-CERTC）。在INCLEN支持下，以双语教学的模式培养了大批临床流行病学骨干，现在已经成为全国的循证医学骨干。

1996年王吉耀教授首次将"evidence-based medicine"翻译为循证医学。2002年王吉耀教授主编《循证医学与临床实践》，是国内第一本系统介绍循证医学与临床实践的专著。中华医学会临床流行病学和循证医学分会进一步推动了循证医学在国内的发展。循证医学学科的发展，在国内经历从单一学科专家参与，到以解决临床问题为核心、多学科合作、有机整合的专业化团队。以四川大学华西医学中心、兰州大学等为代表的循证医学中心，方法学专家为主导，更强调循证医学的方法学建设与拓展；以复旦大学上海医学院、北京协和医学院等为代表的循证医学中心，临床专家为主导，更关注循证医学理念在临床实践与科学研究中的推广应用与评价。

循证医学是临床医学的基础学科，掌握循证医学方法才能更好地开展临床实践，服务患者，并不断提高自身的诊疗水平和能力。

本 章 小 结

循证医学通过综合最佳研究证据、医师临床经验和患者个人价值观，为最佳临床决策的制定提供可靠的依据。经过长期医学及公共卫生事业的发展，循证医学也逐步得到完善和改进，为个体化精准医疗实践创造可能性。

（陈世耀　刘天舒）

第二章

提出临床问题

学习目标

1. **掌握** 如何清晰地提出临床问题。
2. **熟悉** 临床问题的来源及种类。

做出决定及临床实践需要健康保健知识。首先需要提出恰当的、可回答的问题,这是实践循证医学的起点。下面将举例说明临床问题是如何产生及形成的。

例如,一位 58 岁的男性胃癌患者,接受了胃癌 D2 根治术,术后病理为腺癌,病灶累及浆膜,清扫的淋巴结共 32 枚,有 4 枚阳性淋巴结,切缘(−),病理分期为 pT3N1M0(ⅢA 期)。患者可能会询问以下问题:

1. 我为什么会得胃癌? →病因
2. 我手术后是否需要辅助化疗? →治疗
3. 我能活多久? →预后

据此,可以提出许多重要的临床问题,找到答案有助于更好地选择诊断或治疗手段。因此,构建一个好的问题是十分重要的。提出问题不但是查找证据的第一步,而且提出一个好的、可回答的临床问题本身就是循证医学实践的第一步。

第一节 临床问题的来源及分类

一、临床问题的来源

临床问题常常来源于临床实践。寻求重要问题的答案首先要求对基础知识有所掌握,明确已知和未知的部分。没有对目前知识的基本了解,很难知道下一步该如何进行。因此,临床医生应该随时保持好奇心,善于在临床实践中认真观察、发现问题并解决问题。

二、临床问题的分类

临床问题包括目标人群(例如:成人、儿童、急诊患者、长期治疗者等)、重要的干预措施、重要的结果等,并且可能有进行比较的内容(例如:比较标准治疗与可供选择的新治疗),以及临床经济学的影响等。形成临床问题时需要明确临床问题的类型。临床问题的类型将决定选择何种研究设计方法(表 2-1)。

表2-1　回答各类临床问题时推荐的研究类型

问题分类	研究类型
病因	随机对照试验＞队列研究＞病例对照研究
诊断	前瞻性、盲法与金标准进行比较
预后	队列研究＞病例对照研究
治疗	随机对照试验＞队列研究＞病例对照研究＞病例报告
预防	随机对照试验＞队列研究＞病例对照研究
经济效益	成本效益分析
生活质量	生活质量评估

注:＞这里指"优于"。

1. 病因　怎样判别患者可能的病因、危险因素?

2. 诊断　怎样基于精密度、准确度、可接受性、费用及安全性等因素来选择和解释诊断性试验,以便确定或排除某种诊断?(精确度包括精密度和准确度)

3. 治疗　怎样为患者选择利大于弊且价有所值的治疗方法?

4. 预后　怎样估计患者可能的结局和预测可能发生的并发症?

5. 预防　怎样通过识别和纠正危险因素来减少疾病的发生及通过筛查实现早期诊断疾病?

6. 经济效益　与其他干预措施相比,此项干预措施的经济效益如何?

7. 生活质量　干预措施带来的生活质量会是什么?

第二节　如何提出临床问题

一、临床问题的构建

构建良好的临床问题通常包括背景问题及前景问题两大部分。

提出可回答的问题能够帮助获得新的知识。发现新的及有用的问题的前提是需要对相关疾病有基本的了解。这些"背景"问题可以包括任何疾病或健康状态、治疗或干预、健康保健的其他方面、心理社会因素等。

1. 背景问题　关于疾病的一般常识问题,由以下两部分基本成分。

(1)疑问词(谁、什么、何时、哪里、怎样、为什么)＋动词。

(2)一种疾病或疾病的某个方面的问题,例如病因、检查、治疗或其他医疗保健等。

例如:我为什么会得胃癌?

2. 前景问题　主要关注与疾病直接相关的特殊知识,可包括生物的、心理的及社会性的问题。前景问题是对处理患者的特殊知识形成问题提供临床决策,由以下四个部分组成。

(1)患者及其所处的具体状态:思考你所诊治的患者,如何准确地描述患者的类型?尝试确定所有会影响问题的临床特征。有时,患者的年龄、性别或种族也会与诊断或治疗相关。

(2)干预措施:主要干预措施是什么?主要干预措施的定义很宽泛,包括暴露因素、诊断试验技术或方法、预后因素、治疗方法,等等。

（3）对照措施：相对于所研究的干预措施，其对比的主要措施是什么？可以为空白或者标准治疗。直接比较两者可以获得更多有用的证据。

（4）结局：希望得到什么？需要花时间弄清楚什么才是对你及患者较为重要的结局。

3. 临床问题构建举例

（1）问题1：（构建不好的问题）

胃癌患者术后是否需要**辅助化疗**？

患者类型　　　　干预措施

（2）问题2：（构建良好的问题）

辅助化疗与**不化疗**相比能使**胃癌患者（pT3N1M0）**的生存时间延长吗？

干预措施　　　　对照措施　　　　　患者类型　　　　临床结局

问题1缺乏对照措施及临床结局两个内容，且患者类型不清楚（缺乏术后分期）。问题2则包括了4个基本成分，是一个内容完整、比较清楚的临床问题。

临床医生既需要背景知识也需要前景知识，随着时间的推移及医生经验的积累，两者的比例也在发生变化（图2-1）。这取决于医生对某种疾病的经验。当医生经验较为缺乏时，如图2-1中的A点，医生的多数问题属于背景问题。当医生的责任和经验增加时，如图2-1中的B点，怎样正确处理患者的前景问题比例增大。当医生的经验继续增加至C点时，医生的多数问题是前景问题。图中斜线的位置提示医生永远既有背景问题，又有前景问题，只是不同时期两者比例不同。

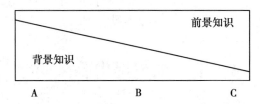

图2-1　背景知识和前景知识的比例随时间的推移及医生经验的积累而发生变化

A. 医生经验较少时，背景问题占较大比例；B. 随着经验增多，前景问题的比例增大；当医生的经验继续增加至C点时，医生的多数问题是前景问题。

二、选择需要回答的临床问题

当医务工作者面对很多问题而时间较少时，需要确定如何开始。由于患者的疾病通常牵涉较广，一次可发现很多问题。因此推荐对诸多问题进行选择。选择意味着决定诸多问题中哪些是医务工作者必须探寻的。这个决定需要全面评估患者疾病及医生需要的知识。面临众多问题的情况下，可以根据以下因素选择优先回答的问题。

1. 哪个问题对患者的生命健康最重要？

2. 哪个问题最可能得到满意的答案？

3. 哪个问题和临床实践相关性最大？

4. 哪个问题最令人感兴趣？

5. 哪个问题最有可能在临床实践中再次出现？

优先回答的问题是关系生命、健康、临床工作需要等实际需求的问题。同时，应该从患者的角度提出问题，这样可以帮助收集或提供真正有利于患者的证据，从而提高疾病治愈率及医疗服务的质量。

三、确定问题的范围

问题范围的宽窄对于临床研究人员非常重要。确定问题的范围，使提出问题所确定的范围尽可能恰当，提出的问题太宽或太窄都会对提供证据进行研究和使用证据用于个体患者治疗参考带来不利的影响。确定研究范围应考虑所拥有的资源和条件、临床意义和研究质量等。临床研究实践中常有以下几种情况。

1. 提出问题范围太宽 范围太宽的问题可能对处置患者没有帮助。例如，"化疗对癌症患者有好处吗？"这一问题范围太宽，不明确何种癌症及何种化疗，不能为特定患者提供有用信息。范围太宽的问题可能导致纳入的患者样本量或研究异质性增大。但另一方面，范围宽的研究可以提供较多的信息，实用性较好，但消耗更多的资源。

2. 提出问题范围太窄 范围太窄的问题因所获得资料较少而容易出现机遇的作用，增加了出现假阳性和假阴性结果的情况，导致结果不可靠。一个范围太窄的问题可以作为一个范围较宽问题中的一个亚组，因此，可以视为与亚组分析相同的问题。范围太窄的问题还存在着结果推广价值受限制的桎梏，但范围窄的问题可能提高研究对象的同质性。

本 章 小 结

临床问题来源于临床，提出问题的目的是为临床决策服务。提出一个好的临床问题，应深入临床实践，需勤于思考，了解构建良好临床问题的要素，弄清这个临床问题属于哪类问题，清楚地知道问题相关的知识（包括了解的和未知的）。提出好的问题是循证医学实践的基本技能，构建良好的问题则有助于直接聚焦患者的临床需要。

（刘天舒 陈世耀）

第 三 章

如何得到有用的证据

学习目标

掌握 文献分析方法；循证医学数据库的运用。

　　循证医学的一个重要特征是依据高价值的证据做最优化的医学决定，因此如何获得可信度高且意义重大的证据就显得尤为重要，这也是在本章中将要重点学习的内容。这里所指的证据通常来自设计和实施均非常优秀的科学研究，从中获取有用信息的方法主要有以下几种：其一是文献分析，主要针对较前沿或者小众的研究内容，包括对原始临床研究文献的数据可信度进行评价后整合分析，还包括对定性和定量系统综述的分析；其二是对循证医学数据库的运用，主要针对按照数据结构组织、存储和管理的已整合的医学信息资源，是获取可靠科学依据的重要手段。

第一节　医学文献概述

　　记录和传播知识的所有出版物都属于文献。其中涉及医药知识的文献即称为医学文献。按照文献的级别进行分类可将文献划分为一次文献、二次文献和三次文献三大类。

　　一次文献也称作原始文献，一般包括直接记录的研究成果，报道的新发明创造以及知识见解等文献，如期刊、学位及会议论文、专利说明书、科技报告等；二次文献是通过鉴别和筛选原始文献，进行加工处理而形成的文献，包括文摘、索引、目录等文献类型；而三次文献是基于二次文献材料，根据目的，筛选一次文献，进行整理加工和综合处理形成的文献，包括综述、年鉴、指南、教科书等形式。

一、原始临床研究

　　原始临床研究根据能否进行随机分配划分为观察性研究和试验性研究。观察性研究针对的研究对象携带各种客观存在的特征，不能对研究对象按照需要研究的因素进行随机分配，而只能对观察对象的研究因素进行系统性的客观描述，或对设计细致的研究方案分析比较获得研究结果。这种研究方法不涉及医学伦理学方面的问题，同时操作较为方便，但是这种研究方法存在多种偏倚，因此不能确保研究的真实性。

　　按照有无设立相应的对照组，将观察性研究划分为描述性和分析性两种研究形式。描述性研究未提前设立对照组，顾名思义，主要用于描述某种疾病或性状在不同人群、地域或时间的分布情况，同时研究其发生发展的可能规律，如病例报道及横断面研究等。描述性研究方式只能提出病因假说，而不能鉴定出暴露与效应的联系。分析性研究以描述性研究为基础，其最重要的特点是根据研究的需要设立了可以互相比较的两个组，如病例对照研究和队列研究。分析性研究主要用于探索可能的致病因素与疾病及健康状况之间的关联，通过分析、筛选其中的致病因素，进而形成或验证病因假说。

与观察性研究相对应的试验性研究，通过将研究人群进行随机分配，划分为试验组和对照组，在相同的条件下给予两组不同的处理，其中试验组给予需要观察的措施，而对照组不给予措施或施加安慰剂，随后比较两组的结果，分析给予的措施所产生的效果。由于在实验过程中处理因素是通过研究者随机分配的，即研究者能够控制各种因素的影响，故而能够得到可靠的结论。

二、综述和述评

综述和述评都属于三次文献范畴。这二者之间既有联系，也有区别。综述是对一个时间段内某个研究领域相关研究课题所报道的成果进行的搜集和分析，从中整理出具有参考价值的数据和资料，形成的综合和叙述性文献。综述通过将一次文献中的相关研究数据及产生的结果进行汇总及浓缩，并从中归纳出具有科研价值的信息，能够较全面地反映某个研究课题在一定时间段内的研究进展，进而引导读者能够快速而高效地掌握这个时间段内该课题领域的整体情况，有助于认识有待进一步解决的科研问题以及国内外研究水平及差距。

述评是对某一研究领域内的相关研究课题等专题内容在国内外研究中报道的文献进行系统性搜集、整理和分析，进而进行叙述并进行评论的文献形式。述评的目的是纵观某个研究课题在既往和目前所取得的科研成果以及目前所达到的研究水平，并就现在尚未克服的科研难题以及今后可能的研究热点和前景提出自己的观点和意见，以供其他科研工作者参考，从而更有利于该课题的进一步研究。

二者相比较，综述注重于文献的综合和叙述，而述评除了注重于综合、叙述，还注重于评论，因此综述的适用范围较述评广泛，而述评的学术价值要高于综述。

三、系统综述和 meta 分析

系统综述是通过搜集、整理原始文献，分析和归纳其中的信息并进行客观评价和对研究结果综合的二次研究，故而又称为系统评价（systematic review）。系统综述能够形成更为可靠的科研信息和数据，并对相关研究课题产生深远的影响。

虽然也称为综述，但是其与一般的叙述性综述有着明显的不同。系统综述要求十分严格，通常是集中于某个有待解决的具体科研问题，通过详尽的文献检索策略介绍（包括检索式及检索工具等），尽可能全面地搜集所有已经发表及尚未发表的文献及数据资料，同时要结合检索之前已经明确的标准进行整理及严格的评审。系统综述主要针对文献的真实性、成果的应用价值情况以及对实验结果产生影响的因素等内容进行盲审或者多人评审，从而降低选择偏倚。并且需要持续搜集新的原始数据，从而更新和补充新的信息。

系统综述根据统计学处理分为定性和定量两种类型。定性系统综述是搜集和整理的原始研究结果，没有进行统计学方法处理和合并；而定量系统综述则是通过对搜集的原始研究结果统计学处理、进行数据合并的分析方法，也称为荟萃分析，即 meta 分析。

meta 分析可以对同一个研究方向的多个研究结果进行综合分析,从而避免单个原始研究样本量偏小而造成的统计效能不足,同时能够解释对相同研究方向不同团队不同样本研究出现的不一致的结果,并能够对原来各原始研究没提出的科研问题进行解答。目前 meta 分析在医学科研领域备受关注,是循证医学的高级证据,主要用于随机对照研究结果的合并。而在原始观察性研究中主要用于病例对照及队列研究检验病因假设及应用于医学干预。

系统综述在准备过程中,首先要明确拟综述的内容,制订确切的检索策略和文献排除及纳入标准,运用 meta 分析对入选研究的所有合格样本进行合并分析,并对合并后的结果进行敏感性检测,各入选的独立研究质量与 meta 分析结果的可靠性关联密切。为了获得高质量的合并结果,需要确保入选文献的质量。meta 分析注重异质性检验,若入选文献一致性较好,采用固定效应模型运算;存在异质性,但合并后仍存在临床意义的采用随机效应模型计算;异质性严重者,不能采用 meta 分析。

第二节　临床研究报告格式

一、概述

临床研究报告包括临床研究的全过程、结果、研究者对临床研究结果的评价、对研究完成工作的深化和总结及后期继续深化研究的展望。临床研究报告是临床研究工作的深化和总结,高度概括了研究工作的全过程,充分反映了研究的成果和价值,其报告内容全面、详细、真实可靠。临床研究的结果为临床医生提供了临床医疗和决策的证据,并在伦理和科学性方面保证了其传达信息的精确性。

临床研究报告包括生物医学科研论文等,是对临床研究内容的高度凝练。1978 在加拿大温哥华起草的《温哥华宣言》对生物医学杂志论文格式提出了统一要求。我国也在 1987 年颁布了科学技术报告、学位论文、学术论文编写格式的国家标准(GB 7713—87)。

医学科研论文的一般格式要求:标题、署名(作者、单位等)、摘要(中英文)、关键词、引言、正文、结论、参考文献、附录及英文缩略词表等,正文主要为 IMRAD 格式,分别代表前言(introduction)、材料与方法(materials and methods)、结果(results)和讨论(discussion)。

本节将对研究报告的正文撰写进行重点阐述。

二、正文格式

1. 前言　对于一篇科研论文来说前言即是研究的目的,在论文的一开始说明要进行的研究是要解决什么样的科学问题及问题的重要性。然后,回顾过去到现在关于这个问题已经进行过的研究,最后说明这次研究相较于过去的不同之处、研究的侧重点。

2. 材料与方法　这个部分应提供详细的实验细节,包括:实验设计、实验对象、实验材料、实验处理方法等,并严格按照实验方案中的内容详细地描述,让其他人有办法根据这些信息复制实验,具有可复制性应该是所有实验的必要条件。如药物研究报告中通常使用随机、对照、盲法等设计方法对研究对象进行分组归类,详细描述分组的治疗方案,随后完整列出试验方案中的评价疗效、安全性指标等,最后阐述数据的采集、处理方法及过程,所使用的统计软件及方法。

3. 结果　在结果中，不需要进行评论和说明，理论上来说，这个部分可能是最简短的，可以适当地使用图表来辅助。临床试验结果报告的表现形式主要包括临床试验结果的文字描述、经统计处理过的数据、导出的公式、效果比较的图表、影像资料、病理照片和模式图(直条图、线图、散点图等)。文字叙述和图表要合理配合，不要重复，以清楚表述为原则。数据要有机结合，层次鲜明，以突出主要内容和创新性结果。数据是研究的论据，对于临床试验结果应全面真实报告，即使与研究预期结果有矛盾的现象、结果及数据，如无效、恶化、不良反应、失访情况等，也应客观反映。阴性或与预期相反结果可能就是真实结果，其中包含着真理，可以提示设计、实施等方面的缺陷。

4. 讨论　临床实验报告的讨论部分是对临床试验结果的分析提炼，是为了寻找研究结果和理论之间的内在联系，是从理论上对实验和观察结果进行的分析和综合，为得出研究结论提供理论依据，并通过理性分析、归纳综合以及合理的推理，进而探索新的研究方向。临床试验结果讨论内容必须依据本文的实际结果，紧紧围绕提出的科学问题和研究假说展开。合理分析、解释结果要有充分的理论依据，不可主观臆断。在讨论研究结果时，不仅要解释阳性结果，还要解释阴性结果或者和预期相反的结果，即使研究未得出结果，也要进行讨论，分析原因。

三、报告其他部分内容的撰写

1. 结论　结论指将研究结果和讨论分析后的认识以简明的形式归纳总结起来，指明理论和实际意义，对文章内容进行高度概括。

2. 参考文献　参考文献是科研论文必不可少的组成部分，参考文献应该是对了解和进行该课题研究有帮助的、最重要的、能够反映研究领域现状动态和发展方向的、国内外公开出版发表的有关文献资料。参考文献仅限于作者亲自阅读过的、需要引用参照的文献。

参考文献的格式有期刊、图书、会议文献、科技报告、学位论文、专利文献等。如期刊：

HALPERN S D, UBEL P A, CAPLAN A L. Solid-organ transplantation in HIV-infected patients[J]. The New England Journal of Medicine, 2002, 347(4): 284-287.

四、临床研究报告问题案例分析

通过对关于儿童特异性皮炎的临床特征性研究分析来进一步了解临床研究报告格式。

张莉梅. 298 例儿童特应性皮炎临床特征分析[D]. 重庆：重庆医科大学，2010.

1. 前言　在论文的一开始说明为什么要进行儿童特应性皮炎(AD)患者临床特征地域性差异研究及研究的重要性。随后，回顾关于儿童 AD 患者临床特征地域性差异研究已经完成的研究，最后说明这次的研究相较于过去的不同之处，研究的侧重点。

2. 材料与方法

(1)病例资料收集，如选定 298 例 AD 患儿，且须符合 1980 年 Hanifint-Rajka AD 诊断标准。

(2)临床特征定义，如主要特征及次要特征参见诊断标准；疾病严重程度根据特应性皮炎评分(SCORAD)和特应性皮炎客观评分(OSAAD)进行评分。

(3)研究方法，如由患者本人或者其合法监护人签订知情同意书后，由经过专门培训的流行病学调查员记录患者的临床特征及实验室检查资料。调查的内容一般包括：姓名、性别、出生年月、年龄、家庭住址、联系电话、发病年龄、首发症状、疾病进展中的临床表现及诱因等。

（4）资料收集及录入过程中的质量控制方法，如调查表的设计经反复检查、修改，可操作性强；调查员经统一培训并进行调查结果的一致性检验，合格后上岗；所有患者均由皮肤科专家通过病史辅助检查后确诊；资料的重复录入及核对，减少人为误差；数据的一致性核对；抽样进行电话回访。

（5）分析患儿的发病年龄、加重及缓解季节、AD 对生活质量的影响，并根据年龄分组，分析不同年龄段儿童 AD 的皮损类型、严重程度、好发部位、次要特征、发生率等临床特征。最后进行统计学处理，如采用 SPSS 26.0 统计软件进行分析，χ^2 检验进行分类资料的比较。

3. 结果　在结果里，对儿童患者的年龄分布、男女比例、首次发病时间、好发部位、好发季节等以及发生情况、疾病严重程度及患者次要症状及其他症状发生率的对比进行描述。最后，依据研究调查的实际结果展开结果讨论：合理分析、解释结果，如果结果有差异性，就按照有差异性讨论；如果无差异性，就按无差异性讨论，并分析当下结果的原因。

4. 讨论　对结果进行分析提炼，为得出研究结论提供理论依据。合理分析、解释结果，得出以下结论：①特应性皮炎发病年龄早，半岁以内为发病高峰，首次发病率随着年龄增加而下降。②特应性皮炎具有明显的季节性，多于冬季加重，夏季缓解。③特应性皮炎患儿多伴有过敏性疾病家族史；食物过敏在 AD 患儿中的发生率显著高于普通人群。④不同年龄段的特应性皮炎在皮损类型、皮损累及面积、AD 严重程度以及好发部位等方面有差异。

第三节　循证医学数据库

循证医学是遵循科学证据的临床医学，提倡将临床实践和经验与客观的科学研究证据结合起来，强调任何医疗决策应建立在最佳科学研究证据的基础上，为患者做出最佳的医疗决策。因此，针对临床工作中遇到的问题，需要不断查寻新的文献资料，掌握学科发展的前沿与趋势、更新知识结构。

从最初的手工检索，循证医学证据资源发展经历了漫长的过程。随着计算机及网络技术的高速发展，逐渐摆脱了耗时费力的手工检索时代，转变为快速高效的检索时代，极大地提高了获取最新信息的能力。含有临床科学证据的数据库即循证医学数据库，按照数据结构来组织、存储和管理医学信息资源，是获取可靠科学依据的重要工具。

循证医学数据库是以临床证据数据为核心的数据库检索系统，旨在建立一个完整的临床证据数据获取体系，最终目的是要实现以科学的方法收集和整理临床医学证据，为临床工作者和研究人员提供获取和利用最佳临床证据的平台。从 20 世纪 90 年代创立 Cochrane 协作网、Cochrane Library 以及《英国医学会杂志》（*BMJ*）推出的 Clinical Evidence，越来越多的循证医学资源供临床医生选择。这些资源严格评估原始临床研究，采用系统评价或 meta 分析方法总结与整合，极大地方便了临床医生开展循证临床实践。常用循证医学数据库有下几种。

1. 循证医学图书馆（Cochrane Library）　是国际 Cochrane Collaboration 的主要产品，由英国 Wiley InterScience 公司出版发行，收录年限从 1996 年至今。Cochrane Library 是循证卫生保健的"金标准"——在循证医学系统评价的基础建立起来，汇集了众多数据库。可以帮助参与卫生保健决策的人员及时了解所有最新证据，为他们提供有关现有治疗方法和新治疗方法的最高品质信息。Cochrane Library 主要面向对循证卫生保健感兴趣的广大人群，包括临床医生、决策者、研究人员、教育者和学生等。Cochrane Library 是一个提供高质量证据的数据库，是临床研究证据的主要来源，包括：Cochrane 系统评价数据库（Cochrane Database of Systematic Reviews，CDSR）、疗效评价文摘库（Database of Abstracts of Reviews of Effects，DARE）、Cochrane 临床对照试验中心注册库（Cochrane Central Register of Controlled Trials，CENTRAL）、Cochrane 协作网方法学文献注册数据库（Cochrane Methodology Register，CMR）、卫生技术评估数据库（Health Technology Assessment Database，HTA）、英国国家卫生服务部卫生经济评价数据库（NHS Economic Evaluation Database，NHS EED）。

2. DynaMed 数据库　　是全球内容最全面、使用最广泛和知名度最高的循证医学数据库之一。DynaMed 数据库将最有用的医学信息提供给临床医生，以适合的方式得到最需要的信息，创建最有用的临床潜在资源。DynaMed 数据库的独特优势包括：系统评估当前所有相关的研究，力求呈现给临床医生最小偏倚的证据；持续更新，在第一时间整合新的证据到 DynaMed 数据库；可采用网址（本地和远程）和移动设备等多种方式进行检索和阅读。DynaMed 数据库根据纳入研究的内部真实性与外部真实性，将证据按质量分为 3 级，同时基于证据进行分级，其中一级证据为最有效且以患者为中心的研究结论。

3. UpToDate 数据库　　于 1992 年创建，现隶属于荷兰威科（Wolters Kluwer）出版集团，涵盖 20 多个医学领域的 1 万多个医学主题。UpToDate 的理念是给临床医师提供即时、循证的临床医药信息，快速解答临床专业人员提出的相关临床疑问，并提供临床治疗建议与决策、继续教育服务，同时为患者提供更好的医护信息。UpToDate 的编辑流程主要包括反馈意见、评价分级、证据分析、推荐建议、专家审稿、完成更新等过程。UpToDate 不仅将所有医学主题的内容分成专业与非专业版本，为保持自身受到持续关注，还直接提供全部免费的最具个性化的医疗咨询和继续教育服务。

4. MD Consult 数据库　　由全球最大的医学出版集团爱思唯尔（Elsevier）于 1997 年出版发行的临床医学在线咨询平台，为医疗保健专业人员提供权威和不断更新的循证临床信息资源。其内容涵盖 15 个学科领域的 1 000 多个临床实践指南和 15 000 多个患者教育讲义。在全球，超过 2 000 家卫生机构订阅了 MD Consult 数据库，95% 的美国医学院校订阅了 MD Consult 数据库。MD Consult 数据库是医学教学、科研和临床工作的高效资源配置方案数据库。MD Consult 编辑流程主要包括检索论文、信息分类、编辑审稿、修改完善、跟踪监测、整合更新。MD Consult 首次将数据库做成专业的交流互动平台，针对用户提出的问题，选定不同的临床主题。

5. Clinical Evidence 数据库　　由《英国医学会杂志》（BMJ）出版集团于 1999 年正式推出的循证临床实践资源，2009 年，其对 Clinical Evidence 数据库进行全面改进，并推出其升级版 Best Practice 数据库。升级版数据库不仅完全整合了 Clinical Evidence 中的临床诊疗证据，还增添权威学者和临床专家执笔撰写的，并且涵盖基础、预防、诊断、治疗和随访等各个关键环节的内容。升级版数据库收录 660 多个临床主题、3 250 余种治疗方法以及 3 000 多项诊断性检测和 4 000 多篇诊断和治疗指南。Clinical Evidence 主要为临床医生提供不同疾病病症的概述，以及用于病症的预防和治疗干预手段的总结，重在为患者带来最佳的诊断和治疗结果。Clinical Evidence 的编辑流程主要包括专家委托、同行评审、质量评价、在线发布、定期更新等步骤。Clinical Evidence 是第一个包含中文版的国外循证医学数据库，也是第一个将数据库核心内容编辑成图书在全球发行的数据库。

6. ACP Journal Club　由美国内科医师学会出版,主要针对内科及其亚专科,编辑人员定期筛选 50 余种核心临床医学期刊涉及的临床问题、临床结局的高质量原始研究和系统评价,以结构摘要的形式进行总结,提出具有临床实践价值的建议。主要通过纸质或网络发行,有助于临床医生了解内科领域的新进展。

7. PIER(Physicians' Information and Education Resource)数据库　主要包括疾病诊治、筛选与预防、伦理与法律、药物信息等内容,其优点是采用多层次结构指导临床医生应用研究证据,临床医生可以通过该数据库得到临床和实践上有效的建议。PIER 的信息是以"资料层层下掘"(drill down)的格式展示,即从汇总数据深入到细节数据,用户点击开放的指导说明,逐步获得更多的详细信息。新的疾病模组每个月都会增加及更新,提供最新的资讯用于医师的诊断。

第四节　循证医学检索策略

检索策略,就是在正确分析检索信息需求的基础上,选择合适的检索系统、确定检索途径和检索词、明确各检索词之间的逻辑关系与检索步骤、编制符合检索要求的检索式。检索策略制订的原则是全面性和可重复性。在临床医生日益繁忙的临床工作中,了解并掌握如何制订循证医学检索策略,如何直接从浩瀚的生物医学数据库中获取最新、最有价值的信息数据,可以为临床医生节省很多时间,同时提高检索的效率。

一、循证医学检索策略制订方法

1. 根据检索需求确定检索范围。

2. 选择合适的检索数据库。

3. 选择合适的检索途径,主要采用主题词与自由词检索相结合的方式。

4. 确定 2~3 个精炼和符合检索需求的检索词,如分类途径以分类号作为检索词,主题途径以标题词、关键词等作为检索词等。

5. 充分利用布尔逻辑运算符、位置运算符、截词符、限制符等将检索词进行合理组配。

6. 预检索,根据临床问题对检索出的文献的数量和质量进行分析评价。

7. 根据预检索情况进行修改并完善检索词和检索式,直至检索结果符合检索需求。

二、如何制订一个相对较好的检索策略

1. 针对疾病应该尽可能选用该疾病的所有病名作为检索词,并用"OR"连接。

2. 针对干预措施选用多个同义词作为检索词,并用"OR"连接。

3. 针对纳入试验的设计类型也要尽可能地选用多个检索词,用"OR"连接。

4. 使用逻辑运算符"AND"连接以上三套检索式。

5. 如果三套检索式同时检索不到任何文献,可以考虑省略其中一套检索式重新检索。

三、循证医学检索策略的编制

在 MEDLINE 数据库中检索符合循证医学系统综述要求的有关治疗、诊断、病因、预后、系统评价和指南方面最新、最全的医学信息资源,检索步骤如下所示。

1. 先通过主题词、自由词或两者相结合等方式检索出所需的不同主题的内容。

2. 根据需要调整保证查全率的检索（检出的文献量较多，但有些文献可能不相关）或保证查准率的检索（检出的文献量较少，但相关文献多，不过可能会有一些漏检文献）。

查准率＝（检索出的相关信息量／检索出的信息总量）×100%

查全率＝（检索出的相关信息量／系统中所有的相关信息总量）×100%

使用泛指性较强的检索语言（如上位主题词）能提高查全率，但查准率下降。

根据不同的检索目的对于查准率和查全率要有所侧重：要应用证据作出临床决策时，应尽可能提高查准率；要基于证据开展临床研究时，应尽可能提高查全率。

3. 检索策略举例

（1）有关治疗方案的检索模式 ①保证较高查全率的检索策略：（diabetes）AND（randomized controlled trial［PTYP］OR drug therapy［MESH］OR therapeutic use［MESH：NOEXP］OR random*［WORD］）；②保证较高查准率的检索策略：（diabetes）AND（（double［WORD］AND blind*［WORD］）OR placebo［WORD］）；③查全与查准均衡时的检索策略：（diabetes）AND（randomized controlled trial［PTYP］）。

（2）有关诊断方案的检索模式 ①保证较高查全率的检索策略：（diabetes）AND（recall and precision［MESH］OR recall［WORD］OR（diagnosis［MESH］OR diagnostic use［MESH］OR precision［WORD］））；②保证较高查准率的检索策略：（diabetes）AND（recall and precision［MESH］OR（predictive［WORD］AND value*［WORD］））；③查全与查准均衡时的检索策略：（diabetes）AND（diagnosis）。

（3）有关病因的检索模式 ①保证较高查全率的检索策略：（diabetes）AND（cohort studies［MESH］OR risk［MESH］OR（odds［WORD］AND ratio*［WORD］）OR（relative［WORD］AND risk［WORD］）OR（case control*［WORD］OR case-control studies［MESH］））；②保证较高查准率的检索策略：（diabetes）AND（case-control studies［MH：NOEXP］OR cohort studies［MH：NOEXP］）；③查全与查准均衡时的检索策略：（diabetes）AND（risk［TW］）。

（4）有关预后的检索模式 ①保证较高查全率的检索策略：（diabetes）AND（incidence［MESH］OR mortality［MESH］OR follow-up studies［MESH］OR mortality［MESH］OR prognosis*［WORD］OR predict*［WORD］OR course［WORD］）；②保证较高查准率的检索策略：（diabetes）AND（prognosis［MH：NOEXP］OR survival analysis［MH：NOEXP］）；③查全与查准均衡时的检索策略：（diabetes）AND（prognosis）。

（5）有关系统评价和指南的检索模式 ①系统评价的检索策略：（diabetes）AND（meta-analysis［PTYP］OR meta-analysis［MH］）；②指南的检索策略：（diabetes）AND（Guidelines［MH］OR consensus development conferences［MH］）OR（Guideline［PTYP］OR consensus development conferences［PTYP］）。

四、调整检索策略

检索策略制订好后并不是说检索任务就完成了，在实际的检索过程中往往并非一次检索就会获得理想的检索效果，此时就需要对检索策略进行调整。检索策略的修改和调整，在实际操作上主要指数据库的选择和检索表达式的编写，前者取决于现有的数据库资源，后者则直接反映检索目标。一般情况下，检索结果过多，就应在提高查准率上下功夫，主要从缩小检索入手；如果检出篇幅过少，就应在提高查全率上下功夫，主要从扩大检索入手。

1. 缩小检索时调整检索式的主要方法

（1）选用专指性更强的检索词，如词表中更专指的下位词或副主题词。

（2）增加"AND"运算符，提高检索的准确率。

（3）使用"NOT"运算符，排除不相关的检索结果。

（4）选用词表中的主题词代替文本中的自由词。

（5）使用字段限定检索范围，如篇名、年份、出版物类型、主要主题词等。

2. 扩大检索时调整检索式的主要方法

（1）减少"AND"运算符的使用，拓宽检索范围。

（2）选全同义词、相关词和近义词，降低检索词的专指性并多用"OR"算符。

（3）采用分类号进行检索。

（4）同时选用主题词和自由词，或选用所有副主题词。

（5）减少或去除某些过严的限制符。

本 章 小 结

综上所述，获取有用证据的主要途径有文献分析和循证医学数据库。其中文献主要针对较前沿或者小众的研究内容，临床医师可以根据具体的临床问题检索原始临床研究，还可以参考已发表的系统综述分析。此外，类似 Cochrane Collaboration 的计划已经完成了大量的系统综述分析，并以此为基础建立了众多数据库，其中很多优秀的数据库能提供系统的高质量证据，是临床研究证据的主要来源。尽管获取证据非常重要，对已有证据质量进行评价和分级也是有用证据搜集过程中的重要一环，尤其是在参考原始临床研究时。此外，在循证医学决策的过程中，还包括医师和患者两个环节，因此需要依据当前最佳证据，结合医师的临床经验和患者意愿综合考虑，做出最佳决策。

（孙良丹）

第四章

如何评价证据

学习目标

掌握 证据真实性的评价；证据重要性的评价；证据适用性（实用性）的评价。

医学需要批判性思维。具备批判性评价证据质量的能力是循证实践的基础。在医疗实践中，批判性评价是对科学研究结果（即证据）进行有效性、重要性和实用性三个方面认真而系统的评价的过程。如果不对证据进行客观和全面的评价，医疗保健将无证可依。评价证据需要医生具备临床研究设计和统计学的相关知识，同时还需要能够根据当前的患者情况对研究数据进行分析和思考。医生应该不断学习和培训，成为知识广博、具有评判性思维的人。

在检索获取到最能回答 PICO 问题的相关文献后，就要对这些文献证据进行评价。现代的医疗保健不仅仅取决于个人的医疗技能，而且有赖于医务工作者不断获取各种干预措施的有效性和安全性方面可靠的信息资料。因此，对科学研究论文证据的质量和实用性进行批判性评价是循证实践的关键步骤。批判性评价证据的目的在于确定研究真实性，研究结果的重要性以及其适用性。

第一节　证据分级与推荐

可以回答一个问题的研究证据往往有很多，但各种证据其实是有等级之分的，也就是说，不同级别的证据其价值各异。不过还要强调一下，各种级别的证据都很重要，并都具有其各自独特的价值。

证据分级最早出现在 1979 年加拿大定期健康检查工作组的一份报告中。此后，许多作者、组织机构和期刊提出了一些证据分级系统，其中的证据级别一般分为 4 级或 5 级。这些证据分级系统大多大同小异：它们大多根据偏倚风险（risk of bias），即系统误差（systematic error）对研究进行分级。对于各种流行病学和临床研究类型的相对论证的强度，人们有着广泛的共识。随机对照试验（randomized controlled trial，RCT）和 / 或基于随机对照试验的系统综述的证据等级高于观察研究（observational study）。而另一方面，专家意见和病例经验位于证据金字塔的底部。在各种证据分级系统中，牛津（英国）循证医学中心（CEBM）证据分级系统传播广泛，并广为接受（表 4-1）。牛津 CEBM 证据分级首次发布于 2000 年，并于 2011 年修订，通过对患病率、预后、诊断、治疗效果和危害，以及筛查等各种研究目的的证据进行级别划分，旨在以更简单的形式（更少的分类和备注）帮助临床决策。

表 4-1　牛津循证医学中心 2011 证据分级系统

问题	1级[*]	2级[*]	3级[*]	4级[*]	5级[*]
该问题有多普遍？	当前当地的随机抽样调查（普查）	对调查研究的系统综述，可以匹配当地的具体情况[**]	当地非随机抽样调查[**]	病例系列分析[**]	不适用
诊断、监测试验准确吗？（诊断）	均采用了金标准和盲法的横断面诊断试验研究的系统综述	单个横断面研究，采用了金标准和盲法	研究对象非连续入组，或未能一致采用金标准的研究[**]	采用病例对照研究设计，或者没有很好的金标准或非独立地进行金标准检查对比[**]	根据机制进行推理
如果没有治疗，结果会如何？（预后）	基于早期队列研究（inception cohort study）的系统综述[***]	早期规整的队列研究[***]	队列研究或随机对照试验中的对照组[*]	病例系列分析或病例对照研究，或者质量不佳的预后队列研究[**]	不适用
治疗措施有用吗？（治疗带来的获益）	单病例随机对照试验，或基于随机对照试验（RCT）的系统综述	RCT，或者具有非常显著效应的观察性研究	非随机、设置对照的队列/随访研究[**]	病例系列分析，病例对照研究，或历史性对照研究[**]	根据机制进行推理
治疗措施带来的常见危害是什么？（治疗的风险）	基于 RCT 的系统综述，基于巢式病例对照研究的系统综述，考虑到该问题的单病例随机对照研究，或有显著效应的观察性研究	单个 RCT 研究，或者特别情况下具有显著效应的观察性研究	如果有足够的事件数来明确是否为常见危害，非随机、设置对照的队列/随访研究（上市后监测）（对于长期危害，随访时间必须足够长。）[**]	病例系列分析，病例对照研究，或历史性对照研究[**]	根据机制进行推理
治疗措施带来的罕见危害是什么？（治疗的风险）	单病例随机对照试验，或基于 RCT 的系统综述	单个 RCT 研究，或者特别情况下具有显著效应的观察性研究			
该（早期检测）试验是否值得？（筛查）	基于 RCT 的系统综述	RCT	非随机、设置对照的队列/随访研究[**]	病例系列分析，病例对照研究，或历史性对照研究[**]	根据机制进行推理

注：[*] 根据研究的质量、不精确性、间接性（研究 PICO 与临床问题 PICO 不能对应）、各研究间不一致性，或绝对效应很小，证据的级别要下调；如果效应量大或非常大，则级别可上调。

[**] 系统综述通常优于单个研究。

[***] 早期规整的队列指的是一个队列人群，其中所有个体进入研究之时均处于某种状态的早期，例如症状初发期、初诊期、某种病理状态的临床表现期等。对早期规整的队列进行随访研究是疾病自然病程、预后研究的重要方法。

　　大多数证据的分级方案简单易用；然而十多年来它们一直面临一些批评和质疑，其主要原因是过于简单：在这些分级体系中，RCT 被赋予过多的信任。其实，观察性研究有的时候也能提供非常好的证据；而 RCT 设计可能并不适于回答某些问题（例如患病率、预后或罕见危害的问题），或因为伦理原因而无法开展。在某些情况下，即使是病例系列分析和病例报道也能提供明确的证据。而 RCT 或系统综述也会出现不确定的结果。此外，并非所有的 RCT 都经过精心设计，并且良好执行，故而应该审慎检查。

　　因此，证据推荐分级的评估、制定与评价（grading of recommendations assessment, development and evaluation, GRADE）工作组开发了一种更全面的证据分级系统，该系统问世后得到了广泛的关注，并得到了许多组织的认可和采纳。GRADE 工作组以多种维度的方式定义了"证据质量"（表 4-2 和表 4-3）和"推荐强度"（表 4-4）。在对证据体（body of evidence）进行评价时，需要综合考虑偏倚风险、效应量、一致性、间接性、精确性等因素，因而在进行系统综述、卫生技术评估（health technology assessment, HTA）和临床实践指南（clinical practice guideline, CPG）时能更准确地对证据进行评价，从而也在世界范围内广为接受。但鱼与熊掌不可兼得，GRADE 系统准确的同时，也较为复杂。需要花较多的时间学习才能掌握 GRADE 系统，运用它对证据进行分级同样也要耗费较多时间。

表 4-2　GRADE 四个级别证据的意义

证据质量级别	定义
高	非常确信真实的效应值接近效应估计值
中	对效应估计值有中等程度的信心：真实值有可能接近估计值，但仍存在二者大不相同的可能性
低	对效应估计值的确信程度有限：真实值可能与估计值大不相同
极低	对效应估计值几乎没有信心：真实值很可能与估计值大不相同

表 4-3　GRADE 证据资料评定标准和定义

研究设计	证据体初始质量	如果符合如下条件，降级	如果符合如下条件，升级	证据质量等级
随机试验	高	偏倚风险	效应量大	高（++++）
		-1 严重	+1 大	
		-2 非常严重	+2 非常大	中（+++-）
观察性研究	低	不一致性	剂量 - 反应梯度	低（++--）
		-1 严重	+1 有剂量 - 反应梯度证据	
		-2 非常严重	所有可能的残余混杂因素	差（+---）
		间接性	+1 可降低所显示的效应	
		-1 严重	+1 研究未观察到效应时	
		-2 非常严重	可提示其为假效应	
		不精确		
		-1 严重		
		-2 非常严重		
		发表偏倚		
		-1 可能		
		-2 非常可能		

表 4-4 GRADE 系统中推荐的强度和方向

强度	其他名词	描述	因素	方向
强		所有或几乎所有知情的人都会作出此推荐以支持该干预或反对该干预。强推荐提示个人之间或地区之间临床实践的变异程度很小。强推荐并不一定意味着优先推荐	1. 与备选方案相比，该方案在理想和不理想的后果间的平衡性。越是平衡，强推荐的可能性就越小	支持
			2. 对效应估计的信心（证据质量）。信心越低，强推荐的可能性就越小	反对
弱	条件性、斟酌性或保留性	此类推荐可根据患者的价值观和偏好、可用的资源，或干预措施的实施环境而变；或由患者和临床医师酌情决定；或者因为对其中一些问题的解释不一而将导致不同的决策，故而持一定的保留态度	3. 价值和偏好的不确定性或变异性。所估计的价值和偏好越低，变异越大，强推荐的可能性就越小	支持
			4. 资源耗用。资源占用越高，强推荐的可能性就越小	反对

在应用任何分级方案对证据进行分级时都应该注意以下几点。

1. 证据级别不会显示提出的问题是否正确合理。所谓最佳的证据也无法回答一个含糊的、不明确的问题。

2. 不应该仅仅根据研究设计类型来判断证据的质量高低。

3. 证据等级并不能直接转化为推荐意见。

第二节 证据评价的原则与方法

证据评价也称为批判性评价（critical appraisal）或文献评阅，是指对已发表的研究进行审慎、系统地阅读评价，对其研究方法是否能反映客观事实、研究问题和结果是否重要以及是否能应用于临床实践做出合理判断。

尽管现在有很多文献评价的标准，但并没有被普遍接受的唯一的"金标准"评价工具。不过，在文献评价过程中采用结构化的方法和清单或可提高评价质量，并有助于筛除低质量或相关性不高的一些研究。下面列出了一些使用较为广泛的清单：CASP、牛津 CEBM、SIGN、SURE。

与此同时，现在还有各种研究论文报告书写指南，以促进研究论文能准确、透明地报告研究的情况。CONSORT 声明适用于各种证据，对 RCT 研究报告提出了最低限度的要求和建议。该声明包括了一个由 25 个条目组成的清单和一张流程图。清单条目涵盖了研究报告中应该如何报道研究设计、数据分析和结果解读。流程图则要求显示所有试验受试者进入、参与和离开试验的全过程。此外，还有针对观察性研究（STROBE）、系统综述（PRISMA）、诊断试验研究（STARD）、临床实践指南（AGREE）等的报告和评价指南。这些声明和指南不仅可以指导科学论文报告的撰写，还有助于批判性地评价相关类型的论文和报告。EQUATOR 网站全面收集了这些报告、指南和声明，同时提供了与研究报告相关资源的网络链接。

一般来说,在评价一项研究时,应从以下4个主要问题着手。

1. 这项研究是否必要,是否有临床意义?

2. 该研究选用的方法是否能正确地反映客观事实并且回答临床问题?(这项研究可信吗?)

3. 如果该研究方法真实可信,其结果是否重要?(这项研究的结果有重要的临床意义吗?)

4. 如果该研究真实可信、结果重要,是否能将其应用于患者或人群?(可以使用该研究提供的信息吗?)

文献评价中,首当其冲的是该研究所提出的问题是否清晰明确、是否在该专业领域中得到大家的关注。如果一项研究没有针对重要的问题、增加新知,或者与当前想解决的PICO问题无关,不管它采用了多严格的研究设计、执行得多完美,从当前来说,该研究也没有多大的价值。

评价研究问题的必要性和相关性时,不可避免地会有一定程度的主观性,因为有的问题对于某些人来说至关重要,但对另外一些人来说则无关痛痒。但不管怎么说,评价任何一项研究,首先要问的就是其研究目的和假说是否有意义。

首先,需要明确开展这项研究的必要性,作者在研究报告中对此是否阐述清楚。一般情况下,可以在文章的引言部分看到研究问题是如何提出来的,有哪些证据说明问题形成的原因。一个好的研究问题通常由3个或4个部分组成(PICO):患者群或人群、研究的因素(如干预)、结局以及必要的对照。

如果研究问题具有必要性和重要性,接下来需要对研究的真实性、重要性和适用性进行评价。下文将依次对这些内容进行解释、介绍。

第三节　证据的内部真实性评价

在科学研究中,内部真实性又称内部效度(internal validity),指的是一项研究对效应或效果的估计是真实可靠的。从理论上讲,内部真实性代表了研究反映客观事实的程度。研究中系统误差越小,内部真实性越高。内部真实性有时简称为真实性(validity);还有一种真实性称为外部真实性,又称外部效度(external validity),指一个研究结果在其他条件和环境下仍能适用的程度。

下面的几个问题有助于评价一项研究的内部真实性。

一、其研究设计是否适合回答该研究问题?

不同的研究问题应该通过不同的研究设计得到解决和回答(见表4-1,图4-1)。一般来说,常见的研究问题分为2大类,一类是测量事件的频率,另一类评估事物和因素间的关联(例如一项干预措施的效力或效果)。对于第一类问题,最合适的研究设计是采用观察性研究,而不是RCT设计;而对于后者来说,单个RCT或者基于高质量RCT的系统综述也许能更好地回答研究问题。在RCT不可行或不符合伦理要求的情况下,可以依次考虑非随机对照试验、队列研究、病例对照研究以及其他观察性研究。

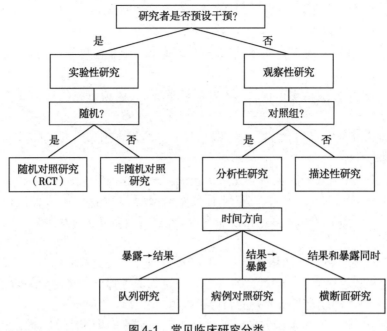

图 4-1　常见临床研究分类

二、研究方法是否能应对解决潜在的各种偏倚来源?

偏倚是研究结果或推论与客观事实之间系统性的偏离,常可分为 3 大类:选择偏倚、信息偏倚和混杂偏倚。选择偏倚源于选择受试者的过程,以及通过影响受试者参与研究而使得研究结果发生偏离的各种因素,比如,有区分性地挑选一部分潜在合格的受试者进入研究或区分性地将受试者分配进入某一组就会给研究带来选择偏倚。信息偏倚是研究中对需要检测的信息的一种测量误差,将导致夸大或低估所研究的效应或频率。而混杂偏倚可导致对暴露因素和结局之间关系的错误估计,其发生原因是另外有别的混杂因素,该因素既与暴露因素有联系,又可影响结局的发生。

Glasziou 等人建议通过以下问题来评估原始研究的内部真实性:

招募对象(recruitment):研究中的受试者能代表目标人群吗?

分配或调整(allocation or adjustment):在随机分组之前做好了随机分配序列的隐藏吗?各组在试验开始时(基线)具有可比性吗?

维护(maintenance):各组平等对待和管理,并有足够的随访时间,从而保持研究各组间的可比状态?

测量(measurement):测量结局时,采用对受试者和评价者设盲(blinding)和 / 或客观(objective)结局?

可以利用以上问题关键词的部分字母,组成 RAMMbo 这个词来帮助记忆。

此外,研究设计不同,容易导致的偏倚种类也不一样。因此在设计和实施研究时,研究者需要根据不同情况采取一些方法和策略以尽量减少偏倚。而在文献评阅时,也需要按不同的研究设计类型具体分析,采用一些针对性清单进行评价。

1. 系统综述与荟萃分析　系统综述是一种二次研究,该研究根据一个特定的主题,采用细致、标准化的方案获取所有相关的研究,进行批判性评价并综合证据信息。如果可能的话，还可以用荟萃分析将各个研究的结果合并成单一结果。系统综述的偏倚风险可源于对原始研究的选择、评价以及原始研究本身的质量。其中有一种偏倚称为发表偏倚（publication bias）。发表偏倚是由于选择性地发表和报道阳性的试验结果所致的。因为发表偏倚的存在，人们对于某一问题的认识就会发生总体偏差。

系统评价和荟萃分析优先报告的条目（preferred reporting items for systematic reviews and meta-analyses，PRISMA）是基于证据的条目精简集，是对于干预措施有效性和安全性的荟萃分析和系统综述。PRISMA 为大家提供了一个全面的框架以评价此类研究报告，它强调了研究报告的透明性、完整性。此外，CASP 系统综述评价清单也非常实用，可以作为快速评价的工具。系统综述和荟萃分析也不局限于 RCT。流行病学观察性研究的荟萃分析（meta-analysis of observational studies in epidemiology，MOOSE）指南针对的是非 RCT 的荟萃分析。

2. 随机对照试验　在 RCT 中，研究者更应该关注随机化的完整性、各组同等对待、盲法或客观地评价结局、受试者流失或失访率等问题。在试验中受试者通过随机分配的方式进入到不同的组别，这样就消除了选择偏倚，并能确保各组之间在所有已知和未知的混杂因素方面是均衡的。如果各组间在某些基线特征（即潜在危险因素）上存在任何差异，均只能归因为机遇。这样的话，各组在结局方面的差异就应该归因于干预因素加上机遇的结果。基于某些概率分布模型就可以对效应进行描述和推断了。如果结局是采用盲法或客观的方法进行的评估，则信息偏倚也可以消除。

然而，研究设计本身并不能保证零偏倚。研究方案的关键部分有纰漏和瑕疵，或者研究未能很好地实施，都会给研究带来偏倚。如果大家知道或者能够猜测到下一例患者将被分配进入哪一组，那么就可能会出现选择性地将患者纳入研究的情况，从而导致明显的偏倚。随机分配序列的隐藏是保护随机化完整性的重要方法，做好了隐藏就能确保每位患者进入研究之前无法知道或猜到其入组的方案。有许多方法可以有效地隐藏随机分配序列。例如，使用顺序编号的、不透明的密封信封（sequentially numbered, opaque sealed envelopes，SNOSE），既便宜又有效。使用计算机生成的随机分配序列在中心随机化（centralized randomization）中，能有效地做到分配方案隐藏，在多中心试验中尤为便利高效。如果不能隐藏分配序列将导致结果严重偏离真实。意向性治疗（intention-to-treat，ITT）分析是基于最初的随机分组、而非实际治疗的情况来分析试验结果的。ITT 分析的目的在于避免受到各种假象的误导，例如受试者非随机地离开试验，或接受其他组的治疗方案。因此在数据分析阶段，ITT 保持了随机化的完整性。

在 RCT 中，除了所研究的干预措施，各研究组都应该被同等地管理和对待。所有的结果都应该客观地或盲法测量，以避免信息偏倚。

试验报告的强化标准（consolidated standards of reporting trials，CONSORT）声明非常全面，可以作为评价随机对照试验的标准和工具。CONSORT 的清单和流程图，以及前述的CASP、牛津 CEBM、SIGN 和 SURE 等评价随机对照试验的清单均非常有用。

3. 队列研究　队列研究中，研究者对两组或两组以上的受试者进行随访，最终观察和比较各组在研究者所感兴趣的结局方面的差异。队列研究可以是前瞻性的，也可以是回顾性的，或者双向性的。

从方法学上来说，队列研究的最主要的问题是有较高的选择偏倚和混杂风险。特别在研究治疗性的干预措施时，这些问题尤为突出。此时，某个患者接受什么样的治疗取决于患者或医生的偏好、当前的常规治疗模式或当地政策因素。不同组的研究对象在许多方面都可能不一样。因此，研究者观察到各组结局上的差别，很可能是因为这些差异，而非治疗措施本身所致。这里特别要介绍一下所谓的适应证混杂（confounding by indication），该混杂指的是那些容易发生预期结局的人选择性地使用或者不使用干预措施。这种情况下，干预措施与疾病结局之间的因果关系不能确立。虽然一些潜在的混杂因素可以在数据分析时进行考量和定量，但是在队列研究中无法处理残存混杂（residual confounding）。所谓的残存混杂是指通过研究设计考虑和/或数据分析排除各种潜在混杂因素之后仍然残存的混杂因素。残存混杂主要有三个来源。

（1）未被考虑进去的其他混杂因素。

（2）对混杂的校正不充分。

（3）受试者在混杂因素变量的分类上存在错误。

在队列研究中采用客观或设盲的方法、独立于暴露状态测量结局，也是减少信息偏倚的关键。

强化流行病学观察性研究报告（STROBE）声明是观察性研究的报告书写指南，包括队列研究、病例对照研究和横断面研究。STROBE声明和其他清单（例如，CASP、牛津CEBM、SIGN和SURE）都可用于队列研究的评价。

4. 病例对照研究　病例对照研究中，研究者首先选择有某种结局（例如疾病）的人作为病例组，没有该结局的则作为对照组。然后回顾性收集潜在暴露因素的数据，比较病例组和对照组的暴露情况。对于罕见结局（如罕见病）的危险因素研究，是一种理想的研究设计。

方法学上来说，病例对照研究最主要的困难是选择合适的病例和对照，以及如何处理可能的"回忆偏倚"（人们会对造成其结局的原因做出一些主观解释，这将影响其对潜在危险因素的回忆）。为了减少选择偏倚，对照和病例均应从同源人群中抽取，对照和病例之间的唯一的区别应该是对照没有出现该结局状态（换句话说，一个人出现在病例组还是在对照组，唯一的原因即是其有或无该结局状态）。除了结局状态之外，病例组和对照组有相同的排除标准；病例和对照的定义清晰，区分明确。为了减少信息偏倚，应以标准、有效和可靠的方式测量暴露因素；同时，病例的确认不应受暴露因素的影响。最后，在研究设计和数据分析中，应该考虑和测量潜在的混杂因素。前文介绍的那些清单亦可用于评价病例对照研究。

5. 横断面研究　横断面研究同时测量人群中的暴露因素和结局状态，是该人群的"快照"。同样，研究者也可以通过STROBE声明和其他清单来评价横断面研究的真实性。

6. 诊断试验准确性评价的研究　诊断试验准确性评价的研究通常采用横断面设计，但该类研究有许多特别之处，包括招募入组受试者、诊断试验评价的金标准、诊断试验准确度的评价参数等。

诊断准确性研究的报告标准（standards for the reporting of diagnostic accuracy studies，STARD）包括详细的流程图和30个条目的清单，是诊断试验准确性研究的标准报告和评价标准。同样，前文提及的其他清单也有类似作用，只是更简单。

综上所述，研究者一旦明确了一篇论文的研究设计，就可以用针对该研究设计类型的评价清单来检查它的偏倚风险，包括前文介绍的批判性评价技能项目（critical appraisal skills programme，CASP），牛津循证医学中心（Oxford Center for Evidence-Based Medicine，Oxford

CEBM)、苏格兰校级指南网（Scottish Intercollegiate Guidelines Network，SIGN）等各个组织开发的各种清单。针对系统综述、RCT、队列研究、病例对照研究、诊断试验研究、经济学评价和定性研究等各种研究的特定评价清单都可在上一节提到的网站上找到。这些清单中的大部分条目都源于最初发表在《美国医学会杂志》（*JAMA*）上的题为"医学文献读者指南（Users' Guides to the Medical Literature）"的系列文章。

三、这项研究是按照原来的方案进行的吗？

偏离方案会影响研究的真实性或相关性。常见的方案偏离包括样本量的变化、纳入和排除标准的变化、治疗或干预措施的变化、技术或设备的改变以及随访时间的变化。评价证据时，研究者应该仔细查看并思考所有方案的偏离，要考虑这些偏离是否会损害内部真实性和外部真实性。

四、统计分析是否正确，能通过数据得到结论吗？

由临床医生判断一项研究的统计分析是否正确，并不太容易，不过可以判断论文的方法部分，作者对统计分析方法和工具的描述是否恰当。特别需要注意，作者是如何处理数据缺失的。在论文的结果部分，作者应该详细说明失访和数据缺失的情况，最好以流程图的形式展示。

论文的结论必须基于研究数据而得，需要合理、符合逻辑。有的作者将一个亚组的结果放大到更广泛的人群中去。还有的作者将两者的相关性误解为因果关系。

五、存在利益冲突吗？

当一些个人因素有可能会影响专业角色或责任时，就存在利益冲突，应该公开披露。当然，潜在的利益冲突并不意味着一定会出现实际的利益问题，也未必说明研究质量不佳。在批判性评估的过程中，研究者应该了解研究可能的资金来源、其对研究的影响以及利益冲突是如何处理的、是否有相关声明等。

第四节　证据重要性评价

如果一项研究是可信的（具有内部真实性），接下来就要问该研究是否重要，或者具体来说，某项治疗措施或诊断试验到底有多好、多重要。很多时候，研究者总是想简单地用一句话或一个数字来说明研究有多重要，但实际上，一个数字远远不够。有些人只看假设检验，他们一看到 $P<0.05$，也就是所谓的具有统计学意义，就大为振奋，认为这是一个重要的结果，但其实，$P<0.05$ 虽具有统计学显著性却不能衡量影响的大小或结果的重要性。

以下四个问题将有助于评价研究结果的重要性。

一、研究的主要结局是什么？临床上有意义吗？

结局是各种可能的结果之一，或是因暴露于某个因素之后引起的变化，或是接受预防性或治疗性干预措施之后发生的变化。主要结局（primary outcome）是研究者认为研究最重要的结果参数，与研究中许多的其他结局，即次要结局（secondary outcomes）不一样，主要结局决定了研究的总体结果和结论。在研究设计阶段即要确定该研究的主要结局指标，以根据其来确定研究所需样本量。一个合适的样本量应有足够的统计把握度,以避免研究出现假阴性错误。主要结局和研究假设均应事先确定,这样也减少了对多个结局进行多次统计学假设检验而导致的假阳性错误。特别值得注意的是,每个 RCT 都只有一个主要结局,区分主要结局和次要结局是非常重要的。对次要结局进行统计学检验,其假阳性和假阴性的风险均可能增加。

在临床试验中,"终点"是对试验中受试者的结果的测量和评价。终点有两种类型:临床终点和替代终点。根据美国食品和药品管理局(FDA)的相关文件,临床结局是最可靠的临床试验终点。临床结局测量的是人们认为最重要的内容和参数,比如是否不适的感觉好转了、功能提高了或者是活得更长了等。当临床试验采用的是临床结局,且试验显示治疗利大于弊,研究者就可以有信心地推荐该治疗方案。

有些临床试验也用所谓的替代终点(surrogate endpoint)来代替临床结局。如果采用临床结局可能需要相当大的样本量或花费很长的时间进行研究时,或者当替代终点(如血压控制)和临床获益之间的关系很明确时,人们常常采用替代终点来开展研究。有时候,如果采用临床结局需要有创检查或不符合伦理,也可采用替代终点。在药物的评价中,常用的替代终点包括:药代动力学测量、体外(即实验室)测量、组织的形态观察、所谓的"疾病的生物标志物"的水平变化检测以及影像学表现等。

明确替代终点可以可靠地预测临床获益,或说明两者相关,需要通过临床试验来证实。通过临床试验证实的替代终点被称为经过验证的替代终点(validated surrogate endpoint),FDA 也认可这样的替代终点。然而,即使是经过验证的替代终点有时也会产生误导。例如,在控制糖尿病患者心血管危险行动(ACCORD)试验中,与标准治疗相比,强化治疗显著降低糖化血红蛋白水平,但它却并没有明显降低心血管事件的发生率,强化治疗组的死亡率甚至更高。如果一项研究的主要结局没有明显的临床意义、不能代表临床实际获益或者风险,对其结果的解释要特别小心。理想的替代终点应该具备以下特征。

1. 替代终点应该可靠、可重复、可行、容易定量、支付得起、有剂量 - 效应关系。

2. 替代终点能可靠地预测疾病(或疾病风险),而不仅仅是暴露因素的一种协变量。替代终点与临床结局的关系,可以从生物学机制上做出很好的解释。

3. 替代终点应该具有高灵敏度和高阳性预测值,即:最终会出现某临床结局者,全部或者绝大部分人的替代终点都是阳性;替代终点阳性者,全部或绝大部分人最终都会出现某临床结局。

4. 替代终点应该具有高特异度和高阴性预测值,即:最终不会出现某临床结局者,全部或者绝大部分人的替代终点都是阴性;替代终点阴性者,全部或者绝大部分人最终都不会出现某临床结局。

5. 替代终点如果是连续变量,应该有明确的临界值以区分正常和异常结果。

6. 替代终点能快速、准确地反映治疗效果。

7. 可以通过质量控制监察等对替代终点进行调整、修改。

复合结局(composite outcome)是指将多种结局(如多个不同的严重病症)组合成一个单一的结局。在随机对照试验中常常将复合结局作为主要结局指标。如果正确使用的话,复合结局可以提高统计效率和精度,但同时也会使结果的解释更为复杂,并带来更大的不确定性。复合结局的组成可能不合理、不统一,报道时不完全、不充分。发表在 BMJ 上的一项系统综述发现采用复合结局作为主要结局的 16 个"阳性"(即具有统计学意义)临床试验中，其中有 11 个研究在其摘要中错误地暗示读者：研究发现复合结局中最重要的组成部分有统计学意义。

二、研究结果的效应量有多大？有临床意义吗？

效应或效果具有两个含义：其一是因果关系中的果（例如：艾滋病是 HIV 感染的效应）；其二是指某一个因素发生变化之后在某个人群中某些特征（如某个人群中的疾病频率）发生的变化。疾病频率常用指标包括危险度（在某一时段，疾病的发生概率）、发病率（某个易患人群在某一时段中的新发病人数与易感人数及其随访时间乘积之比）和疾病比数（在某一人群中，患病人数与没有该疾病的人数之比）等，因此效应可以是疾病危险度、发病率或疾病比数的变化。效应量是研究各组间疾病危险度、发病率或疾病比数的算术绝对差值或比值（不过，比数的算术绝对差值实际上几乎不用）（表 4-5）。确定效应量的大小是定量研究的主要研究结果，应该在论文的摘要和结果部分进行报告。对于效应量，研究者始终要考虑的是其大小是否具有临床意义。在临床上，死亡率降低 0.2% 或中位生存时间增加 12 天真的有意义吗？血压下降 1mmHg 对高血压患者真的有好处吗？研究者需要基于科学认识和背景知识，对效应量大小的临床意义进行合乎逻辑的推理和判断。

表 4-5　效应测量常用指标

指标	计算方法	备注
相对危险度（RR）	EER/CER	RR=1 代表两组危险度一样； RR<1 代表试验组事件发生率低于对照组； RR>1 代表试验组事件发生率高于对照组
比数比（OR）	（EE/EN）/（CE/CN）	罕见病时，OR 近似 RR（罕见病假设）
相对危险度降低（RRR）	|CER-EER|/CER 或 1-RR	与对照组相比，试验组事件发生率下降的相对幅度比值。如果试验组导致事件发生率上升，也可用相同公式计算相对危险度增加（RRI）
危险度降低（RD） 绝对危险度降低（ARR）	|CER-EER|	RD 即 ARR，是试验组与对照组事件发生率之差。当试验组导致事件发生率上升，该值即为绝对危险度增加（ARI）。当事件代表"好"的结局时，该值即为绝对获益增加（ABI）
需要治疗的患者数（NNT）或导致伤害的治疗人数（NNH）	1/RD	NNT 和 NNH 分别是 ARR 和 ARI 的倒数。NNT 代表平均需要采用试验组治疗方案治疗多少位类似的患者才能避免一个不良结局。同样，当试验组导致某个不良结局发生率增加时，NNH 代表采用某治疗方案治疗多少人会导致一个不良结局的发生

注：CE 代表对照组事件数；EE 代表试验组事件数；CN 代表对照组无事件人数；EN 代表试验组无事件人数；CER 代表对照组事件率；ERR 代表试验组事件率。

相对危险度（relative risk，RR）或相对危险度降低（relative risk reduction，RRR）是基于危险度的比值来计算的（表 4-5），如果研究的效应量的大小是用 RR 或 RRR 表示的，应该特别当心。因为 RR 和 RRR 不能反映基线风险（即对照组中的事件率），故而不能反映效应量的实际大小。例如，当试验组事件率（experimental event rate，EER）为 20%，对照组事件率（control event rate，CER）为 40% 时，RRR 为 50%（RRR=1-RR=1-0.2/0.4=50%）。在这种情况下，通过治疗实际降低了 20% 的事件风险，即绝对危险度降低（absolute risk reduction，ARR），ARR=40%-20%=20%，治疗带来的改变非常明显，很可能具有显著的临床意义。然而，当 EER 为 0.2%、CER 为 0.4% 时，RRR 仍然为 50%（RRR=1-RR=1-0.002/0.004=50%），但此时，治疗产生的效果非常微小，仅能降低 0.2% 的事件风险（ARR=0.4%-0.2%=0.2%）。由此可见，ARR 作为效应指标在临床上更有意义，因为它保留了基线危险度信息，反映了危险度的绝对变化。

需要治疗的患者数（number needed to treat，NNT）是 ARR 的倒数（1/ARR），即采用某种治疗方案平均需要治疗多少患者才能避免一个额外的不良结局事件。也可以理解为，与临床试验中的对照措施相比，平均需要治疗几位患者，才会有一位患者从治疗中受益。NNT 非常直观，在评价干预措施（特别是药物治疗手段）的效果时是个很重要的指标。在上述例子中，当 ARR 为 20% 时，对应的 NNT 为 5，这意味着平均需要治疗 5 位患者以减少 1 个不良后果。而当 ARR 为 0.2% 时，NNT 变成 500，亦即平均需要每治疗 500 位患者，才能减少 1 例不良结局的发生。

与 NNT 相似，导致伤害的治疗人数（number needed to harm，NNH）表示平均需要有多少位患者暴露于不利的干预措施或危险因素一段时间之后，就会有一位患者遭受损害。NNH 是 ARI 的倒数，即 1/ARI。举例来说，据报道，男性吸烟者补充 β- 胡萝卜素会增加其患肺癌的风险，假设 5 年的绝对危险度增加大约为 0.5%，则 NNH 为 200，意味着平均来讲，如果 200 名男性吸烟者服用 β- 胡萝卜素 5 年，与不服用者相比，肺癌患者会增加 1 例。

综上所述，NNT 和 NNH 可以代表为了防止不良结局的发生，医患所需付出的努力程度，同时 NNT 和 NNH 之间的相对关系可以帮助研究者考虑某一诊疗措施的利弊。要正确、全面地理解 NNT 和 NNH，需要着重考虑以下几点。

1. 通常情况下，NNT 以一个数值的形式呈现，这是点估计（point estimate）。一般来讲，只有当治疗的效果有统计学意义的时候，NNT 的点估计才有意义。可以根据 ARR 的置信区间（confidence interval，CI）对 NNT 进行区间估计（interval estimation）。将在下一个问题对区间估计和置信区间做更多介绍。这里先举个例子，在一项临床试验中发现与氟康唑相比，使用伊曲康唑能使得移植术后 6 个月内的感染率降低 17%（ARR；95%CI，4.7%～29.2%），而死亡率增加了 3%（ARI；95%CI，13.2%～19.8%）。此时，需要平均治疗与试验受试者相似的 6 例患者，就可以预防 1 例感染，其 95%CI 为 3～21 例。这个区间告诉了研究者该估计的不确定程度。另一方面，因为 2 组在死亡率上的差异无统计学意义，NNH 相应的区间估计则有 2 段，95%CI 分别是 -∞～-8 例，和 5～+∞例。

2. NNT 的概念中包含了时间的维度。在前文的例子中，NNT 为 6 意味着与氟康唑相比，在移植术后的前 6 个月里面，伊曲康唑平均每治疗 6 人就可预防 1 例感染。要预防移植术后 1 年内的感染，其 NNT 肯定不再是 6 了。所以，在比较不同随访时间的 NNT 时，研究者要做一些假设，并将随访时间校正一致。

3. NNT 基于试验组和对照组的比较，故而患者的基线风险因素及对照组所接受的治疗对其有显著影响。当前的患者可能有不一样的基线因素（例如血糖控制不佳的糖尿病患者可能有更大的感染风险），他们发生结局事件的风险就可能高于或低于临床试验中患者的平均水平。所以，在日常临床工作中，应该根据每一位患者自身的基线风险而对预期的 NNT 做出调整。

三、结果有多精确?

开展一项研究的目的是估计真正的效应。然而实际上,研究者永远无法知道真正的效应。研究者所能做的是通过开展一个严格控制的研究,观察研究中的效应,用以估计真正的效应。这个单一的估计值即是所谓的点估计,它是样本的观测值,用以估计总体值或参数。虽然研究者一般认为点估计与真实值相差不大,但它不太会恰好与真实值一模一样。如果研究结果是真实可信的,估计值和真实值存在多大的差别是精确性的问题,该差别也就意味着在研究中存在一些随机误差(random error)。随机误差的误差方向和误差大小是不确定的,其产生原因包括生物或社会学方面的内在变异性、测量仪器的精确度差异、不同的研究者或医生对患者数据解释上的变异性等。原则上讲,内部真实性优先于精确度。然而,一个内部真实性很好的研究,如果其结果是高度不精确的、似是而非,也无法得出任何可靠的结论。

测量精确度常用置信区间来表示,如 95% 置信区间。该区间范围内的一系列数值均符合常规统计学检验中有统计学意义的值。置信区间的两个端点,即置信区间的下界和上界,称为置信限(confidence limit)。置信区间是区间估计的一种。如果统计模型正确,没有偏倚,则在无限次重复研究中采用正确的统计学方法产生的置信区间包含真实参数的频率不低于其置信水平。例如,95%CI 表示如果没有偏倚,进行 100 次重复试验,该种方法产生的100 次区间中,至少有 95 次包含真实值。简单来说,置信区间是一段数值范围,在 95% 的信心水平上研究者可以认为总体参数位于其间。

构建置信区间的过程涉及统计假设检验。例如,如果相对危险度 RR 的 95%CI 包含 1 这个无效值(null value),则在 $\alpha=0.05$ 的水平上无法拒绝 RR=1 这个无效假设(null hypothesis)($P>0.05$)。又如,如果绝对危险度降低 ARD 的 95%CI 不包含 0 这个无效值,则在 $\alpha=0.05$ 的水平上研究者可以拒绝 RD=0 这个无效假设($P<0.05$)。然而,区间估计比 P 值提供了更多的信息。P 值仅仅表示统计学假设与所观察到的数据之间的一致和相容程度。但置信区间同时提供了效应可能的方向和大小,以及效应值点估计的随机变异程度。但对于双侧检验的 P 值而言,它仅表示观察到的数据与统计学假设之间的一致性程度,无法提示效应的大小和方向以及点估计的随机变异程度。

置信区间的宽度不仅取决于数据的随机变异程度,而且往往也取决于研究的样本大小。一般来说,样本量越大,统计把握度越大,越能检测微小的效应,相应的置信区间也越窄。换句话说,越大样本的研究,有着越高的精确度。

置信限(即置信区间的下界和上界)也有助于研究者认识研究结果的重要性。假设在一项 RCT 中,研究人员发现青光眼患者使用一种眼药水能够比传统的抗青光眼药物多降低 1mmHg 的眼压。一般认为,多降低 1mmHg 眼压还是有临床意义的。然而,如果眼压降低的 95% 置信区间的下限仅为 0.1mmHg,即使其结果具有统计学意义(因为 95%CI 未包含0mmHg 这个无效值),考虑到 0.1mmHg 并没有什么临床意义,故而在 95% 置信区间的水平上,该结果可能未必有足够的临床意义。

四、对假设检验有其他可能的解释吗(例如假阳性、假阴性或机遇)?

一般认为,研究中的假设检验结果和置信区间都是真实可信的。但实际情况并非如此。除了第三节提到的偏倚和混杂会造成结果偏离真实之外,研究者始终应该牢牢记住,统计学假设检验存在两种类型的错误：Ⅰ类和Ⅱ类错误。Ⅰ类错误是拒绝一个正确的无效假设（即"假阳性"），而Ⅱ类错误是不能推翻错误的无效假设（即"假阴性"）。换言之，Ⅰ类错误是把不存在的东西错当存在，而Ⅱ类错误是把存在的东西错当不存在。

波考克（Pocock）等人详细介绍了当研究的主要结果为阳性或阴性时应该问的一些关键问题（表4-6）。

表4-6 研究主要结果为"阳性"和"阴性"时分别需要考虑的关键问题

"阳性"结果时需要考虑的问题	"阴性"结果时需要考虑的问题
1. P值仅仅小于0.05就能提供足够强的证据吗（是否需要更小的界值）？	1. 是否存在一些潜在的获益提示？
2. 疗效显著吗？	2. 试验是否把握度不够？
3. 主要研究结局在临床上重要吗？如果使用替代结局指标、组合结局指标，可靠吗？	3. 主要研究结局的选择和定义是否合适？
4. 次要研究结局能支持治疗的有效性吗？	4. 人群选择是否合适？
5. 该结果在各主要亚组都一致吗？	5. 治疗方案是否合适？
6. 试验的样本量是否足以令人信服？	6. 试验的执行是否存在缺陷？
7. 研究提前结束了吗？	7. 是否可以根据事先定义的非劣效界值，进行非劣效性试验？
8. 是否可能存在安全性问题以致弊大于利？	8. 亚组分析是否能提示一些信息？
9. 是否提供进行利弊平衡、个体化考虑的信息？	9. 次要结局是否有一些阳性结果？
10. 试验设计或执行是否存在缺陷瑕疵？	10. 换一种分析方法是否有一些新的提示？
11. 该结果是否能适用于患者？	11. 是否有更多阳性结果的外部证据？
	12. 是否有强有力的生物学依据可以支持疗效的存在？

在明确了效果的大小和精确度之后，临床医生进而可以考虑最后一个问题，即如何将研究结果应用于患者身上。

第五节 证据的适用性

证据通过真实性和重要性的评价之后，下一步研究者需要做的是确定可否将其应用于当前的患者。在这一步，需要将该证据、医生自身的临床经验和专业知识，与患者的价值和偏好结合起来以做出决定。下列问题将有助于评估证据的适用性。

一、该证据是否可以应用于本医疗单位和当前环境？

首先，研究者需要考虑是否可以将该证据应用于当前的条件和环境。有一些新药可能在当地并未上市，或医疗保险尚不能覆盖；有时候，如果本医疗机构缺少特殊的检查设备或者试剂盒，某些诊断试验也无法开展。

二、当前的患者是否与研究受试者类似？

临床诊疗工作中，如果面前的患者符合该研究中所有的纳入标准，不符合任何排除标准，而且该患者的人口学特征与研究中的受试者相似，之前又通过文献评阅证明了该研究可信且结果重要，那么研究者就可以放心地应用该证据了。但实际上，面前的患者往往不会与研究中的受试者完全相同。通常情况下，他们在某些方面有些相似，而在另外一些方面又存在一些差异。此时，该研究结果还能应用吗？一般而言，这些所谓差异往往是量变（例如年龄差距、不同程度的风险水平等），而不是质变（例如对感染的不同免疫状态和反应、绝对禁忌证存在与否等）。因此可以考虑一下，所面对的患者是否在社会人口学特征或病理学特征上与研究受试者差别太大，从而导致其研究结果完全不能应用。如果的确是这样，那么只有继续查找其他更为相关的研究文献。如果不是的话，则该证据仍然可以应用，只不过研究者需要估计该证据应用于该患者时，其预期的个体化效果到底如何。

三、如果将证据应用于当前患者，预期效果如何？

每一位患者都有其独特的危险因素，因此同一个治疗方案用于不同的患者其预期效果就可能不一样，其预期的获益和预期的风险均可能不一样。如果某一治疗方案在研究中被证实是有临床意义的，但是如果估计其用于当前患者时预期效果不佳，则不应该应用。

要估计患者的预期效果，第一步可以先估计患者的预期事件率（patient's expected event rate，PEER）。PEER 指的是如果当前患者未被治疗，最后出现某种结局事件的发生率；第二步是将 PEER 与某项干预措施的 RRR 或者 RRI 相乘，其结果的倒数就是个体化的 NNT 或 NNH。

NNT $_{个性化}$=1/（PEER×RRR）或 NNH $_{个体化}$=1/（PEER×RRI）。

PEER 是患者的个体化基线风险参数，可以根据以下方法来进行估计。

1. 研究论文中的 CER。

2. 研究论文中与患者特征相似的亚组的 CER。

3. 根据一些已经验证过的临床风险预测指南（公式）进行计算。

4. 其他可信的研究论文中的数据。

估计了某一措施在当前患者中的预期效果之后，研究者可以通过患者被帮助和被伤害的似然比（the likelihood ratio of being helped and harmed，LHH）来考虑该措施在该患者中的利弊关系：

LHH=（1/NNT）/（1/NNH）=NNH/NNT 或

LHH=ARR/ARI

例如，含有 β- 胡萝卜素的年龄相关性眼病研究（AREDS）膳食营养配方可以使得老年性黄斑变性的进展风险降低 28%。如果当前的患者是一个吸烟者，根据 AREDS 研究，其 PEER 达到 43%。而另一方面，有研究提示 β- 胡萝卜素使得吸烟者罹患肺癌的风险增加 0.5%。此时，NNT $_{个体化}$=1/（PEER×RRR）=1/（0.43×0.28）=9；而 NNH $_{个体化}$=1/ARI=1/0.5%=200。因此，LHH=200/9=22.2，这提示使用 AREDS 膳食补充剂后患者虽然有一定的罹患肺癌的风险，但患者的获益是风险的 20 余倍。

四、患者对干预和结果的价值和期望是什么？

医生应该始终铭记，循证医学是最好的研究证据与临床专业知识和患者独特的价值观和期望的结合。俗话说，萝卜青菜各有所爱。每个人对好和坏的价值判断不一，一个好的结局有多好，一个坏的结局有多坏，每个人的理解和要求都不一样。因此，医生需要与患者进行很好的沟通，了解患者独特的价值观和偏好，确保患者能理解相关的知识和细节、结局的好坏及其可能性的大小，并将其整合在一起进行决策。在这一过程中，即医患的共同决策（shared decision making，SDM），医务人员和患者一起根据最好的科学证据、临床专业知识以及患者的价值和偏好做出医疗保健决策。

本 章 小 结

现代的医疗保健需要医务工作者不断获取各种干预措施的有效性和安全性方面可靠的信息资料，对科学研究论文证据的质量和实用性进行批判性评价是循证实践的关键步骤。批判性评价证据的目的在于确定研究的真实性、研究结果的重要性以及其适用性。

（袁源智）

第 五 章

临床研究设计

学习目标

1. **掌握** 临床研究设计的内容和原则。
2. **熟悉** 临床研究设计的不同类型。
3. **了解** 如何利用临床研究设计的不同类型解决实际临床问题。

【案例 5-1】 如何利用临床研究设计解决临床实际问题

马某某，女，21 岁，北京某重点大学大三学生，患者于 2016 年 4 月 19 日以下腹痛为主诉就诊，血常规提示白细胞总数 14.51×10⁹/L，中性粒细胞比例 74.5%，C 反应蛋白 10mg/L（正常低于 0.5mg/L），提示存在感染或炎症。B 超检查提示：盆腔两处占位性病变，宫底偏右性质待定，考虑来源于卵巢、盆腹腔大量积液。进一步经腹壁及经阴道超声提示双侧卵巢体积增大，内呈囊实性改变，囊性区域呈蜂窝状排列，超声血流探测实性区可见较丰富的血流信号，腹腔内游离液体，最大深度 5.6cm，考虑卵巢癌可能。进一步查肿瘤标志物 CA125 升高至 151.5μl/ml（正常范围小于等于 35μl/ml），凝血及肝肾功能均正常。同时为患者完善了甲状腺及乳腺超声，发现双侧甲状腺多发结节伴点状钙化，双侧乳腺增生，腺体结构紊乱。腹腔核磁共振检查提示双侧卵巢囊性占位性病变，考虑囊腺癌或囊腺瘤可能性大。PET-CT 提示腹盆腔积液，盆腔子宫周围片状低密度影，轻微高代谢，局部可见出血密度。肝、胆、胰、脾及双肾未见明显异常。

临床专家如何处理这一患者：

（1）该患者的诊断结果是卵巢癌吗？诊断依据是什么？

（2）什么原因造成了这种变化？应该怎样取得循证医学证据？

（3）怎样进行有效干预才能解决患者痛苦？

临床医学属于应用科学的范畴，服务对象是患者。医生的工作是查找病因、明确诊断并采取适当的治疗手段，从而最大限度地帮助患者恢复健康或改善预后。临床问题是在医疗实践活动中需要解决的问题。临床研究问题来源于临床实践，问题的解决有利于提高对疾病的认识并有望对疾病的诊治提供帮助。对疾病的诊断是临床医生面对患者时首先要解决的问题，正确的诊断是合理治疗的基础，而正确的诊断首先依赖于对特定病因、病理机制及临床表现的正确认知。随着医学的发展、人类社会的进步及自然环境的变化，新的未知疾病不断出现，即使对已知疾病的病因的认识也存在一个不断深化的过程。生活环境的改变使得人类的疾病谱也发生了很大的变化，因此病因诊断在不断地变化及深化。流行病学中病因学研究探索的是疾病发生的原因及相关因素间的相互作用。在病因学研究中，需要强调的是与结局（疾病）相关的暴露都必须发生在结局之前，但这些因素不一定是结局的真正原因（病因）。绝大多数的慢性病，如肿瘤、原发性高血压、糖尿病、动脉粥样硬化等，均是遗传因素与环境因素共同作用的结果，对病因学的探讨有利于为疾病的临床诊断、治疗和预防提供依据，从而获得疾病防治的最大效益。本章以病因探索为例，介绍临床常用的研究设计类型（表 5-1）。

表 5-1　常用病因学研究设计类型简表

研究类型			特点	用途
观察性研究	描述性研究	病例报告	快，无对照，无设计	用于提供病因线索
		横断面研究	有设计，无对照	描述分布，寻找病因线索
	分析性研究	病例对照研究	由果及因，按有无疾病分组	初步诊断因果关系
		队列研究	由因及果，按暴露状况分组	验证因果关系
实验性研究		随机对照试验	随机化分组，人为干预	验证病因，研究药物疗效及副作用

本章以案例 5-1 中的青年女性患者的诊治经过为例探讨、介绍常用的病因学研究方法。

第一节　临床问题的提出：病例报告

病例报告（case report）是有关单个病例或少数几个病例的详细的临床报告。包括患者的临床表现、有鉴别意义的查体结果、实验室化验及检查结果、疾病的治疗及转归，通常包含了作者对患者病因及诊治经过的分析及探讨。病例报告都是从这些异常病例中提出某些可疑的假设，通过异常的发现探讨可能的原因，在实际临床工作中经常是发现某药物临床应用中严重或罕见不良反应的第一线索。

以案例 5-1 中疑诊卵巢癌的患者为例，这是一例不典型的疑诊为卵巢癌的青年女性患者，卵巢超声及核磁共振均高度怀疑卵巢癌，存在多个内分泌器官变化的表现，但 PET-CT 未发现明显的高代谢灶、无晚期卵巢癌患者常见的恶病质表现，通过对该例患者的临床特征、化验检查进行详细检查和报告，发现卵巢改变及腹水等类似于卵巢癌的表现的可能是患者其他原因造成的，但临床特点与常见的卵巢癌的表现存在明显差异。进一步追问病史，了解到患者近期应用了推迟月经周期的药物，考虑不除外与用药有关，建议停药，并于 2016 年 4 月 21 日复查妇科超声结果提示双侧卵巢增大似排卵后改变，盆腔积液较前减少。继续随访，5 天后再次复查妇科超声提示双侧卵巢增大，子宫声像图未见明显异常。血常规恢复正常，腹痛症状消失。

通过查阅相关文献，未发现这种表现的药物副作用在临床上的报道，该病例报告提示该调节月经周期的药物可能存在一种严重的不良反应，提出的研究问题引起了研究者的关注，随后，对患者生活环境类似的人群进行横断面研究，从而探讨不良反应的发生是患者个体差异导致的，还是在人群中存在一定的患病率，进行深入的病因学探讨。

在实际的临床及科研工作中，医生常常接触到各种大量特殊的病例，将这些病例的诊治经过加以整理分析，也就是病例报告，病例报告往往会提供一定的思路。类似这例患者：该患者在临床上非常容易误诊为卵巢癌，但存在多个内分泌系统受累改变，临床一般状况好，无一般卵巢癌患者的恶病质改变。与既往接触到的卵巢癌患者存在差异，患者诊断准确性引起医师的怀疑，临床上的个别或者系列病例可获得最初的临床线索，但仅仅个案报道在临床研究方面受到个体差异的限制，因此需要进行描述性研究的另一种常见类型：横断面研究。

第二节　横断面研究

横断面研究（cross-sectional study）又称现况调查或患病率研究。按照事先设计的要求，采取整群或抽样的方式对特定时间点（时间段）和特定人群的相关因素与健康状况进行调查，为进一步病因研究提供线索和病因假设。横断面研究的主要特点包括：在进行横断面研究时，疾病或健康状况与发现的某些因素的存在是同时获得的，无法判断病因发生在疾病前还是疾病后，因此无法判断因果关系，仅能提供患病率。横断面研究无事先确定的对照组，初步统计分析是按照是否发病分组，且因患者病程的长短不同导致调查时获得的患病率存在差异，如一种观察结局持续时间短，即使在病因作用下发生了，但可能在进行横断面研究的时间段内没有发现，导致低估患病率，从而产生较大的偏倚。

横断面研究可帮助研究者通过收集研究因素及疾病状态在整个人群中的分布及其特征，进而进行整体描述，也可为进一步研究疾病病因、危险因素提供线索。如前述病例，研究者进一步设计调查表对与患者生活环境类似的该校同专业女生进行横断面调查，调查的内容包括患者的基本信息（包括年龄、生活方式、是否用药及用药方式、有无其他合并用药）、体格检查和辅助诊断检查（如对接受调查的研究对象完善妇科超声检查）等，假定发现存在用药史的研究对象存在上述卵巢改变的比例增高，且与无药物暴露组存在统计学差异，则通过分析性研究初步考虑服用改变月经周期的药物可能与卵巢变化有关（表 5-2）。

表 5-2　应用及未应用改变月经周期的药物卵巢变化的发生情况

是否用药	接受调查人数 / 人	卵巢变化比例 /%
是	128	6.25
否	128	0

研究者同时对用药频次展开调查，查找不同剂量药物对卵巢变化发生率的差异，发现应用频率越高，发病率越高（表 5-3）。

表 5-3　应用改变月经周期药物频次与卵巢变化的关系

用药频次	接受调查的人数 / 人	卵巢变化比例 /%
大于 5 次	32	15.625 0
3～5 次	32	6.250 0
小于 3 次	64	1.562 5

根据以上横断面研究的结果，可以看出这种不良反应在应用该药物 3 次以上的患者中患病率较高，提示其病因可能与应用频次及累计剂量有关。

如上所述,对不同班级、年级、学校等既往健康状况、用药情况进行大规模调查,通过询问患者周围有无类似情况及发病前有无用药史,了解到患者同学中存在类似情况,近期服用推迟月经周期的药物后,出现卵巢变化。一方面对该患者进行去除干预因素后的随诊,结合该患者的转归,更高度提示患者的近期服药史与患者的卵巢表现存在相关性,另一方面通过设计的调查表对与患者生活方式接近的同专业的女性同学这一特定人群进行整群抽样调查,从人群、地区及时间几个维度对卵巢变化这一疾病状态进行描述可以较为全面地了解这一特定人群的整体患病情况。

什么原因导致了疾病的表现?下面就介绍病因研究常见的分析性研究方法:病例对照研究和队列研究。

第三节 病例对照研究

病例对照研究(case-control study)是分析性流行病学研究中的重要方法之一,基本原理是以一组已经确诊的有某种特定疾病的患者作为病例组,以一组未患该病但在某些方面与病例组具有可比性的个体作为对照组,搜集患者既往各种可能的危险因素的暴露情况及患者的临床资料信息,测量并比较病例组与对照组中危险因素的暴露比例,并进行统计学检验,若两组之间某暴露因素的比例差异有统计学意义,则可初步认为该因素与疾病之间存在着统计学上的关联。在评估了各种偏倚对研究结果的影响之后,再对某个或某些暴露是否为疾病的危险因素进行推断,从而对最初假设做出解释。病例对照研究属于回顾性研究,是由结果探索可能的病因的研究方法。病例对照研究的关键是对照的选择,一方面,对照选择既要保证具有代表性,即代表可能产生病例的一般人群。另一方面还要求病例与对照之间存在可比性,即除外研究因素,病例组与对照组的其他因素尽可能地平衡。以便提高病例对照研究的检验效果。

以前述的卵巢变化患者为例,按照病例对照研究设计,对患者同专业的女同学161人进行整群抽样调查,发现发生类似卵巢变化的32人,无卵巢变化的女同学为对照组,收集所有上述研究对象的一般资料、用药史、用药季节、进食习惯、运动习惯、辐射暴露情况(应用微波炉、吹风机等的频次)等进行分析。测量并比较病例组与对照组中各因素的暴露比例,计算相关指标(如OR)并进行统计学检验,从而判断哪些因素的暴露可能与卵巢变化的发生有关。

值得注意的是,病例对照研究设计是按照患者周围同学是否存在卵巢改变分组,进而比较既往这类药物的暴露情况,包括用药频率、剂量、既往的生活习惯等,提示病因线索。如果进行验证,就要进行队列研究设计。

第四节 队 列 研 究

队列研究(cohort study)是分析性流行病学研究中的另外一种重要方法,其基本原理是将特定人群按照是否暴露于某因素或按照不同暴露水平对人群进行分组,追踪观察期内各自的发病结局,并比较不同分组间疾病结局的差异,从而判定暴露因素与发病有无关联,并进一步判断关联程度大小的一种研究方法。队列研究在验证病因假设方面的效能优于病例对照研究。但队列研究仍属于观察性研究,因素的暴露不是随机分配的,而是研究之前客观存在的。类似上述例子，按照是否服用药物及服用药物的剂量、频次分组，对上述患者进行随访观察。因队列研究是由因到果的研究，检验病因假设的能力较强，可用于深入研究、验证病因假设。

按照是否用药及用药频次进行分组，进行队列研究，随访用药后 6 个月内的卵巢变化情况，计算发病率的结果见表 5-4。

表 5-4　女性用药情况及随诊结局

是否用药	卵巢发生类似变化人数 / 人	发病率 /%
是	120	5.0
否	240	0.2

第五节　随机对照试验

随机对照试验（randomized controlled trial，RCT）属于实验性对照研究范畴，是在人群中进行的、前瞻性的、用于评估医学干预措施效果的研究。它把研究对象按照随机原则分配到不同组，采取不同的干预措施，通过适当时间段的随访观察，比较组间观察结局发生频率的差别，以评估不同措施效果的差别。随机对照试验属于前瞻性研究，有人为的干预措施，受试对象按照随机的原则被分配至实验组或对照组，实验组和对照组之间具有可比性，采取的盲法设定可有效地减少观察者偏倚及患者心理因素带来的偏倚，在随访中准确记录观察结局，提高依从性和随访率，提高因果验证的效率。随机对照试验是目前评估医学干预措施效果及判断因果关系的最严谨、最可靠的研究方法。

病例报告提供了线索，应用横断面研究、病例对照研究及进一步的队列研究为疾病的流行特征及病因研究提供一定的证据及思路，因患者服用的是已经上市的药物，结合目前的分析性研究的结果，高度怀疑该药物应用与卵巢改变有关，可按照 RCT 原理，遵循随机、设立对照组和盲法的原则进行上市后的大规模临床试验，将用药后发生卵巢改变的患者随机分为继续用药组及安慰剂组，随访观察卵巢的变化情况，进而验证药物作用与卵巢变化的关系，也就是进行临床试验。若继续使用药物的受试人群卵巢无明显变化，而应用安慰剂的受试者卵巢逐渐恢复正常，则证明药物对卵巢的影响的确存在，需要及时上报有关部门，采取进一步应对措施。

为了进一步证明改变月经周期的药物与卵巢变化之间的因果关系，选择在临床上应用该药物并出现卵巢变化的人群为研究对象，按照随机的原则进行分组，对照组继续应用该药物，实验组停止用药、改服与药片性状相似的安慰剂，受试者和研究人员均不了解研究对象的真实用药情况，追踪观察其卵巢的变化情况，并对队列进行长达 1 年的随访，观察、记录临床结局，比较好转率，从而对研究结果进行判断，结果如表 5-5 所示。

表 5-5　用药组及安慰剂组卵巢变化的恢复情况

分组	观察例数 / 人	卵巢恢复例数 / 人	好转率 /%
用药组	60	2	3.33
安慰剂组	60	10	16.67

本 章 小 结

　　综上所述,临床研究的范围涉及诊断、治疗及预后等方方面面,常见的病因学研究方法包含了临床流行病学所有的设计类型,就因果论证强度而言,实验性研究大于观察性研究,有对照的研究大于无对照的研究。但研究设计类型的选择常由面临的临床问题的不同阶段和研究者的需求决定,病例报告常是第一步,为研究者提供一定的临床思路、发现一定的临床问题,但是否有实际意义有赖于进一步设计的研究方案的结论。观察性研究因不涉及人为的干预措施,仅需签署知情同意及注意隐私保护,无需考虑其他医学伦理问题,因而更容易操作,接近真实生活环境,但研究本身较容易受到混杂因素的干扰,得出结论的可靠性可能会受到一些影响。实验性研究控制偏倚的能力远大于观察性研究,研究结论本身更可靠,但实验性研究常涉及伦理学问题,有时很难实现真正意义上的随机、盲法及对照等,实验性研究可能与临床实际存在较大差异而在实际临床工作中出现推广受限的状况。

　　针对不同的临床问题,研究者可根据实际条件和需要,选择适宜的设计类型进行临床问题的探索。每种设计类型与它的验证强度(证据级别)存在密切关系,较严谨科学的设计可尽可能地控制各类偏倚的干扰,所获结论不易被后来的研究否定,可信度高。由浅入深、由弱到强地开展临床研究,合理选择不同类型的临床研究,依据不同的验证得出恰当的结论,也有利于对疾病的病因探讨做出合理的解释,进而指导疾病预防及诊疗处置。

(赛晓勇)

数据测量：准确性和精确性

学习目标

1. **掌握** 结局变量的测量和一致性检验方法。
2. **熟悉** 数据的类型与描述方法、随机误差与系统误差的概念和控制措施。

【案例 6-1】 开展研究需要数据测量

某课题研究一药物对急性脑梗死的临床疗效及安全性，需要测量的指标包括基线资料：性别、年龄、身高、体重、体温、脉搏、呼吸、血压、血常规、肝肾功、心电图、头颅 CT、脑卒中相关临床评分（如：NIHSS 评分，Barthel 指数和改良 Rankin 量表），主要结局指标为 3 个月时的改良 Rankin 量表评分，次要指标为 8 天和 15 天时的 NIHSS 评分、Barthel 指数、改良 Rankin 量表评分以及 3 个月时的 NIHSS 评分、Barthel 指数。

数据测量是指对研究的个体、群体健康及疾病状态的相关指标的数量化。如在脑卒中的临床研究中，研究对象的身高、体重、体温和血常规等指标均可通过仪器进行测量，疾病的严重程度则可通过国际公认的卒中量表进行量化。定性指标可以根据一定的原则进行分类量化，如性别分为男、女，预后依据相关的评分分为良好和不良等。测量结果经过量化后，方能采用合适的统计方法处理并进行分析比较。数据测量贯穿科研工作的始终，而真实可靠的测量是高质量研究的重要保证。

第一节 数据类型与描述

一、临床数据的类型

在临床工作中，临床症状、体征、实验室检查、临床疗效和预后等测量结果需要按数据类型进行分类，主要分为以下三类。

1. 定量资料 又称计量资料、数值资料或尺度资料，是测量观察对象相关指标的数值所得的资料，数据值可表示为在数轴一定区间内的连续数值，一般有度量衡单位。例如：身高（cm）、体重（kg）、血红蛋白（g/L）、白细胞计数（×10^9/L）等。

2. 定性资料 又称计数资料，是按观察对象的某种属性或特征进行分类，分类值结果本身并无数量的含义，无法在数轴上表示出来。如性别、血型等。

3. 等级资料 按观察对象的某种属性或特征进行分类，但分类之间有强弱、轻重、大小、程度的区分，既非连续分布的定量资料，也不是按性质属性归属于独立若干类别的定性资料，等级之间既非等距，也不能度量。例如临床疗效分为治愈、好转、无效、死亡，教育程度分为文盲、小学、初中、高中、大学、研究生，尿蛋白表示为 −、±、+、++、+++ 和 ++++ 等。

二、数据类型的转换

在临床研究中，有时要结合临床的实际意义对几种资料类型进行转换。例如，三位患者血压的测量值分别为 125/78mmHg、143/98mmHg、175/110mmHg，血压为定量资料，根据高血压定义，可分为血压正常和高血压，这样就将定量资料转化为定性资料。在进行结局影响因素分析时，若将血压以连续性变量进行多因素分析，得出的是 1mmHg 血压变化对结局的影响，这在临床工作中并无实际意义，一般观察 10mmHg 或 20mmHg 变化的临床意义，可按收缩压分为 <120mmHg、≥120mmHg 且 <140mmHg、≥140mmHg 且 <160mmHg、≥160mmHg，将定量资料转化为等级资料。在进行相关转换时，需依据国内外公认的标准或相关文献。

三、软测量指标的量化

软测量指标是指临床上没有客观定量测量方法的指标，如疼痛、恶心、乏力、失眠等。这类变量多数情况下只能用定性描述，如有与无、是与否、轻与重等，与患者的主观感受密切相关，缺乏客观的、度量衡精确的标准，容易产生较大的测量误差。在临床科研中，此类指标要尽可能向定量化发展。目前，一方面采用新的定量测量方法替代软指标，例如采用多导睡眠图对失眠进行客观评估，通过入睡潜伏期、觉醒次数和时间、两种睡眠时相、各期睡眠比例和睡眠总时间的记录对失眠进行精确客观的评价。另一方面是采用心理学、社会医学、性格测量、生活质量测量等方法，对软指标进行量化处理，用数值表示，以便分类进行统计学处理。例如疼痛的测量，以前多依赖患者的主观表述，目前国内外已采用分级评定法，将疼痛分为 5 级，即轻微疼痛（1 分）、引起不适感的疼痛（2 分）、具有窘迫感的疼痛（3 分）、严重的疼痛（4 分）、剧烈的疼痛（5 分）。

第二节　系统误差和随机误差

在实际工作中，受主观或客观因素的影响，测量值和真实值之间会有差异，称之为测量误差。按其产生的原因和性质可分为随机误差和系统误差。

一、随机误差

随机误差也称偶然误差，是指在测定过程中一些因素微小的随机波动而形成的具有相互抵偿性的误差。随机误差是一类不恒定的、随机变化的误差。其产生的原因是一些不稳定的随机因素，如室温、相对湿度和气压等环境条件的不稳定，分析人员操作的微小差异以及仪器的不稳定等。随机误差的特点是大小和方向都不固定，但误差的分布服从统计规律，表现为单峰性、对称性和有界性。单峰性，即误差小的多于误差大的；对称性，即正误差与负误差概率相等；有界性，即误差很大的概率几乎为零。随机误差随测定次数的增加，正负误差可以相互抵偿，误差的平均值将逐渐趋向于零。由于随机误差影响因素多、原因复杂，因而无法避免、不能测量，但其呈正态分布，可用统计学方法进行分析。

二、系统误差

系统误差指由于测量工具的局限性、测量方法理论的缺陷、实验人员操作不规范等原因造成的误差。它具有重复性、单向性、可测性等特征。即在相同的条件下，重复测定时会重复出现，使测定结果系统性地偏高或偏低，其数值大小也有一定的规律。仪器的零点不准、仪器未调整好、操作者的方法不当、试剂纯度不够等情况均会引起系统误差。如在测量血压时，采用不同厂家生产的血压计、水银柱是否含有气泡、束臂带过宽或过窄等均可引起测量误差。另外初次使用血压计的护士在测量血压的过程中，未熟练掌握测量血压的规范操作，存在充气不足或放气过快等均可导致血压测量不准确。

三、误差的控制

在临床研究中，由于随机误差无法避免，因此要尽可能控制系统误差。测量者需对所用测量工具、环境条件、测量方法等仔细地进行分析研究，找出产生系统误差的根源，进而采取措施加以控制。

1. 消除被测量者误差　向被测量者说明测量目的，争取积极配合，提供真实可靠的情况；统一测量时间和方法，严格控制测量条件。

2. 消除测量者误差　测量者在研究前进行相关培训，严格统一测量方法和技术；疗效评价时，尽量采用客观评价指标和方法，如生存和死亡。而对于非客观指标，一定要进行严格的定义。如在进行脑梗死的预后研究中，根据改良 Rankin 量表评分将预后分为良好（0～2 分）和不良（3～5 分）及死亡；并尽可能采用盲法测量。

3. 测量过程中的误差　在测量之前，统一测量仪器、试剂，仔细检查仪器仪表，正确调试和安装，必要时可利用中心实验室进行测量。

第三节　结局指标和测量工具的选择

一、结局指标

临床结局是疾病在干预措施下发生的、与患者直接相关的、有临床意义的重要临床事件，如生存、死亡、残疾等。在一定时间点测量的反映健康或疾病临床结局的变量称为结局指标。一项干预措施对于目标疾病的治疗是否有效，结局指标的选择是十分重要的因素之一。良好的结局指标应具备以下几个特点：能较好地反映干预措施对症状的改善程度，体现治疗前后的变化情况；有严格统一的标准，定义明确，不易引起歧义；不同研究有良好的一致性，便于比较。

结局指标可根据研究目的进行分类，从信息来源角度分为基于医生的结局评价和基于患者的结局评价。从干预措施角度可分为主要结局指标和次要结局指标。主要结局指标是指临床研究中要评价的测量的主要目标，根据干预措施所产生的主要效果来确定。次要结局指标根据干预措施辅助的或次要效果确定。从反映患者的健康状况角度可分为终点指标和替代指标。终点指标是指对患者影响最大、患者及研究者对于疾病的发展最为关注的临床事件，如死亡、骨折、复发等，对临床决策最具有参考价值。替代指标是在终点指标的测量不可行（如需要很长时间）的情况下评估干预措施的效果，建立在流行病学、治疗学、病理生理学等基础上，能代替重要临床结局、实验室或影像学测量指标，如血脂水平、肿瘤大小等。采用替代指标必须有足够证据支持其与临床终点指标的关系，并可预测疾病结局。

结局指标的选择应当根据干预措施的特点、治疗目标和疾病性质综合考虑。例如研究某种药物治疗失眠的有效性，结局指标可采用相关的量表，包括匹兹堡睡眠质量指数（PSQI）、失眠严重程度指数（ISI）、睡眠功能障碍等级量表（SDRS）等，以总分或各项分值作为结局指标。还可根据《中药新药临床研究指导原则》，将疗效分为 4 个等级，即临床治愈：睡眠时间恢复正常或夜间睡眠时间在 6h 以上，睡眠深沉，醒后精力充沛；显效：症状明显好转，睡眠时间增加 3h 以上，睡眠深度增加；有效：症状减轻，睡眠时间较前增加不足 3h；无效：治疗后失眠无明显改善或加重者。

二、测量工具的选择

临床结局的测量工具包括技术测量、临床测量和患者导向的测量。技术测量方法包括实验室检查、影像学检查和电生理检查。临床测量方法包括身体和认知损伤检查、活动如步行的评定方法。患者导向的测量方法包括患者和代理人对健康状况、生活质量和健康主观感受的自我报告。

第四节　一致性检验

一、一致性检验

在实际临床工作中，不同医务人员对各种特殊检查、疾病诊断等都可能出现判断不一致的情况。一是同一医务工作者对多个对象进行两次观察不一致；二是两个医务工作者对多个对象进行观察做出的判断不一致；三是多个医务工作者对多个对象进行观察做出的判断不一致。特别是在大型的多中心研究中，有必要了解观察或判断的一致程度，若一致性较差，说明结果的可靠性受到重复检查判断不一致的影响，应采取必要措施控制测量误差；若一致性较好，说明重复检查的结果是可靠的。在实际工作中由于重复观察造成的判断不一致很难避免，一方面要采用适当的统计方法评价其判断的一致性，另一方面采取措施把这种不一致控制在最低限度，这就涉及一致性检验。

一致性检验方法根据资料的分类而有所不同。对于定量资料，如血压的测定结果，可采用组内相关系数评价。对于定性资料分为两种情况。

1. 二分类变量，例如：症状的有或无，检测结果的阳性或阴性。

2. 多分类变量，如疗效（分为治愈、显效、有效、无效）。定性资料的一致性检验较为常用，主要采用 Kappa 值作为评价判断一致性程度的指标。

二、Kappa 检验

Kappa 检验是一种旨在校正机遇、衡量一致性的方法，适合于两名或多名调查人员对诸如调查结果、诊断结果、检测结果等一致性进行评价，一致性越高，则表明结果的可靠程度越高。

Kappa=$(P_0-P_c)/(1-P_c)$，其中 P_0 称为观察一致率，P_c 称为机遇一致率，即两次检验结果由于偶然机会所造成的一致率。

例如，两名放射科医生阅 100 例患者头颅 CT 判断其是否有脑梗死，结果见表 6-1。

表 6-1　两名放射科医生对头颅 CT 诊断脑梗死的判断结果

甲医生	乙医生		合计 / 人
	阴性 / 人	阳性 / 人	
阴性 / 人	74（a）	2（c）	76（a+c）
阳性 / 人	4（b）	20（d）	24（b+d）
合计 / 人	78（a+b）	22（c+d）	100（n）

观察一致率（P_0）=（a+d）/n=（74+20）/100=0.94。

机遇一致率（P_c）=［（a+b）（a+c）/n+（c+d）（b+d）/n］/n=（78×76/100+22×24/100）/100=0.65。

实际一致率 =P_0-P_c=0.94-0.65=0.29。

非机遇一致率 =$1-P_c$=1-0.65=0.35。

Kappa= 实际一致率 / 非机遇一致率 =0.29/0.35=0.83。

Kappa 值取值范围一般为 -1～+1。如果观察一致率大于机遇一致率，则 Kappa 值在 0～+1 之间，反之，则其值在 -1～0 之间。Kappa=-1，为完全不一致；Kappa=0，说明观察一致性完全由机遇造成；Kappa=+1，即完全排除机遇一致后的观察一致，但实际中出现的可能性极小。Kappa 值的大小划分为六个区段，分别代表一致性的强弱程度。Kappa<0，一致性极差；0.00～0.20，一致性微弱；0.21～0.40，一致性弱；0.41～0.60，中度一致性；0.61～0.80，高度一致性；0.81～1.00，一致性极强。

本 章 小 结

临床测量贯穿临床和科研工作的始终，是高质量研究的重要保证之一。测量数据类型包括定量资料、定性资料和等级资料，应根据临床研究的实际情况进行相应转换，并尽可能用定量测量方法替代定性指标。

测量误差分为随机误差和系统误差，应尽可能找出产生系统误差的根源，进而采取措施控制。

结局指标的选择是判断干预措施对于目标疾病的治疗是否有效的重要因素之一，应当根据干预措施的特点、治疗目标和疾病性质综合考虑。

一致性检验用于判断不同医务人员对各种特殊检查、疾病诊断等发生判断不一致的情况，Kappa 检验用于定性资料，其值一般在 -1～+1 之间，值越大，代表一致性越强。

（刘学东）

第七章

偏倚发现：内部真实性判断

学习目标

1. **掌握** 选择偏倚、信息偏倚及混杂偏倚的基本概念。
2. **熟悉** 三种偏倚的控制方法。
3. **了解** 三种偏倚的测量。

任何科学研究包括医学研究的目的是揭示事物发生的本质及内在规律，使其研究结果与真实结果一致。研究收集的数据、分析的结果和所得的结论与客观实际的一致程度，称为研究的真实性（validity）。真实性也是研究发现并能准确反映"真实世界"的程度。真实性分为内部真实性和外部真实性。内部真实性是研究结果与源人群真实情况的符合程度，是指研究自身的真实性。真实性高的研究结果更有信心被认为是真实的研究结果。外部真实性是指研究结果能够外推到受试对象以外的不同时间、不同地区及不同人群的程度。内部真实性是外部真实性的前提，但内部真实性好，由于样本代表性差，外部真实性不一定就好。

误差（error）是研究的结果与真实值之间的差异。流行病学研究中常见的误差包括随机误差和系统误差。随机误差是指随机抽样所得的均值与总体参数的差异。随机误差普遍存在于随机抽样的研究中，可通过使用正确的抽样方法、增加样本量等措施减小随机误差。系统误差，亦称偏倚（bias），是指在研究设计、实施、数据处理和分析以及结果解释、推论中的片面性，使得研究结果系统地偏离真实值，从而得出错误的结果或结论。系统误差是可以避免的，而且必须被控制。

一般将偏倚分为选择偏倚、信息偏倚和混杂偏倚。

第一节 人群选择中发生的偏倚

一、概念

选择偏倚是指被选入到研究中的研究对象与没有被选入者特征上的差异所导致的系统误差。此种偏倚在确定研究样本、选择比较组时容易产生，在资料收集过程中的失访或无应答等也可能产生。选择偏倚在各类流行病学研究中均可发生。

二、种类

主要包括以下几种。

1. 无应答偏倚（non-response bias）　在特定研究样本中，无应答者的患病状况以及对某些研究因素的暴露情况与应答者可能会不尽相同，由此而导致的偏倚称为无应答偏倚。主要发生在横断面研究和实验流行病中。在队列研究中的失访是无应答的另一表现形式，是指由于某些原因，研究对象未能按照研究设计方案的计划被随访，从而导致此类偏倚。公认的应答率最低为80%。

2. 易感性偏倚（susceptibility bias）　在研究因素与结局（包括发病、疾病复发、死亡等）的关系时，有些因素可直接或间接影响观察人群或对照人群对所研究结局的易感性，从而夸大或缩小了暴露因素与结局的关联强度，由此而导致的偏倚称为易感性偏倚。

3. 入院率偏倚（admission rate bias）　也称伯克森偏倚（Berkson bias），指当以医院患者为研究对象时，由于不同暴露及结局的患者入院率的不同所导致的系统误差。如在病例对照研究中，如果病例或对照与以人群为基础的病例或对照的暴露不同，则会导致OR值低估或高估。

4. 现患病例 - 新发病例偏倚（prevalence-incidence bias）　也称奈曼偏倚（Neyman bias）。病例对照研究以现患病例为对象时，同时纳入新旧病例，而不包括病情重、病程短而很快死亡的病例，或轻型、不典型病例；由此而形成的病例样本与单纯由新发病例构成的样本相比，其病情、病型、病程等不尽相同，既往暴露史也可能不同；另一方面，旧病例可能由于患病而改变影响因素的暴露情况，从而歪曲了影响因素与疾病的关系。

5. 检出症候偏倚（detection signal bias）　是指某因素与所研究的疾病在病因学上没有关系，但该因素的存在可导致所研究的疾病相关症状或体征的出现，促使患者及早就医，以至于具有相关症状或体征的人群比一般人群对于该病的检出率高，从而得出该因素与该疾病相关联的错误结论。该偏倚在以医院为基础的病例对照研究中容易出现。

三、选择偏倚的控制

选择偏倚一旦发生，很难消除。主要是通过恰当的研究设计与实施来控制。在设计阶段，明确目标和样本人群，如果需要随机抽样，一定确保做到真正的随机，使抽到的样本具有代表性。若研究需随机分组（实验性研究），确保研究对象通过随机分组后，各组间具有均衡性。病例对照研究的病例尽可能从多个医院获取，也可以同时选择医院和社区或住院和门诊病历。研究对象的选择须有严格、明确的纳入和排除标准，以使其能较好地代表其所出自的总体。在研究过程中要积极采取措施，尽量取得研究对象的合作，以降低无应答、随访性研究中的失访以及实验性研究中的不依从等情况的发生。

第二节　测量过程中发生的偏倚

一、概念

研究实施过程中，获取所需各种信息时所产生的系统误差，称信息偏倚（information bias），也称观察偏倚（observation bias）、测量偏倚（measurement bias）。信息偏倚在各类流行病学研究中均可发生，可来自调查者，可来自研究对象，也可来自用于测量的方法、仪器、设备、环境等。信息偏倚可使研究信息被错误分类，按其所致错误分类在观察组与对照组分布的异同，分为无差异错误分类（non-differential misclassification）和有差异错误分类（differential misclassification）。前者是指错误分类等同地发生在用于比较的两组之中；后者是指错误分类不等同地发生在用于比较的两组之中。

二、种类

主要包括如下几种。

1. 测量偏倚（measurement bias）　指研究者对研究所需数据进行测量时所产生的系统误差。包括研究所使用的仪器设备、方法、试剂、条件等不标准、不统一，研究指标选择、设定不合理，操作人员的操作误差，数据记录错误、不完整等。测量偏倚可发生在各种流行病学研究设计中。

2. 回忆偏倚（recall bias）　指研究对象在回忆以往研究因素的暴露情况等信息时，由于回忆的准确性或完整性，在比较组间的差异而导致的系统误差。多见于病例对照研究。

3. 报告偏倚（reporting bias）　指在收集研究信息时，由于某些原因，研究对象有意夸大或缩小某些信息而导致的系统误差。

4. 暴露怀疑偏倚（exposure suspicion bias）　指调查者事先了解研究对象的患病情况或某结局，可能会在各比较组间采用不可比的方法探寻某病或某结局有关的因素，由此而引起的系统误差。如多次认真地询问病例组某因素的暴露史，而不同样认真地询问对照组，从而导致错误结论。

5. 诊断怀疑偏倚（diagnostic suspicion bias）　研究者若事先了解研究对象的暴露情况，在主观上倾向于其出现某种结局，在做诊断或分析时，有意无意地倾向于自己的判断，使得诊断或分析在暴露组和非暴露组不可比，从而导致错误结论，由此而导致的系统误差称为诊断怀疑偏倚。

三、信息偏倚的控制

1. 严格信息标准　对研究内容包括结局、暴露及混杂因素要有公认、明确的定义和标准，并力求量化或等级化。要制订严格、明细的资料收集方法。使用的仪器、设备应予校准；试剂等应符合测试要求。要设计统一的信息收集用表，调查员要予以培训，统一调查标准和调查方法。采取适当措施取得研究对象的合作，使其提供研究所需的客观、准确的信息。

2. 盲法收集信息　收集研究所需信息时尽可能地采用盲法，避免或消除研究对象或调查者主观心理因素的影响，避免信息偏倚。

3. 采用客观指标　研究信息尽量采用客观指标。

4. 调查技术的应用　对敏感问题进行调查时，应尽量采用敏感问题调查的技术或方法，如设计适当的问卷，应用随机应答技术等，以获得可靠的信息，避免报告偏倚。对某些信息的问卷调查，询问时可同时收集一些与调查内容看似无关的变量来分散调查人员或被调查者的注意力，以减少主观因素对信息客观性的影响。

5. 统计学处理　对研究资料的信息偏倚可应用错分分析予以分析与评价。

第三节　混　杂　偏　倚

一、概念

混杂偏倚或称混杂（confounding）是指在研究中由于一个或多个潜在的混杂因素（confounding factor）的影响，掩盖或夸大了研究因素与研究疾病（事件）之间的联系，从而使两者之间的真正联系被错误地估计，它是一种系统误差。

混杂因素亦称外来因素（extraneous factor）、第三因素、混杂因子或混杂变量，指某因素与研究因素和研究疾病（事件）均有关，若该因素在比较的人群组中分布不均衡，则可以歪曲（缩小或夸大）研究因素与疾病之间的真实联系。

二、混杂因素的基本特点

1. 混杂因素是所研究疾病（事件）的危险因素。
2. 混杂因素与所研究的因素有关。
3. 混杂因素不是研究因素与研究疾病因果链上的中间变量。

如果某因素具备以上三个基本特点条件，而且在比较的人群中分布不均匀，即可导致混杂偏倚产生。

三、混杂偏倚的控制

1. 限制（restriction）　指在研究设计时针对某些潜在的混杂因素，通过研究对象的入选标准予以限制，得到同质的研究对象，可避免这些混杂因素的混杂作用，有利于对所研究因素与研究疾病之间关系的正确估计。但会大大减少样本量，结果外推时受到限制。

2. 随机化（randomization）　指以随机化原则与技术使研究对象以等同的概率被分配在用于比较的各组之中，使潜在混杂变量在各组间分布均衡，从而排除其混杂作用。

3. 匹配（matching）　指在为指示研究对象（病例、有某特征者等）选择对照时，针对一个或多个潜在的混杂因素，使其与指示研究对象相似，从而消除这一（些）混杂因素对研究结果的影响。对某因素予以匹配可以消除该因素的潜在混杂作用，提高研究效率，但同时也失掉了对这一因素予以分析的机会。因此一般认为，匹配因素不宜太多，以只列入主要的混杂变量为宜。

4. 统计学处理　混杂偏倚在资料分析阶段可通过一定的统计学处理方法予以识别与控制。如标准化法、分层分析、多因素分析等。其中分层分析可用 Mantel-Haenszel 分层分析方法进行分析，得到将该混杂变量调整后的结果。若控制的混杂因素较多，可应用多因素分析方法进行分析，如协方差分析、多因素逻辑回归分析等。

第四节　偏倚的影响

偏倚是影响流行病学研究真实性的重要问题。选择偏倚和信息偏倚在观察性研究及实验性研究过程中均存在，但在回顾性研究中信息偏倚（回忆偏倚）影响更大。实验流行病学通过随机分组将已知的及未知的混杂因素均衡地分配到各组，从而控制了混杂偏倚。

一、选择偏倚的影响及其测量

一项研究是否存在选择偏倚，理论上可通过比较总人群与研究样本所研究疾病（事件）与暴露因素分布两个四格表的数据及其效应值予以评价。总人群与实际抽样样本（研究样本）疾病与研究因素的分布及样本选择概率如图 7-1 所示。

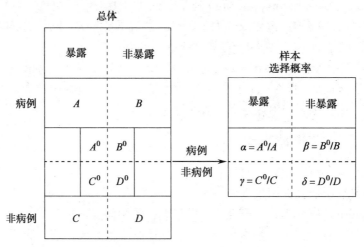

图 7-1　总体与研究样本中疾病与研究因素分布示意图
α、β、γ、δ 分别为各组样本选择概率。

由图 7-1 可见：

总人群比值比 $OR = \dfrac{A \cdot D}{B \cdot C}$。

样本比值比 $OR^0 = \dfrac{A^0 \cdot D^0}{B^0 \cdot C^0}$。

根据选择概率 $OR^0 = OR \cdot \dfrac{\alpha \cdot \delta}{\beta \cdot \gamma}$。

选择偏倚的大小与方向可用下式表示：

选择偏倚 $= \dfrac{OR^0 - OR}{OR}$ 或 $\dfrac{\alpha \cdot \delta}{\beta \cdot \gamma} - 1$。

若得值等于 0，即 $\dfrac{\alpha \cdot \delta}{\beta \cdot \gamma} = 1$ 则不存在选择偏倚。

若得值大于 0，即 $\dfrac{\alpha \cdot \delta}{\beta \cdot \gamma} > 1$，则存在选择偏倚，此时 $OR^0 > OR$。

若得值小于 0，即 $\dfrac{\alpha \cdot \delta}{\beta \cdot \gamma} < 1$，则存在选择偏倚，此时 $OR^0 < OR$。

若以 RR 作为研究因素与疾病的关联指标（如在队列研究中），那么：

总人群相对危险度 $RR = \dfrac{A \cdot (B + D)}{B \cdot (A + C)}$。

研究样本相对危险度 $RR^0 = \dfrac{A^0 \cdot (B^0 + D^0)}{B^0 \cdot (A^0 + C^0)}$。

根据图 7-1 所示的选择概率 $RR^0 = \dfrac{\alpha \cdot A \cdot (\beta \cdot B + \delta \cdot D)}{\beta \cdot B \cdot (\alpha \cdot A + \gamma \cdot C)}$。

此时，RR^0 与 RR 差异（偏倚）的大小与方向可用下式表达：

选择偏倚 $= \dfrac{RR^0 - RR}{RR} = \dfrac{\alpha (A+C)(\beta \cdot B + \delta \cdot D)}{\beta (B+D)(\alpha \cdot A + \gamma \cdot C)} - 1$。

若 $\alpha = \gamma$，$\beta = \delta$，则偏倚等于 0，即不存在选择偏倚，否则，存在选择偏倚。

二、信息偏倚的影响及其测量

1. 一致性 常用评价信息偏倚的方法是对调查获得的信息进行重复调查（测量），根据重复调查数据计算 Kappa（κ）值（具体计算方法请参考相关书籍），评价重复检测的一致性，同时也可作为研究结果内部真实性评价的依据。以 κ 值判断一致性强度的标准，一般认为：κ>0.8 为很好；0.6<κ≤0.8 为较好；0.4≤κ≤0.6 为中度；κ<0.4 为较差。

2. 偏倚程度与方向 某研究是否存在信息偏倚及其方向与程度，可用调查所得信息计算的 OR 值（OR_O）与根据实际情况（如客观检查、记录等）计算的 OR 值（OR_T）的差异予以估计：

信息偏倚 $= \dfrac{OR_O - OR_T}{OR_T}$。

得值的大小即表示偏倚的程度。

若得值等于 0，则不存在信息偏倚。

若得值大于 0，则存在信息偏倚，此时 $OR_O > OR_T$，为正偏倚。

若得值小于 0，则存在信息偏倚，此时 $OR_O < OR_T$，为负偏倚。

一般来说，当发生无差异错误分类时，调查所得资料的效应估计值（OR 或 RR）低于实际效应值，使效应估计值趋于无效假设，低估研究因素与研究疾病（事件）之间的联系。当发生有差异错误分类时，所得资料的效应估计值高于或低于实际效应值，很难判断偏倚的大小和方向。

三、混杂偏倚的影响及其测量

1. 测量某潜在混杂因素对研究因素与事件之间关系的混杂作用，可以通过比较存在该因素时研究因素与疾病的效应估计值（如 RR、OR 等），与调整了该因素后的效应估计值来实现。

若存在某混杂因素（f）时，研究因素与研究疾病的效应估计值在队列研究和病例对照研究分别为 cRR 和 cOR，称作粗 RR 或粗 OR；将该混杂因素（f）调整后的效应估计值，即排除该因素的混杂作用后的效应估计值为 aRR（f）或 aOR（f），称作调整 RR 或调整 OR。aRR（f）或 aOR（f）可用 Mantel-Haenszel 分层分析等方法进行计算。以队列研究的效应估计值 RR 为例，说明混杂因素测量如下。

若 cRR=aRR（f），则 f 无混杂作用，cRR 不存在 f 的混杂偏倚。

若 cRR≠aRR（f），则 f 有混杂作用，cRR 存在 f 的混杂偏倚。

若 cRR>aRR（f），则为正混杂（positive confounding），由于 f 的混杂作用，使 cRR 高估了研究因素与研究疾病之间的联系。

若 cRR<aRR（f），则为负混杂（negative confounding），由于 f 的混杂作用，使 cRR 低估

了研究因素与研究疾病之间的联系。

2. 混杂偏倚的程度与方向可用下式测量：

$$混杂偏倚 = \frac{cRR - aRR_{(f)}}{aRR_{(f)}}。$$

若得值等于 0，为无混杂。当得值不等于 0 时，若为正值，为正混杂；若为负值，为负混杂。值的大小为混杂的程度。

本 章 小 结

研究所收集的数据、分析的结果和所得的结论与客观实际的一致程度，称为研究的真实性。真实性的反面就是误差，包括随机误差和系统误差，后者又称为偏倚。误差越大，真实性越低。

流行病学研究中一般将偏倚分为三类，即选择偏倚、信息偏倚和混杂偏倚。选择偏倚是指被选入到研究中的研究对象与没有被选入者特征上的差异所导致的系统误差，主要包括无应答偏倚、易感性偏倚、入院率偏倚、现患病例 - 新发病例偏倚、检出症候偏倚。信息偏倚是指在研究实施过程中获取所需各种信息时所产生的系统误差，主要包括测量偏倚、回忆偏倚、报告偏倚、暴露怀疑偏倚、诊断怀疑偏倚。混杂偏倚是指在研究中，由于一个或多个潜在的混杂因素的影响，掩盖或夸大了研究因素与研究疾病（事件）之间的联系，从而使两者之间的真正联系被错误地估计，它是一种系统误差。当怀疑有偏倚发生的时候，应该对偏倚的程度、方向加以测量，并评估其对研究结果可能产生的影响。在研究的设计、实施和资料分析阶段均可以采取多种措施控制偏倚。

（赵亚双）

病因与危险因素研究

学习目标

1. **掌握** 病因与危险因素的基本概念、因果推断研究的评价原则。
2. **熟悉** 病因与危险因素研究的基本过程。
3. **了解** 病因模型及有向无环图等应用工具。

发现疾病的原因、对疾病进行有效的治疗和预防，是人类千百年来孜孜以求的目标。天花病毒的发现及其疫苗的研制，使天花成为全世界第一个被人类消灭的传染病。低密度脂蛋白胆固醇对心血管系统危害的认识及降胆固醇药物的研制，使西方国家冠状动脉疾病的发生率与死亡率大幅下降。医生怎样去发现疾病的病因或危险因素？又该怎样对病因与危险因素的研究进行评价？这些都是在本章中需要回答的关键问题。

第一节 基 本 概 念

病因是导致疾病发生的原因。病因学研究是医学研究中的重要内容，因为只有真正理解导致疾病发生的原因，才能有效地对疾病进行预防、诊断和治疗。一直以来，人们都对疾病发生的原因抱有浓厚的兴趣，发现病因也是医学科研工作者孜孜以求的目标。病因学研究需要基础、临床和预防医学研究等多学科的多角度探索，阐明病因需要多个学科的综合研究与相互印证。临床流行病学正是从群体的宏观角度，对疾病的病因进行研究，通过认识疾病发生和流行的规律，有效地对疾病进行预防、诊断和治疗。

一、充分病因和必要病因

从逻辑上讲，原因分为充分条件和必要条件，病因也分为充分病因和必要病因。

充分病因（sufficient cause）是指如果该病因存在，则必然导致某疾病的发生。对大多数疾病而言，充分病因往往并不是一个因素，而是由若干个因素共同组成的，即便是病原学明确的感染性疾病也是这样，比如肺炎链球菌是导致肺炎链球菌肺炎的病原体，但仅仅接触肺炎链球菌并不足以致病，只有在人体抵抗力低下的同时接触肺炎链球菌，才会罹患肺炎链球菌肺炎。在这个例子中，肺炎链球菌和人体抵抗力低下共同组成了肺炎链球菌肺炎的充分病因。

必要病因（necessary cause）是指如果发生某疾病，在发病之前必然有该因素存在，如果没有该因素就不会发生某疾病。比如在上面的例子中，如果没有肺炎链球菌存在，就不会出现肺炎链球菌肺炎，因此肺炎链球菌是肺炎链球菌肺炎的必要病因，而不是充分病因。

如果某个因素存在必然导致某疾病的发生，且该疾病发生之前必然有该因素存在，这个因素就是该疾病的充分必要病因，如 21 号染色体三体是唐氏综合征的充分必要病因。如图 8-1 所示，因素 A 是疾病 X 的充分必要病因。

如果某个因素存在必然导致某个疾病的发生，但该疾病发生之前不一定有该因素存在，这个因素就是该疾病的充分病因，但不是必要病因，如人体

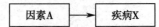

图 8-1　因素 A 是疾病 X 的充分必要病因

暴露于大剂量放射线必然导致白血病发生，但并非所有白血病患者都曾经暴露于放射线之下。在这种情况下，还存在其他导致该疾病发生的充分病因。如图 8-2 所示，因素 A 是疾病 X 的充分病因，但不是必要病因，因素 B 或因素 C 也是疾病 X 的充分病因，而不是必要病因（本例中，疾病 X 没有必要病因）。

如果某疾病发生之前必然有某因素存在，但该因素存在却不一定导致某疾病的发生，这个因素就是该疾病的必要病因，但不是充分病因，如宫颈癌患者既往都有人乳头瘤病毒（HPV）感染，但并非所有感染了 HPV 的女性都必然发生宫颈癌。在这种情况下，还存在其他因素与 HPV 共同组成宫颈癌的充分病因，导致宫颈癌发生。如图 8-3 所示，因素 A 与因素 B 和因素 C 共同组成疾病 X 的充分病因，因素 A 是疾病 X 的必要病因，但不是充分病因（在本例中，因素 B 或因素 C 分别也是疾病 X 的必要病因，而不是充分病因）。

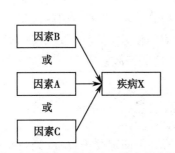

图 8-2　因素 A 是疾病 X 的充分病因，但不是必要病因

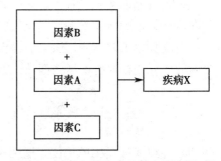

图 8-3　因素 A 是疾病 X 的必要病因，但不是充分病因

如果某因素是某疾病发生的病因之一，但疾病发生之前不一定非要有该因素存在，而该因素存在也不一定导致该疾病的发生，这个因素就既不是必要病因，也不是充分病因，如高血压是导致冠心病的诸多原因之一，但并非所有高血压患者都会发生冠心病，而冠心病患者在得病之前也并非都患有高血压。在这种情况下，高血压与某些因素的组合构成冠心病的一个充分病因，但同时还有高血压以外的其他因素的组合也构成冠心病的充分病因。如图 8-4 所示，因素 A 与因素 D 共同组成疾病 X 的充分病因，但同时还有因素 B 和因素 E 以及因素 C 和因素 F 分别组成疾病 X 的另外两个充分病因，因素 A 既不是疾病 X 的充分病因，也不是必要病因。

在临床上，大多数传染性疾病和职业病等都有一个比较明确的必要病因。而大多数慢性非传染性疾病是多因素致病的，其充分病因可能不

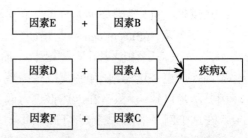

图 8-4　因素 A 既不是疾病 X 的充分病因，也不是必要病因

止一个，而可能有多个充分病因，只是各充分病因的组成因素可能不同，另一方面迄今为止尚未发现哪一个因素是其必要病因，这类慢性非传染性疾病可能不存在一个必要病因，或是必要病因仍然有待进一步探索。实际上，目前大多数疾病的充分病因并未明了，一般只是证实或初步证实其充分病因中的一个或几个因素。

二、直接病因和间接病因

对于某些疾病，导致疾病发生的因素很多，其中某些因素直接导致疾病的发生，称之为直接病因或近因，而另一些因素并不直接导致疾病的发生，而是通过一些其他因素的作用间接导致疾病的发生，称之为间接病因或远因。直接病因往往是一些生物、物理、化学等因素，直接导致疾病的发生，如结核分枝杆菌是结核病的直接病因、烟草中的有害物质是肺癌的直接病因、高血压是冠心病的直接病因等；间接病因往往是社会、经济、文化等方面的因素，它们与疾病的发生间接关联，通过直接病因的作用促成或加速疾病的发生，如社会经济条件差、卫生保健体系不健全、文化程度低等都可能造成疾病易感性的增加，促进疾病的发生。如图 8-5 所示，因素 A 是疾病 X 的直接病因；而在图 8-6 中，因素 A 是疾病 X 的间接病因，它需要通过因素 B 和因素 C 的作用导致疾病的发生。

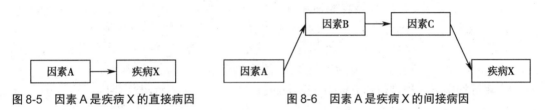

图 8-5　因素 A 是疾病 X 的直接病因　　　图 8-6　因素 A 是疾病 X 的间接病因

直接病因和间接病因都不是绝对的，它们只是用来帮助理解不同因素与疾病发生之间的关系，有些因素直接一些，有些因素还要通过一些中间环节才能发挥作用。随着科学研究的进展，人们对疾病的发生机制理解得更加深入，还会有更多的因素被包括进来，引起致病因素格局的变化，如随着新的中间环节被发现，某些以前被认为是直接病因的因素就成为了新格局中的间接病因。

三、危险因素

很多疾病，尤其是慢性非传染性疾病，病因复杂，需要不同学科从不同的角度对病因进行探索，病因的确立也需要多个学科的研究结果相互印证。流行病学以人群作为研究对象，从宏观的角度研究疾病的病因，由于方法学的局限，流行病学本身并不能够充分阐明和确定疾病的病因，而是用"危险因素"来表示其与疾病发生之间存在的因果关系。一般认为，危险因素是流行病学层面的病因，疾病的发生与该因素有一定的因果关系，但是尚无可靠的证据能够证明该因素的致病效应。当该因素存在时，人群中疾病发生的概率随之上升；当消除该因素时，疾病发生的概率也随之下降。

除了上面提到的病因种类外，危险因素还可以是某种行为或生活方式、环境暴露、遗传特征等。

四、寻找病因的清单

在研究疾病的病因时，为了便于实际操作，人们总结了具体的寻找病因的清单，见表 8-1。

表 8-1　寻找病因的清单

种类	病因
宿主	
先天性	基因、染色体、性别
后天性	年龄、发育、营养状况、体格、行为类型、获得性免疫、既往病史
环境	
生物性	病原体、媒介昆虫、食入或接触的动植物
化学性	营养素、天然有毒动植物、化学药品、微量元素、重金属
物理性	电离辐射、噪声、振动、气象、地理
社会性	社会、人口、经济、家庭、生活方式、饮食习惯、嗜好兴趣、教育、文化、医疗保健、职业、政治、宗教、风俗

五、病因模型

　　病因模型是病因学研究中经常会用到的一种工具，它是在已有理论和经验的基础上构建不同因素与疾病发生之间的概念关系，为研究病因提供一种简洁的思维框架。由于疾病特点以及研究侧重不同，研究者曾经构建过许多不同类型的病因模型。有一定代表性的病因模型有生态学模型（流行病学三角模型和轮状模型）、网络模型和充分 - 成分病因模型等。

　　生态学模型的特点是将机体与环境作为一个整体来考虑，它给出了寻找病因的分类框架，整体性强，其代表性的模型有流行病学三角模型和轮状模型等。

　　1. 流行病学三角模型（epidemiologic triangle）　如图 8-7 所示，模型包括了流行病学研究中致病因子、宿主和环境三个方面，三者相互作用影响疾病的发生。如果三者平衡，则表现为健康状态；如果致病因子作用增强，则发生疾病，如甲型流行性感冒病毒变异导致流行性感冒发生并流行；如果宿主抵抗力下降，同样可以发生疾病，如接受免疫抑制治疗的患者出现感染；如果环境变化，则可加重或减轻致病因素的作用，如贫困地区营养不良、结核病多发。该模型在传染性疾病的病因学研究中应用广泛，较清晰地阐明了病原体、机体和环境三个要素在传染性疾病发生过程中所起的协同作用。

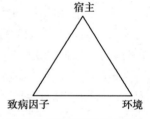

图 8-7　流行病学三角模型

然而随着社会经济的不断发展，现代社会的疾病谱已经发生了很大的变化，慢性非传染性疾病成为当今社会最主要的疾病负担，其病因纷繁复杂，远非流行病学三角模型所能涵盖。

　　2. 轮状模型（wheel model）　如图 8-8 所示，模型由外环和内环两部分组成，内环是机体，包括人的自然特征（如年龄、性别）、营养状况、免疫力、内分泌水平和遗传等，其核心是遗传基因；外环是环境，包括生物环境、理化环境和社会环境，生物环境包括病毒、细菌等各种病原微生物以及作为传播媒介的动植物等，理化环境包括气候、水、大气、土壤、光、辐射和各种化学物质如农药、杀虫剂和职业污染物等，社会环境包括社会经济水平、文化水平、政治制度、职业、居住条件、精神因素、个人行为方式等。轮状模型主要强调机体（宿主）与环境之间相互联系、相互作用，共同导致疾病的发生，

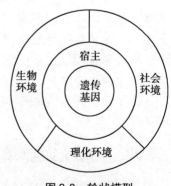

图 8-8　轮状模型

但具体到某一个疾病,则轮状模型中的各个部分对疾病发生的作用或影响又有所不同。

3. 网络模型(web model) 如图 8-9 所示,模型中的病因按时间顺序连接起来构成病因链(chain of causation),多个病因链交错连接构成病因网(web of causation),各种因素之间又存在不同的因果关系或相关关系,反映出现实世界中多病因疾病的复杂性。网络模型的优点是直观、具体,为分析、计算诸多因素之间的关系和作用提供了一个实用的理论框架,具有较强的可操作性,但其分析技术的难度比较大。

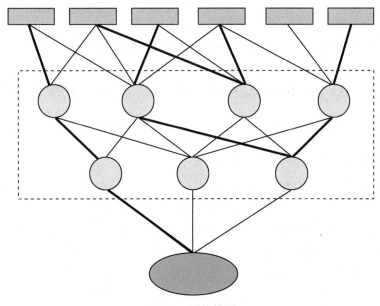

图 8-9 网络模型

4. 充分 - 成分病因模型(sufficient-component cause model) 如图 8-10 所示,某个多因素致病的疾病有若干个充分病因Ⅰ、Ⅱ和Ⅲ,每个充分病因由若干个成分原因构成,充分病因Ⅰ由 A、B、C、D、E 构成,充分病因Ⅱ由 A、D、F、G 构成,充分病因Ⅲ由 A、B、E、H 构成,其中 A 是导致该疾病发生的所有充分病因所共有的成分原因,即必要病因。充分 - 成分病因模型与网络模型有相似之处,但它将充分病因分解成为若干个成分,则更加强调病因的充分性和必要性。

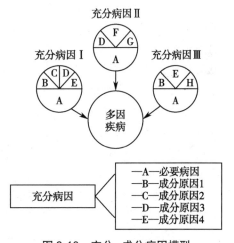

图 8-10 充分 - 成分病因模型

六、有向无环图

有向无环图(directed acyclic graph,DAG)是一种帮助构建病因模型的有用工具,它由若干个线段、箭头、因素和疾病组成,箭头方向代表因果关系,没有箭头的线段代表因果不明的相关关系,箭头还代表发生时间上的前后关系,因此箭头不会形成回路。DAG 能够比较清晰地展现与疾病发生有关的各因素之间及其与疾病发生之间的关系,有利于在此基础上进行因果关系的分析与计算。

如图 8-11 所示，当研究因素 L 对疾病 Y 的致病作用时，还需要考虑其他因素（U 和 A）的影响，其中因素 L 是因素 A 的原因，因素 A 是疾病 Y 的病因，即因素 L 除了对疾病 Y 有直接的致病作用（图中由因素 L 直接指向疾病 Y 的弧线），因素 L 还通过因素 A 对疾病 Y 有间接的致病作用，即因素 A 是因素 L 对疾病 Y 致病作用的中介因素，而因素 U 既是因素 L 的原因，也是疾病 Y 的病因，所以因素 U 是因素 L 对疾病 Y 致病作用的混杂因素。当计算因素 L 对疾病 Y 的致病作用时，需要对混杂因素 U 进行调整，而不需要对中介因素 A 进行调整。

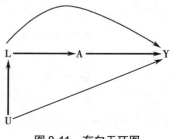

图 8-11　有向无环图

第二节　病因与危险因素研究的基本过程与方法

病因与危险因素的研究遵循一定的科学规律，其基本过程经历以下三个阶段。

一、发现线索，提出病因假设

在实践中发现问题，并根据已知的事实和原理，对其未知的规律提出假定性说明或推测性解释（即假设），是科学研究的通用方法，也是病因学研究的关键一步。迄今为止，许多疾病尤其是慢性非传染性疾病的病因尚未研究清楚，同时新的疾病也在不断涌现，病因不明给这些疾病的正确诊断和有效防治带来了很大的困难，迫使医学工作者必须对这些疾病的发病原因进行研究。病因学研究，必须根据疾病的流行病学史、临床症状和体征、相关的实验室检查结果，应用现代医学的知识和方法提出病因假设。如 2003 年春季肆虐全球的严重急性呼吸综合征（SARS）暴发流行时，其病因不明，但由于其临床表现和传播规律符合急性呼吸道传染病的特点，并在排除了细菌、真菌、支原体、衣原体、常见呼吸道病毒以及流行性感冒病毒感染的基础上，科学家们提出可能是一种毒力很强的新病毒感染所致的病因假设。

从已知的事实和原理出发提出病因假设，往往需要经过一个较为严密的逻辑思维过程，在这个过程中经常会用到以下的一些逻辑方法。

1. 求同法（method of agreement）　又称"异中求同法"，即从不同的现象或关系中找出共同点。如部分肝癌患者虽然其饮食习惯和生活环境有所不同，但他们都有乙型肝炎病毒感染，提示乙型肝炎病毒可能是肝癌的一个病因；食物中毒患者虽然既往病史和行为方式有所不同，但他们大多有近期进食相同食物的病史，提示该食物可能是引起中毒的原因。

2. 求异法（method of difference）　又称"同中求异法"，即从相似的现象或关系中找出不同点。如在病例对照研究中，将同一个村的肝癌患者与其他人进行对比，发现未患肝癌的人中没有或很少有乙型肝炎病毒感染，提示乙型肝炎病毒可能是肝癌的病因之一。

3. 同异并用法（joint method of agreement and difference）　将求同法和求异法并用，相当于在研究中设立对照组以控制干扰因素。

4. 共变法（method of concomitant variation）　是求同法的特例，当某个因素的暴露程度不同时，疾病发生的频率也发生相应的变化，该因素即可能是疾病的病因。共变法受一定条件的限制，只有当某个研究因素是等级变量或连续变量，且与疾病发生的概率呈量变关系时，才可以应用共变法。如在吸烟与肺癌的研究中，随着吸烟剂量的增加，肺癌的优势比（OR）或相对危险度（RR）也增加，呈共变或剂量反应关系，提示吸烟可能是肺癌的病因。

5. 剩余法（method of residues）　是求异法的特例，当人们已知某复合结局事件（A、B、C）的暴露因素仅限于特定范畴（a、b、c），且通过之前归纳又知道 b 说明 B，c 说明 C，则剩余的 a 说明 A。如在肝癌的病因研究中，肝癌的发病率除了乙型肝炎病毒感染和黄曲霉毒素能解释的部分，还有未能解释的部分，其或可归因于暴露因素范畴内的"剩余"因素。

以上这几种方法在逻辑上均属于归纳法，主要是由 19 世纪的哲学家穆勒（Mill）于 1856年在他的著作《逻辑系统》一书中提出的。这些方法可以用于临床流行病学研究，有利于形成假设、设计研究方案并进行病因推断。需要注意的是，如果病因假设清单中没有包括真实的病因，则以上这些方法不仅不能有效地提供指导，而且还可能将病因分析带入歧途。当然，在疾病的病因明了之前，是没有人知道病因假设清单中有没有真实病因的，这里只是提醒大家单纯运用这些方法并不能避免错误的发生。

除归纳法，还有演绎法（类推法），即通过已知规律来推论未知事物的方法。在临床实践中，当发现线索提出病因假设后，根据假设演绎推出需要检验的具体内容或关系，然后用实证的方法进行验证，如果内容或关系经检验成立，则支持该病因假设，如果内容或关系经检验不成立，并不能简单地否定假设，而是需要考虑其他影响因素的存在。通过实证检验的具体证据越多或证据的条件越多种多样，这个假设成立的可能性就越大；反之，则假设成立的可能性就越小（注意：只是越小，而不是排除）。

二、初步验证病因假设

病因假设是否正确，需要通过科学研究进行初步检验。不同学科研究病因的特点和方法有所不同，临床流行病学以患者人群为主要研究对象，涉及的研究方法有描述性研究（如个案报告、病例系列）、分析性研究（如横断面研究、病例对照研究、队列研究）和干预性研究（如随机、双盲、对照）等，其科学性和论证强度依次渐强，如图 8-12所示。描述性研究主要为提出病因假设提供线索，分析性研究和干预性研究是检验病因假设成立与否的主要手段。因为干预性研究所需要的条件（如伦理）较高，所以多数验证病因假设的临床流行病学研究以病例对照研究和队列研究为主。

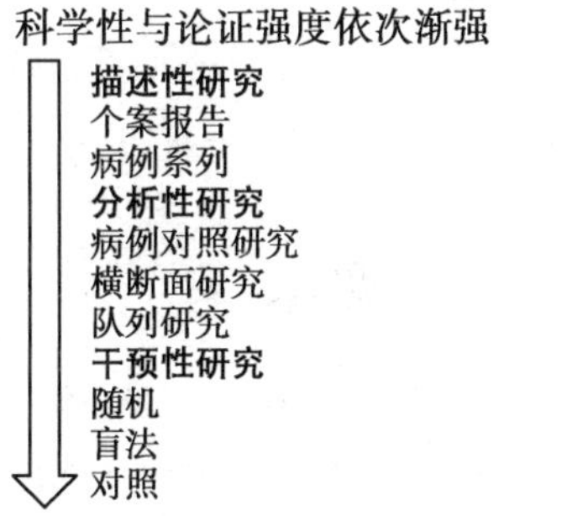

科学性与论证强度依次渐强

描述性研究
个案报告
病例系列
分析性研究
病例对照研究
横断面研究
队列研究
干预性研究
随机
盲法
对照

图 8-12　临床流行病学研究的常用方法

如在 2008 年的三聚氰胺污染婴幼儿配方奶粉事件中，首先是甘肃的儿科医生在临床实践中发现短时期内收治的肾结石幼儿病例明显增多，经了解均曾食用过某品牌的配方奶粉，经检测某集团生产的婴幼儿系列奶粉中有多个批次检出三聚氰胺，于是提出三聚氰胺污染的婴幼儿配方奶粉可能是造成这次婴幼儿肾结石的原因，而随后临床医生和临床流行病学者合作开展的横断面研究初步证实三聚氰胺污染的婴幼儿配方奶粉与婴幼儿肾结石之间存在显著的相关性。在此例，因为前瞻性队列研究和随机对照试验有违医学伦理的要求，所以不会有更高级别的研究对此进行科学检验。

三、综合判断，确定因果关系

在病因研究的过程中，由于偏倚和 / 或混杂的影响，研究结果可能并没有真实地反映出可疑致病因素与疾病发生之间的关系，而是两者之间的关联强度被高估或低估，甚至出现完全虚假的关联或间接关联。

如在研究饮用咖啡是否会导致胰腺癌的病例对照研究中，选取消化科住院的非胰腺癌患者作正常对照，结果发现饮用咖啡是胰腺癌的危险因素，但这个结论被以后的研究否定，因为消化科住院的非胰腺癌患者往往因为有其他消化系统疾病而减少咖啡的饮用，使得这个对照人群饮用咖啡的比例较正常人群低，造成饮用咖啡与胰腺癌发生之间出现虚假关联。

当排除虚假关联后，可疑致病因素与疾病之间存在相关并不一定代表二者之间肯定存在因果关联。当可疑致病因素与疾病发生都与另外一个因素相关联时，即便可疑致病因素与疾病发生之间没有关系，也会出现明显的统计学相关，称为间接关联或继发关联（secondary association）。继发关联是由混杂引起的，如有研究观察到随身携带打火机与肺癌发生相关，但这并非因为打火机本身会导致肺癌发生（因果关联），而是因为随身携带打火机与吸烟相关，而吸烟是肺癌的主要病因之一，这里吸烟是影响随身携带打火机与肺癌发生之间关系的混杂因素，它的存在使二者之间出现了继发关联。

当排除抽样误差、虚假关联和继发关联后，可疑致病因素与疾病发生之间的关联才可能是因果关联，才能进行该因素与疾病发生之间的病因推导。

事实上，单纯的临床流行病学研究对确定疾病的病因是不够的，病因研究还需要其他学科（如基础医学）的广泛参与和支持。动物实验、组织细胞实验以及分子水平的研究都能够为探索某些因素与疾病发生之间的因果关系提供重要的证据，揭示人类疾病在发生过程中某个阶段的变化及其规律，但由于比较极端地控制了研究条件及可能的种属差异，其研究结果往往不可轻易地引申至人。因此，疾病病因的研究很大程度上需要以人为研究对象的流行病学研究和其他学科的研究互相支持和补充，经过反复分析和验证，确定疾病发生的原因。

第三节　因果推断

一、科赫标准

科赫（Koch）在1882年提出以下4点原则对病因和疾病发生之间的因果关系进行推断。

1. 患者体内均能检出引起该病的病原体（必要病因）。
2. 其他疾病患者中不能检出该病原体（效应特异性）。
3. 该病原体能够从患者体内分离培养，易感动物接种该病原体能复制该病（充分病因）。
4. 能从患病动物体内分离到相同病原体。

这些原则比较适用于单病因致病的感染性疾病，但对于多病因致病的慢性非传染性疾病，科赫标准并不适用。

二、希尔标准

对于多病因致病的疾病，希尔（Hill）提出以下9点原则对病因和疾病发生之间的因果关系进行推断。

1. 时间顺序（temporality）　可疑的致病因素必须出现在疾病发生之前，这是因果推断中唯一一个绝对必需的条件。

2. 关联强度（strength of association）　常用相对风险（relative risk）、优势比（odds ratio）或风险比（hazard ratio）等来表示可疑的致病因素与疾病发生之间的关联强度，关联强度越强，该因素是病因的可能性就越大。

3. 一致性（consistency）　不同的研究者在不同的条件下用不同的方法进行不同的研究，发现可疑的致病因素与疾病发生之间的相关性是一致的。

4. 剂量 - 反应关系（dose-response relationship）　可疑致病因素暴露的水平（剂量和时间）越高，疾病发生的风险也越高，或可疑的致病因素与疾病发生之间的关系符合预期的理论形态（如 U 型关系）。

5. 试验证据（experimental evidence）　在人群的试验研究中，对可疑的致病因素进行干预能够预防或减轻疾病发生的风险。

6. 生物可能性（biological plausibility）　可疑的致病因素与疾病发生之间的关联能够用已知的生物学、生理学、病理学等相关的生命科学知识进行解释。

7. 符合性（coherence）　可疑的致病因素与疾病发生之间的关联与已有的理论和知识相一致。

8. 特异性（specificity）　可疑致病因素会产生特异性的效果，如某个疾病的出现而不是多个疾病的出现。

9. 类比性（analogy）　相似的因素会产生相似的结果（疾病发生）。

在以上 9 点原则中，前 4 项原则最为重要，也是病因判断时最常用的几点依据。然而，这些原则的作用不是绝对的，希尔自己也说"我的 9 项观点没有一项可以毫无争议地支持或反对因果假设，也没有一项是不可或缺的"，因果关系的判断还是需要综合考虑。

第四节　病因与危险因素研究的评价原则

在阅读病因与危险因素研究的报告或文章时，需要遵循以下原则对因果关系的真实性和重要性进行评价。

一、病因学研究结果的真实性评价

（一）是否采用了论证强度高的研究设计方案？

不同病因学研究方法的科学性以及因果论证强度是不同的，描述性研究论证强度最弱，病例对照研究论证强度稍强，队列研究论证强度较强，随机双盲对照试验的科学性和因果论证强度最强，因为它通过随机分组保证除干预措施以外的其他已知和未知因素在干预组和对照组都是均衡的，最大程度地减少了混杂的干扰。

（二）除研究的暴露因素外，试验组与对照组其他暴露是否一致？是否存在混杂因素影响？

混杂因素对病因研究的影响很大，除了可疑的致病因素之外，应该注意在试验组和对照组中是否存在混杂以及混杂的程度，是否采用适当的办法对混杂进行控制或消除混杂。混杂因素可能是已知的，也可能存在未知，一般分析性研究（病例对照研究和队列研究）只能对已知的混杂因素进行控制或调整，只有随机对照试验能够真正清除已知和未知的混杂因素。

（三）组间对因果效应的测量方法是否一致？是否采用盲法？

在病因学研究中，对两组研究对象（干预组与对照组、暴露组与非暴露组、病例组与对照组）的暴露和结局应该采用相同的测量方法。采用盲法干预、评价暴露和结局，才能够防止信息偏倚的干扰，增加结果的真实性。

（四）随访观察时间是否足够长？研究结果是否包括了所有纳入随访研究的病例？

任何致病因素引起疾病发生都有一个时间效应关系，急性或自然病程短的疾病其致病效应期短，如急性痢疾，而慢性非传染性疾病其致病效应期长，如冠心病和肿瘤。因此，研究慢性非传染性疾病危险因素的致病效应时，往往需要足够的时间才能观察到结果的发生，观察期过短会获得假阴性结果。

另外，在随访期间研究对象失访过多会影响研究结论的真实性，因为中途退出的研究对象可能在某些特征上与仍然留在研究中的研究对象存在差别，从而带来失访偏倚。一般队列研究或试验的失访率不应大于20%，否则研究结论的真实性将受到严重的质疑。

（五）因果效应的时间顺序是否确切、合理？

致病因素引起疾病发生，必然是因在前、果在后，致病因素与疾病发生之间的时序性是构成因果关系的基础。在评价病因学研究时，如果能明确危险因素的出现先于疾病的发生，则研究结果的真实性就高。试验研究和队列研究因为可以确定因果效应的时间顺序，所以真实性较高，而横断面研究则不能确定因果效应的时序性，所以真实性就较低。

（六）是否存在剂量效应的致病关系？

剂量效应关系是指暴露水平（剂量、程度、时间）与疾病发生之间存在显著的相关关系，如化学性和物理性等有害因素的致病效应与接触的剂量存在相关，接触剂量越大、时间越长，累积剂量越大，致病效应越明显。

（七）病因学研究结果是否符合流行病学的规律？

流行病学在致病因素、机体和环境等方面进行宏观探讨，如果研究中暴露因素的分布与疾病的空间分布、时间分布及人群间分布相符，则暴露因素很可能是疾病发生的危险因素。

（八）不同的研究，结论是否一致？

在不同地区、不同人群中采用不同或者相似的方法对某一疾病的病因进行研究，并采用相关的评价指标进行评价，如果得出的结论较为一致，则该病因致病比较可靠。

（九）病因学效应的生物学依据是否充分？

如果病因学研究提示的因果关系有生物学依据，则可增加其因果联系的论证强度。

二、病因学研究结果的重要性评价

通过上述真实性的分析与评价，如果病因学研究的结果有良好的真实性，则应该进一步地评价该研究结果是否具有重要的临床意义和价值，否则就没有必要再评价其重要性。病因学研究结果的重要性反映在下面的量化指标中。

1. 关联程度 在病因学研究中，有一些反映可疑致病因素与疾病发生之间关联程度的量化指标，如随机对照试验和队列研究中的相对危险度（RR）、归因危险度（AR）、归因危险比（ARR）以及病例对照研究中的优势比（OR）。

在判断 RR 和 OR 的意义时，经常需要进行敏感性分析，即加入不同的混杂因素进行调整后，观察可疑致病因素与疾病发生之间的关联程度是否会发生明显的变化，借以判断因果关联的可靠性。如果调整后的 RR 或 OR 较调整前的 RR 或 OR 明显变小，则应该怀疑原来的结果；如果调整后的 RR 或 OR 与调整前相比保持不变或比调整前明显增大，则应该更加确信该因果关联的真实性。

2. 相对危险度（RR）或优势比（OR）的 95% 置信区间　RR 或 OR 是对因果关联强度的点估计，除此以外还需要了解、评价因果关联强度的精确度，即 RR 或 OR 的 95% 置信区间（CI）。如果 95%CI 的范围较小且不包括 1.0，则其精确度就高，并有显著的统计学意义。

本 章 小 结

病因是导致疾病发生的原因，病因可以分为充分病因和必要病因、直接病因和间接病因；危险因素是流行病学层面的病因，当该因素存在时，人群中疾病发生的概率随之上升；当消除该因素时，疾病发生的概率也随之下降。病因与危险因素研究的基本过程是，首先发现线索、提出病因假设，而后通过不同研究初步验证病因假设，最后综合判断、确定因果关系。因果推断的原则是病因学研究的关键，其重点是时间顺序、关联强度、一致性及剂量 - 反应关系。对具体研究进行评价时，需遵循一定的原则，对结果的真实性和重要性进行分析，以得出恰当的结论。

（刘晓清）

第九章

诊断试验研究证据评价

学习目标

1. **掌握** 诊断试验和诊断性研究的概念。
2. **熟悉** 常用于诊断试验准确性判断的指标：灵敏度、特异度、阳（阴）性似然比、阳（阴）性预测值等；诊断试验研究文献的评价原则。
3. **了解** 验前、验后概率的计算及其临床意义；ROC 工作曲线及其意义。

  临床医师每天都面临着对患者进行诊断的工作，收集患者病史特点和临床体格检查是医师进行诊断的关键步骤，除此以外，为患者选择准确性高的诊断试验以及评价所做检查的临床价值都是临床诊断的关键。为提高临床诊断水平和临床科研质量，临床医师有必要系统地学习和了解临床诊断试验以及诊断研究评价方法，熟悉诊断试验准确性判断的标准。

  诊断试验（diagnostic test）是指应用临床各种试验、医疗仪器等检查手段对就诊的患者进行检查，从就诊者实验室检查结果进行诊断和鉴别诊断疾病的试验。

  诊断性研究（diagnostic study）是研究对疾病进行诊断的试验方法，包括对各种实验室检查、各种影像学检查以及放射性核素、内镜等诊断方法的研究。诊断性研究可以涉及临床医学各领域及环节。在临床工作中，疾病准确且快速的诊断甚为重要。为了提高临床诊断水平和效率，不仅需要发现高水平的诊断试验应用于临床，同时，也需要对现有的诊断试验进行科学的评估和判定，以指导临床医师正确认识和应用。

第一节　诊断试验准确性评价的常用指标及临床应用

一、诊断试验准确性评价的常用指标

  1. 灵敏度（sensitivity，Sen）与漏诊率 灵敏度也称敏感度或真阳性率，指一项诊断试验能将真正患有疾病的人正确诊断为患者的能力，或采用金标准诊断为"有病"的病例中，此项诊断试验检测为阳性例数的比例。

  漏诊率是指一项诊断试验将真正患有疾病的人错误地诊断为非患者的比例，也称假阴性率。

  灵敏度越大，试验发现阳性的可能性越大，而若试验结果为阴性，则更容易排除被检查者患病的可能，即漏诊率越低。

2. 特异度(specificity, Spe)和误诊率　特异度也称真阴性率,指一项诊断试验能将真正无病的人正确诊断为非患者的能力,或采用金标准诊断"无病"的例数中,诊断试验结果为阴性的比例。

误诊率指一项诊断试验将实际无病的人错误诊断为患者的比例,也称假阳性率。

真阴性例数越多,特异度越高,误诊率则越低。

3. 准确性(accuracy, Acc)　准确性指诊断试验中真阳性和真阴性在总检例数中的比例。

灵敏度和特异度是诊断试验的准确性方面的两个基本特征。

一个理想的诊断试验,灵敏度和特异度都应达到100%,即假阳性和假阴性均为零。

【案例 9-1】　诊断试验准确性研究的常用指标计算

研究者以 823 例胸部 X 线提示肺部病变的患者肺 CT 检查结果进行诊断试验准确性研究,下面借用此研究(表 9-1)进行讲解。

表 9-1　肺癌的 CT 诊断研究评价

CT 诊断	真正"肺癌"患者 / 例	非"肺癌"患者 / 例	合计 / 例
阳性 / 例	a(385)	b(17)	a+b(402)
阴性 / 例	c(42)	d(379)	c+d(421)
合计 / 例	a+c(427)	b+d(396)	a+b+c+d(823)

研究者以 823 例胸部 X 线提示肺部病变的患者肺 CT 检查结果进行诊断试验准确性研究,下面借用此研究进行讲解。

各指标计算:灵敏度(Sen)=a/(a+c)×100%=90.16%

漏诊率 =1- 灵敏度 =9.84%

特异度(Spe)=d/(b+d)×100%=95.71%

误诊率 =1- 特异度 =4.29%

在此诊断性研究中,肺部 CT 检查对肺癌的诊断的准确性为:

准确性 =(a+b)/(a+b+c+d)×100%=92.8%

准确性反映诊断试验的灵敏度和特异度,准确性高的试验其灵敏度和特异度也高,但准确性不能反映灵敏度和特异度单方面的特性。在临床实践中,就具体某疾病选择怎样的诊断试验?对于灵敏度和特异度有怎样的要求?

由于恶性肿瘤是一类预后极差的疾病,一旦明确诊断为周围型肺癌,对患者和患者家属来说,无疑带来的是"噩耗"。因此,对于各类恶性肿瘤的明确诊断,势必要求选择特异度高的诊断试验,以降低误诊率。

而如果在 SARS(严重急性呼吸综合征)疫情期间,由于 SARS 的严重传染性和病情发展迅猛,如果出现临床漏诊,将会出现疫情扩散、患者出现生命危险的严重后果。因此,对 SARS 的诊断,就势必要求选择灵敏度高的诊断试验,以降低漏诊率。

二、诊断试验临床应用评估指标及意义

1. 阳性预测值与阴性预测值　预测值是评估诊断试验价值的指标,表示诊断试验的临床意义。预测值是指在已知某诊断试验结果为阳性或阴性前提下,正确评判有无疾病

的概率,分为阳性预测值(positive predictive value,PPV)和阴性预测值(negative predictive value,NPV)。

阳性预测值是指诊断试验阳性结果中真正有疾病的概率;阴性预测值是指诊断试验阴性结果中真正无病的概率。

2. 阳性似然比与阴性似然比 似然比是指在诊断试验中患者出现某种检测结果(如阳性或阴性)的概率与非患者出现此种结果的概率之比,说明患者出现该结果的机会是非患者的多少倍,可分为阳性似然比(positive likelihood ratio,PLR)和阴性似然比(negative likelihood ratio,NLR)。

阳性似然比是诊断试验中,真阳性率与假阳性率的比值,表明该诊断试验阳性时,患病与不患病概率的比值,比值越大,则患病的机会越大。一般认为 PLR≥10 预示该诊断试验具有较高的临床价值。

阳性似然比(PLR)=灵敏度/(1-特异度)=灵敏度/误诊率

阴性似然比是诊断试验中,假阴性率与真阴性率的比值。表明判断阴性的可能性是正确判断阴性可能性的倍数,即该诊断试验为阴性时,患病与不患病概率的比值,比值越小,试验的价值越大,一般认为 NLR≤0.10 预示该诊断试验有较高的诊断价值。

阴性似然比(NLR)=(1-灵敏度)/特异度=漏诊率/特异度

【案例9-2】 示例计算诊断试验临床应用评估指标

患者 A,男,45 岁,因"右侧胸、背疼痛 6 月"门诊就诊。患者 6 个月前无明显诱因出现右侧胸疼痛,呈隐痛,伴有右侧对应部位的背部隐痛,夜间明显,伴有咳嗽,多为干咳,不伴咯血、气促等。起病至就诊体重减轻约 4kg。吸烟近 30 年,15 支/d。既往间常有咳嗽。

门诊医师给予患者肺部 CT 检查,发现"右下肺团块状结节影,周围型肺癌可能性大"。

患者 A 完成 CT 检查并确定为阳性,该患者是真正的肺癌患者的概率有多大呢?以表 9-1 诊断研究的结果对患者 A 结果进行分析。

阳性预测值(PPV)=a/(a+b)×100%=95.77%

阴性预测值(NPV)=d/(c+d)×100%=90.02%

阳性似然比(PLR)=灵敏度/(1-特异度)=21.02

阴性似然比(NLR)=(1-灵敏度)/特异度=0.10

从此研究结果得出结论:

从阳性预测值的结果解释,患者 A 可能患肺癌的概率是 95.77%。

肺部 CT 检查有较高的阳性似然比,患者 A 为患肺癌的概率是不患肺癌的 20 倍。

---

3. 患病率(prevalence,Prev) 诊断试验的全部例数中,真正"患病"例数所占的比例。

灵敏度和特异度提示患病患者和无病对象出现诊断试验阳性和阴性结果的机会分别有多大,但临床医师需要了解的是,诊断试验结果阳性或阴性时,患病和不患病的机会有多大,即诊断试验结果对疾病判断的可靠性怎样。诊断试验的阳性结果并不意味着肯定"患病",阳性结果提示患病的机会取决于诊断试验的灵敏度、特异度以及检测人群中该病的患病率(阴性结果提示"无病"的机会也同样受到这些因素的影响)。但患病率对预测值的影响比灵敏度和特异度的影响更为重要。受试对象的患病率越低，阴性结果提示无病的把握越大，而阳性结果提示患病的把握越小。

当诊断试验用于患病率很低的人群时，即使灵敏度很高，阳性预测值也不会很高，即在阳性结果中可能存在较多的假阳性。同样，当用于患病率很高的人群时，即使特异度很高的诊断试验，阴性结果中仍然会有不少假阴性结果。

因此，临床医师必须注意到，在解释诊断试验阳性或阴性结果时应考虑不同地区、不同人群的区别，估计患病率的高低，因受试对象的差异，其试验结果的意义将存在区别。

【案例9-3】　不同患病率群体的诊断试验评价比较

针对肺癌高危人群126例体检对象肺部CT的结果进行的一项研究。以此结果（表9-2）和表9-1研究结果对比，对影响诊断试验评价指标的因素给予讲解。

表9-2　肺部CT诊断肺癌研究的评价

CT诊断	真正"肺癌"患者/例	非"肺癌"患者/例	合计/例
阳性/例	a（5）	b（8）	a+b（13）
阴性/例	c（2）	d（111）	c+d（113）
合计/例	a+c（7）	b+d（119）	a+b+c+d（126）

表9-3　两个患病率不同的群体肺部CT诊断试验评价比较

不同研究	患病率/%	灵敏度/%	特异度/%	准确性/%	阳性似然比	阴性似然比	阳性预测值/%	阴性预测值/%
研究1	97.2	90.2	95.7	92.8	21.0	0.10	95.8	90.0
研究2	5.5	71.4	93.2	92.0	10.5	0.31	38.5	98.2

从表9-3中结果比较可见，在不同患病率的群体中，肺部CT检查作为一种诊断试验准确性几乎相同的情况下，诊断试验阳性或阴性结果对临床患者诊断的判断，即阳（阴）性似然比、阳（阴）性预测值有很大的差别。

临床医生们应当注意：阳（阴）性预测值是试验阳性（阴性）时患病（不患病）的概率，其受患病率影响。而阳（阴）性似然比是该诊断试验阳性（阴性）时，患病与不患病机会的比值。不受患病率影响。

4. 验前概率（pre-test probability）　是指临床医师在应用某一诊断性试验前估计该疾病的患病概率，即该疾病的患病率，通常可从文献中查找得到。

5. 验后概率（post-test probability）　是指在进行某一诊断性试验后，根据需诊断的疾病的验前概率和该诊断试验的阳性似然比计算而得出，即在不同患病率情况下该试验的预测值。

单纯的灵敏度和特异度不能反映诊断性试验的全貌，而似然比通过比较患病人群和无病人群出现该诊断试验的阳性和阴性结果的概率来反映该诊断试验的特征，不受患病率的影响，较单纯的灵敏度和特异度更全面和更稳定地诠释诊断试验。因此，似然比是诊断性试验综合评价的理想指标，能够依据灵敏度、特异度、试验的阳性或阴性结果，计算出患病的概率（即验后概率），便于在诊断试验后，更确切地对患者作出诊断。

【案例9-4】　如何计算验前概率和验后概率？

1. 患者A为表9-1研究中的一位受试者，那么在肺部CT阳性结果的前提下，该患者可能为真正的患者的概率计算如下：

验前概率（患病率）为97.2%

验前比数 $=0.972/(1-0.972)=34.7$

验后比数 = 验前比数 × 阳性似然比 =729.7

验后概率 = 验后比数 /(1+ 验后比数)×100%=99.9%

结论：患者A在此肺部CT阳性的结果下，患肺癌的概率从验前的97.2%上升至验后的99.9%。

2. 患者A为表9-2研究中的一位受试者，那么在肺部CT阳性结果的前提下，该患者可能为真正的患者的概率计算如下：

验前概率（患病率）为5.5%

验前比数 $=0.055/(1-0.055)=0.058$

验后比数 = 验前比数 × 阳性似然比 =0.61

验后概率 = 验后比数 /(1+ 验后比数)×100%=37.9%

结论：患者A在此肺部CT阳性的结果下，患肺癌的概率从验前的5.5%上升至验后的37.9%。

6. ROC曲线　全称受试者操作特征曲线（receiver operator characteristic curve）。在诊断试验中，通过多次连续分组测定的数据进行制图。制图时以该试验灵敏度（真阳性率）为纵坐标，以1-特异度（假阳性率）为横坐标，依据连续分组测定所得数据，分别计算出的灵敏度和特异度标入图中，连成曲线，即为ROC曲线（图9-1）。曲线上的任意一点代表某项诊断试验的特定阳性标准值相对应的灵敏度和特异度。

以图9-1中ROC曲线为例，A、B、C、D四条曲线分别代表四个诊断试验：由A～D，诊断试验的临床价值逐渐递增。好的诊断试验其曲线远离中间的对角线，并十分接近左上角（如图中所示D曲线）。差的诊断试验则非常接近中间的对角线（如图中所示A曲线）。通常可以通过计算曲线下面积（AUC）来评价试验的准确性，面积越大，表示试验准确性越好。同时，一般选择以曲线距左上角最近的一点为正常值的最佳临界点，这点下的面积最大。用该点区分正常与异常，其灵敏度和特异度均为最高，即误诊和漏诊病例最少。

绘制ROC曲线可用来决定正常值，还可以通过曲线下面积比较不同诊断试验的优劣。

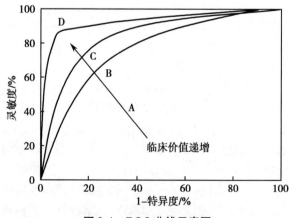

图9-1　ROC曲线示意图

第二节　诊断试验文献评阅标准

为增加诊断试验研究的科学性,提高诊断试验研究结论的可信度,前人从研究实践中总结了具有指导性意义的评阅标准,为后来者检验自身及他人诊断试验研究提供借鉴,以提高诊断试验研究的效率和准确性。诊断试验文献评阅标准(国际通用评价原则)有以下八个部分。

1. 诊断试验与金标准盲法比较和评价。
2. 纳入研究病例的分析与评价。
3. 病例来源和研究工作的安排是否叙述。
4. 诊断试验的重复性及其临床意义是否明确。
5. 诊断试验所确定的正常值是否合理、可靠。
6. 系列试验的应用是否正确。
7. 诊断试验方法叙述及其重复性分析。
8. 诊断试验的实用性如何。

一、是否将研究的诊断试验与金标准进行了盲法比较

诊断性研究中诊断试验的金标准(gold standard)是指当前临床医师公认的诊断疾病最可靠的方法,也称为诊断标准,它能正确区分"患病"与"无病"。临床诊断常用的金标准包括病原学诊断、病理学诊断、外科手术发现、特殊的影像学诊断、临床综合性诊断标准、长期临床随访得出的肯定结果等,但应注意,有些疾病诊断的金标准是相对的,又被称为相对金标准,随着医学的发展以及对疾病进一步深入的认识,相对金标准在不断地进行完善。

金标准的选择及其可靠性直接影响到诊断性研究结论的可靠性,对同一组对象,采用不同的诊断金标准可能对某一诊断试验得出不同的结论,因此,必须严格掌握。

诊断试验的准确性评定,即诊断性试验是否准确反映检查对象患病或无病,是研究的关键。诊断性试验准确性评定主要是与金标准比较而言。为了消除人为偏倚,应用盲法对比则更为科学。因此,被研究的诊断性试验在临床应用之前,应与金标准进行盲法比较,根据四格表计算出灵敏度、特异度、阳性和阴性预测值、准确性和似然比等。

【案例 9-5】　比较诊断试验和金标准

某诊断性研究采用痰培养分离的结核分枝杆菌结果作为诊断肺结核的金标准,对血液结核分枝杆菌 PCR 诊断试验的结果进行评价(表 9-4)。

表 9-4　患者结核分枝杆菌 PCR 诊断试验结果

结核分枝杆菌 PCR 结果	检出结核分枝杆菌 / 例	未检出结核分枝杆菌 / 例	合计 / 例
阳性 / 例	45	5	50
阴性 / 例	8	62	70
合计 / 例	53	67	120

此研究以病原学诊断为金标准,对结核分枝杆菌的血液学诊断试验进行科学的评价。

二、研究中纳入病例的选择是否有代表性

诊断试验的研究对象,应当包括用金标准确定"患病"的研究对象,即病例组,和用金标准证实"无病"的研究对象,其中,所谓"无病"的研究对象,是指没有金标准诊断的目标疾病,而不是完全无病的正常人。

不同应用目的的诊断性研究应选择不同的研究对象,如评价筛选诊断试验价值的,研究对象可选择普通人群;评价临床诊断试验价值的,则应选择病例作为研究对象。同时,病例还应包括不同病程、不同病情程度(轻、中、重)、有无并发症以及典型和非典型病例等,以使研究的结果具有代表性。对照组可选择金标准确认"无病"的其他病例,最好包含由金标准确认无该病,但又易于与该病混淆的其他病例,这样的对照更具临床诊断价值,特别是鉴别诊断价值。正常人一般不宜纳入"无病"对照组,如果在试验的初级阶段将正常人纳入了对照组,则应对其结果谨慎对待。

在案例 9-5 对血液结核分枝杆菌 PCR 诊断试验的评估研究中,纳入研究并接受血液检测的受检人群包括轻、中、重度肺结核患者,也包括原发性、继发性肺结核患者,这样得出对该诊断试验的评价结果才科学可信。

三、研究对象的来源是否正确叙述

患病率对诊断试验的预测值等最后分析结果有很大的影响。不同的研究对象来源,即各级医院不同的就诊患者结构组成,势必出现作为研究对象的某疾病的患病率不同,最后对研究结果产生的影响较大。对于某一诊断试验,其灵敏度和特异度是相对固定的,而在临床工作中,医疗工作者更注重的是诊断试验的阳性预测值,同时又要减少假阳性例数,希望通过该诊断试验提高对疾病诊断的预测,即充分发挥诊断试验的效率。由于患病率对疾病的预测值将产生较大的影响,因此,选择不同患病率的人群应用适当的诊断性试验,是临床医师提高诊断性试验效率的关键之一。

> **【案例 9-6】 诊断性试验在不同人群的应用**
>
> 肺部螺旋 CT 诊断试验在不同患病人群的应用结果有几种不同的预测值。
>
> 在发现肺部结节的人群中,验前估计患病概率为 97.2%,验后阳性预测值为 99.8%,应用肺部 CT 试验后,预测仅增加 2.6%。
>
> 在高危的吸烟体检人群中,验前估计患病概率为 5.5%,验后阳性预测值为 37.1%,应用该试验后,预测增加 32.1%。
>
> 因此,研究中应正确叙述研究对象的来源,以增加研究结果的科学性和论证强度。

四、诊断性试验是否具有很好的重复性

重复性(repeatability)又称精确性(precision)或可靠性(reliability),即诊断试验需重复操作,其重复性是诊断试验临床应用的先决条件。诊断试验要求重复测定值应处于相对稳定状态,即多次测定同一标本,应结果接近,方法才能被认为可靠。

五、诊断性试验的正常值的确定是否合理、可靠

正常值的含义应准确定义及清楚叙述，不同含义的正常值可直接影响正常值的数据。当患病人群和无病人群测定值的频数分布曲线有重叠时，应采取科学的方法（如正态分布数据采用均数±标准差、非正态分布用中位数或百分位数以及应用 ROC 曲线等），正确划分正常和异常的临界点，即找到最佳临界点。是否为最佳临界点直接影响到诊断性试验的灵敏度和特异度以及其他重要指标。

六、联合试验的选择是否合理、科学

诊断试验的联合方式包括平行试验（parallel test）和系列试验（serial test）。

1. 平行试验　为提高诊断的灵敏度，同时做几种目的相同的诊断试验，只要其中一种试验阳性，即可判断为患病者。平行试验的应用可提高灵敏度和阴性预测值，但却降低了特异度和阳性预测值，也就是减少了漏诊率，却增加了误诊率。这种方法在临床应用时，需谨慎考虑鉴别诊断，尽量减少误诊。

平行试验结果的评价方法如表 9-5 所示。

表 9-5　平行试验结果的评价方法

项目	结果		评价结果
	试验 A	试验 B	
平行实验	+	−	+
	−	+	+
	+	+	+
	−	−	−

试验 A：Sen=80%，Spe=60%。
试验 B：Sen=90%，Spe=90%。
平行试验计算：
Sen=SenA+（1−SenA）×SenB=0.80+（1−0.80）×0.90=0.98。
Spe=SpeA×SpeB=0.60×0.90=0.54。

【案例 9-7】 平行试验结果的评价方法

某诊断性研究对胸腔积液患者进行胸腔积液的 LDH 和 ADA 三项指标进行检测（表 9-6），以此诊断胸腔积液患者结核性胸腔积液的可能。

表 9-6　胸腔积液患者胸腔积液诊断试验结果

ADA 试验（A）	LDH 试验（B）	结核性胸腔积液患者	非结核性胸腔积液患者
+	−	8	4
−	+	16	6
+	+	60	2
−	−	16	578
合计		100	590

ADA 试验（A）：

Sen=（8+60）/100×100%=68.0%。

Spe=（6+578）/590×100%=99.0%。

LDH 试验（B）：

Sen=（16+60）/100×100%=76.0%。

Spe=（4+578）/590×100%=98.6%。

平行试验计算：

Sen=SenA+（1-SenA）×SenB=0.68+（1-0.68）×0.76=0.92。

Spe=SpeA×SpeB=0.99×0.99=0.98。

此结果表明，平行试验增加了试验的灵敏度，但降低了试验的特异度。

2. 系列试验　当临床缺乏单一的特异度高的诊断试验时，为提高临床诊断的特异度，需要设计一系列的诊断试验，决定前后顺序进行，一系列试验的结果必须均为阳性，才能作出患病的诊断。系列试验提高了特异度和阳性预测值，但同时降低了灵敏度和阴性预测值，即临床上系列试验降低了误诊率，却可能增加了漏诊率。当临床所用的多项诊断试验特异度都不高时，采用系列试验比较适当。

系列试验结果的评价方法如下。

（1）设计的一系列诊断试验结果必须均为阳性。

（2）计算方法：A、B、C、D……系列试验。

$Sen_{（序列）}$=SenA×SenB×SenC×SenD……计算出序列试验的灵敏度。

$Spe_{（序列）1}$=SpeA+$[$（1-SpeA）×SpeB$]$；$Spe_{（序列）2}$=$Spe_{（序列）1}$+$\{[$1-$Spe_{（序列）1}]$×SpeC$\}$；$Spe_{（序列）3}$=$Spe_{（序列）2}$+$\{[$1-$Spe_{（序列）2}]$×SpeD$\}$……按此规律，最后计算出序列试验的特异度。

准确评价联合试验的灵敏度、特异度和准确性，同时，应和每个单项试验的灵敏度、特异度和准确性进行比较。在一系列同类试验中评比选择最佳联合试验方法。

以表 9-6 中检测结果作为联合诊断试验的计算基础，序列试验后的灵敏度和特异度的计算如下：

$Sen_{（序列）}$=0.68×0.76=0.516 8。

$Spe_{（序列）1}$=0.99+$[$（1-0.99）×0.986$]$=0.999 9。

此结果表明，系列试验增加了试验的特异度，但降低了试验的灵敏度。

七、诊断性试验的操作方法是否仔细叙述

为使被研究的诊断性试验得以在临床上应用，应对其具体操作方法进行仔细地叙述，包括操作步骤、使用仪器及试剂规格、试验前后被检者有何安排或限制（如饮食、药物等限制）以及结果评判方法等。

八、诊断性试验的临床实用性如何

综合评定被研究的诊断试验的临床实用性，包括临床应用是否方便、对患者有无伤害、准确度是否高、结果是否容易判断以及成本效益分析是否好。

本 章 小 结

灵敏度高的试验主要用于排除无病的对象，此时阴性结果最有意义。特异度高的试验主要用于确诊患病的对象，此时阳性结果最有意义。

应用每个诊断试验的似然比，可以计算出验后概率，从而了解该诊断试验结果阳性或阴性时患者患病的概率。对是否需要做进一步诊断，诊断试验还是治疗决策的提供依据。

研究对象的选择直接影响诊断试验的灵敏度和特异度。病例组应包括不同严重程度的病例，对照组应包括由金标准确认无该病，但又易于与该病混淆的其他病例，而非健康正常人。

平行试验的应用可提高灵敏度和阴性预测值，但却降低了特异度和阳性预测值；系列试验提高了特异度和阳性预测值，但同时降低了灵敏度和阴性预测值。

（吴尚洁）

第十章

治疗性研究

学习目标

1. **掌握** 治疗性研究的基本概念及类型。
2. **熟悉** 治疗性研究的评价原则。
3. **了解** 治疗性研究的特点、步骤、设计；影响治疗性研究结果的主要原因。

临床医学的基本目的是了解疾病的发生、发展以及预后转归，逐步主动地采取干预措施，改善和防止疾病的不利结果，提高疾病的治愈率，降低疾病的病残率和病死率，这也是疾病治疗性研究的主要目的。

由于治疗性研究的目的是治疗疾病、改善预后，因而要求研究的结果必须真实可靠，同时具有很好的重复性。真实性是指研究的结果接近事物本身的真值，不受各种偏倚因素的干扰。可靠性或重复性是指研究的结果能被他人引用，可以重复验证其有效性。这两个基本特点是治疗性研究的关键。

第一节 治疗性研究的步骤和研究设计

一、治疗性研究的选题

治疗性研究的核心是选题。选题即临床医师在实际工作中产生的新的想法，而且必须有一定的创意和新颖性。选题往往来源于临床医师在工作中敏锐的观察和大胆的设想，同时，需要临床医师具备对疾病发病机制和流行病学的深入了解。

根据研究目的，通常基于下述依据进行选题。

1. 基于在基因、分子或细胞水平上对疾病的发病机制的认识、考虑进行选题。

2. 基于临床医师对临床现象的仔细观察进行选题，对于尚未明确发病机制的疾病，也能探索出一些有效的临床治疗方法。

3. 基于其他研究的一些结果或结论对拟研究疾病的启发，有些甚至是从错误的结果中得到了启迪。

二、治疗性研究的基本原则

治疗性研究通常是前瞻性研究，为确保研究结果不受已知的或未知的偏倚因素的影响，使研究结果真实可靠,能真正地指导临床实践,在研究设计时一定要遵循随机化、设立对照和盲法三大基本原则。

1. 随机化原则 随机化原则是将纳入研究的个体随机分配到不同的研究组别的方法。研究通常包括实验组也称治疗组,以及对照组。这种方法属于随机分配,需要与随机取样区分。随机取样是指研究者运用一定的方法从人群中选取研究对象的方法,通常用于调查研究。正确地将临床试验对象分配到各研究组是保证各组基线相同,各组间具有可比性的关键。随机化(randomization)原则即要求每一个受试对象都有完全相同的机会被分到试验组或对照组,其目的是保证试验组和对照组患者具有相似的临床特征和预后因素(包括已知的和未知的),从而避免研究人员或试验对象主观意愿的干扰,增加研究结果的正确性。

2. 设立对照原则 评价试验结果的真实性,非常强调研究的对照(control)和比较。因此,设立对照是临床试验的一个重要原则,也是科学研究的一项基本要求。所谓"设立对照",即设立条件相同及诊断一致的一组对象,接受某种与试验组不一样的试验措施,目的是和试验组的结果进行对照性的比较,以证明两组(或多组)间结果的差异及其程度。用以进行比较的这一组患者(又称对照组),除不接受被研究的干预措施外,其他方面的试验条件与观察指标和效应标准都应与试验组相同。因此,设立对照的目的,是使研究的基线情况保持一致而具有可比性,从而消除非试验因素的干扰和影响。对照组的类型包括:同期随机对照(concurrent randomized control)、非随机同期对照(non-randomized concurrent control)、自身对照(self-control)、历史性对照(historical control)和配对对照(matching control)等。

3. 盲法原则 临床试验中,试验的研究者或受试者都不知道试验对象的分配情况,即不知道受试对象分配的组别、接受的是试验措施还是对照措施,这种临床试验方法称为盲法试验(blind trial)。盲法试验的目的是有效避免研究者或受试者的信息偏倚和主观偏见。在评价主观指标时,如判断疼痛缓解、气促缓解等,采用盲法试验可以克服试验者和受试者主观的、暗示性的各种偏倚,得到准确、可靠的评价试验结果。对研究资料进行分析和报告时也可采用盲法试验。

三、治疗性研究的步骤

1. 研究对象的选择 在治疗性研究中,要求对观察的对象、诊断及病情判断十分准确,这是确保研究结果重复性的关键环节。在具体研究中,因为研究对象的复杂病情和研究条件的限制,不可能同时纳入各型患者进行研究,常常只能根据研究课题的特定目的,制订一定的纳入标准和排除标准,使研究对象限定在确定的范围内。然后再通过多层次的研究,积累全面的资料,从而克服单个研究的局限,认识整体规律。

2. 样本大小的估计 临床研究中若样本量过小,往往容易得出假阴性结果;而样本量过大,则会造成不必要的人力、物力、时间和经济的浪费,加大试验的难度。有关样本的估算方法主要根据统计学中样本含量公式进行计算。通常要求把概率的影响而发生错误(包括假阳性和假阴性)的可能性限制在可以接受的范围内,即实验中第一类错误出现的概率(α)和第二类错误出现的概率(β)限制在能接受的范围。通常设定 α 为 0.05,β 为 0.1~0.2,则检验效能为 0.8~0.9,这种犯错误的概率是适当的和为大家所能接受的。同时,治疗措施的效应也是样本大小估算的重要方面,即试验组与对照组出现的结果差异愈大,所需要的样本数愈小。

3. 效果衡量的指标及终点的选择 确定治疗性干预措施的效果,必须要有明确而客观的衡量指标。这些指标要求能准确判定,具有很好的一致性,并最好能做到量化,便于进行有效的比较和分析。

作为治疗性研究的测量指标通常要求包括：能敏感地发现治疗出现的反应；能准确地测量和确定治疗反应的阳性结果；应与治疗措施的特定效果相关；同时，应选择经济及可行性良好的测试方法。通常，测量指标包括软指标和硬指标。临床可靠性差、重复性难以保证的、不易量化的指标称为软指标，如患者的主观症状变化和体征的变化。而将明确、客观、易于判定的指标称为硬指标，如病愈、病残、死亡，以及手术病理发现、实验室测定的定量指标等。

为了观察到治疗措施的真实效果，研究终点的选择也是至关重要的。同时，要求有足够的观察期，要注意近期疗效和远期疗效的观察，以期看到最终结果。如果观察期过短，易造成假阴性或假阳性的结果。当然，随着观察时期的延长，也会对最终观察结果带来更多的影响，增加了研究随访的难度，研究者必须对此加以重视并设法解决。

4. 治疗性研究常用设计方案的选择　要遵循治疗性研究的三大原则，即随机化、设立对照、盲法，治疗性研究的首选设计方案为随机对照研究，但根据不同的研究目的及结合研究者的客观实际，兼顾研究的科学性和可行性，其他的研究方案也是治疗性研究中可以选择的，包括队列研究、自身前后对照研究（before-after study）、半随机对照研究（quasi-randomized control study）以及历史性对照研究（historical control trial）等。

（1）随机对照研究

随机对照研究的设计模式如图10-1，结果分析如表10-1。

1）设计模式

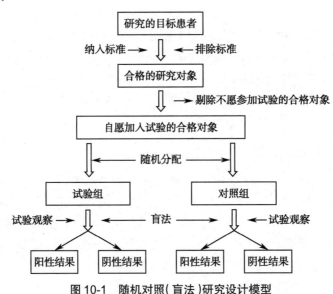

图 10-1　随机对照（盲法）研究设计模型

2）结果分析

表 10-1　随机对照研究结果分析四格表

分组	结果		合计 / 例
	阳性 / 例	阴性 / 例	
试验组 / 例	a	b	a+b
对照组 / 例	c	d	c+d
合计 / 例	a+c	b+d	N

3）实例说明

对于冠心病患者选择内科治疗还是冠状动脉旁路移植术手术治疗，存在不同的意见。某冠心病研究中心进行了 780 例冠心病患者的研究（图 10-2）并做数据分析（表 10-2 和表 10-3）。

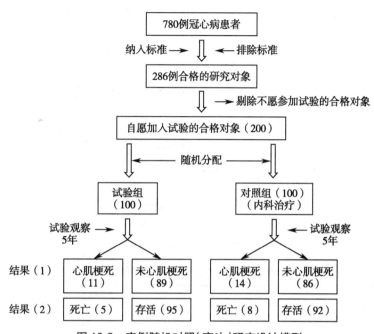

图 10-2　实例随机对照（盲法）研究设计模型

表 10-2　实例随机对照研究结果分析四格表（1）

分组	结果（1）		合计 / 例
	心肌梗死 / 例	未心肌梗死 / 例	
试验组 / 例	11	89	100
对照组 / 例	14	86	100
合计 / 例	25	175	200

表 10-3　实例随机对照研究结果分析四格表（2）

分组	结果（2）		合计 / 例
	死亡 / 例	存活 / 例	
试验组 / 例	5	95	100
对照组 / 例	8	92	100
合计 / 例	13	187	200

结论：根据试验组与对照组 X^2 检验比较，结果（1）和结果（2）均为差异无统计学意义（两个结果均 $P>0.05$）。临床意义：从此研究结果得出结论，冠状动脉旁路移植术手术治疗较内科保守治疗不能减少患者心肌梗死的患病率以及 5 年患者死亡率。

（2）队列研究：在治疗性研究中一般采用前瞻性队列研究，即被观察人群是自然接受而形成的两个队列，干预措施不是由研究者做随机分配入组的，而是自然分组的，且研究者难以控制。前瞻性队列研究最大的特点是能及时地控制试验中出现的干扰，但同时因其不能随机，难以保证两组间人数的平衡和基线情况的一致。队列研究的设计模型如图 10-3，结果分析如表 10-4。

1）设计模式

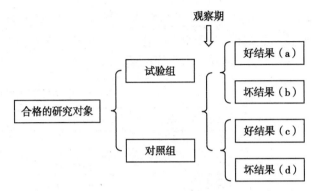

图 10-3　队列研究设计模型

2）结果分析

表 10-4　队列研究结果分析四格表

分组	结果	
	好结果 / 例	坏结果 / 例
试验组 / 例	a	b
对照组 / 例	c	d

采用四格表 X^2 检验，明确是否具有统计学意义。

（3）自身交叉对照研究：自身交叉对照研究是一种前瞻性研究方法，即将两种不同的干预措施应用于受试者前、后两个阶段，最后对两种干预措施效果进行比较分析。在两阶段之间应有洗脱期（wash-out period），其时间的长短以及是否必要，应根据药物的半衰期、采用的措施及目的而定。通常此种方法应用于慢性病或慢性复发性疾病。自身交叉对照研究的设计模型如图 10-4，结果分析如表 10-5。

1）设计模式

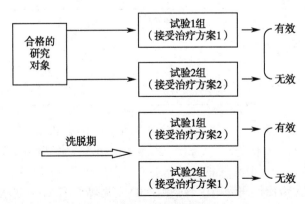

图 10-4　自身交叉对照研究设计模型

2）结果分析

表 10-5　自身交叉对照研究结果分析四格表

方案	有效	无效	合计
治疗方案 1	a	b	a+b
治疗方案 2	c	d	c+d
合计	a+c	b+d	a+b+c+d

（4）半随机对照研究：半随机对照研究与随机对照研究试验设计相似，唯一的差别是研究对象分配是按半随机的方式，即依照被研究者的生日或住院号末尾数字是奇数或偶数，分别分配到试验组或对照组，接受不同的干预措施。因分配的原因，受试者基线状态难以平衡，受到人为的选择偏倚影响的机会比较大。其研究结果的可靠性往往不如随机对照研究。

（5）历史性对照研究：将新的干预措施的研究结果与过去研究的结果进行比较。由于历史性对照非随机分配、非同期对照，其可比性较差，结果论证强度差，但能节省研究成本及时间。

5. 治疗性研究结果的分析和解释　在研究试验阶段完成后，研究结果的分析和解释前，必须确保资料的完整收集，只有资料完整才能进行统计分析和真实的结果评价。结果的分析包括：研究结果受偏倚和概率影响的程度，是否在可以接受的范围内？采取了什么防止偏倚影响的措施，其研究结果的内在真实性如何？应用的统计学分析方法是否适当？

同时，在对研究结果进行解释时，应表明研究结果的可适用的代表人群，结果的科学性和临床方面的意义。治疗性研究只有经过反复实践，扩大试验的范围人群，才能最终完善其结论的真实性。

第二节　影响治疗性研究结果的主要因素

在治疗性研究的进行过程中，研究者除了要注重研究方法的谨慎选择，还要注意到有多种因素的干扰可能影响到研究结果的真实性，研究者必须对有关影响因素加以了解和控制。

一、可比性

可比性是指试验组和对照组除了被观察的干预措施之外，其他特征应具有完全的相似性和一致性，即保证研究基线状况的相对平衡。必须采用严格的纳入和排除标准选择合格的研究对象，同时采用配对、分层、随机分组的方法加强试验组和对照组的可比性，可比性的强弱直接影响到最终结果的真实性。

二、样本大小

样本大小直接反映出概率影响的程度。样本量过小，由概率影响导致的假阳性及假阴性结果的可能性就大，结论的可信度较小。由于临床治疗性研究常常无法达到很大的样本量，因此，应计算并确定一个适当的样本量，控制其产生假阳性和假阴性结果的机会在一个最小的、可以接受的范围。

三、对照及安慰剂效应

对照是治疗性研究判断效果的基本且必需的方法，严格的对照是指同期的、与观察组病例完全相似的对照病例。通过严格的对照组的观察，消除试验组与对照组中出现的非特异性效果，真正的所要观察的干预措施的效果才能显现出来。

治疗性研究中，对照组病例通常给予安慰剂以达到盲法的效果，安慰剂在对照组中出现的效果，甚至是某些副作用，称为安慰剂效应（placebo effect）。它是一种非特异性效应，可以由环境、心理等多种因素引起，其也可以出现在观察组中。因此，可以通过两组对比，确定试验组中特异与非特异的效应以及其出现的比例，去除非特异性效应，得到真实的评价所观察的治疗措施的价值。

四、偏倚与概率

偏倚与概率的影响，可以严重地破坏研究的结果。偏倚可出现在治疗性研究的全过程，包括选择偏倚、信息偏倚以及混杂偏倚，研究者可通过完善、严格的试验设计避免这些偏倚。而概率，即抽样误差，则不可能完全消除，只能通过限制第Ⅰ类误差及第Ⅱ类误差的允许水平，将其控制在可以普遍接受的范围。实际上，所有的临床治疗性研究希望获得的真实可靠的结果，自始至终都是围绕着控制偏倚和概率而进行的。

五、沾染与干扰

当对照组患者意外地接受了试验组的治疗措施，称为沾染（contamination）。沾染的发生会使试验组与对照组产生的疗效差异减小，影响被观察的干预措施真实效果的评价。

当试验组患者在观察期间同时接受了与试验干预措施效果一样的其他处理，称为干扰（co-intervention）。如果没有双盲或者其他处理与干预措施产生极其类似的效果，干扰会使结果偏离真实的情况。沾染与干扰的控制主要依赖研究者的严格管理，特别是治疗性研究中盲法的应用。采用双盲法可有效地避免沾染与干扰的发生。

六、依从性

纳入研究的观察对象对规定执行的医疗措施（如服药次数和疗程）的接受和执行的依从程度，称之为依从性（compliance），多次给药或者患者同时服用其他药物会导致依从性差。通常，在治疗性研究中，被观察对象依从性的高低可用来判断研究质量的水平，如果患者不依从率超过 20%，将导致研究效果无法进行判断与评价。然而，即使失访率不高，但是如果在评估时忽略依从性的影响，也会影响结果的真实性，因为失访的原因可能与治疗措施相关。

第三节　治疗性研究评价的参考标准

一、是否是真正的随机对照研究

这是决定治疗性研究结果是否真实有效的最关键的问题。只有真正的随机对照才能真正实现已知和未知影响预后因素的平衡分布，确保可比性，最终的结论论证强度才高。因此，评价时应注意以下几个问题。

1. 确定其随机分配的具体方法，是否隐藏分组。

2. 注意组间重要临床特点基线状态的可比性。

3. 注意试验组或对照组除了接受各自被观察的干预措施外，是否还接受了其他不同程度的辅助治疗，即注意沾染与干扰偏倚影响研究的结果。

4. 注意研究中是否实施了盲法及其是否正确、合理。

当然，也不排斥其他非随机研究的结果。由于执行随机的可行性的限制，常常不得已选择非随机的队列研究或非随机对照研究等设计方案，但在评价其研究结果时，需对其治疗效果的真实性进行必要的解释和限定。

二、是否观察和报告了全部的研究结果

治疗性研究从设计开始就应有明确的目的、相关的测量指标和最终的判断效果的标准。因此，在评价和应用研究结果时，应报告由被观察的干预措施所产生的正、反两方面的作用，即产生的效应和危害或副作用，这些内容都具备了才能算是全面的研究结果，也才能进行研究结果的最后分析和评价。同时，应评价是否对研究结果进行了盲法分析，因为盲法分析可以有效地排除信息偏倚，从而可确保研究结果判断的重复性和真实性。

三、被研究的对象是否明确

这是治疗性研究结果能否被正确应用的重要环节。报告中研究者应详细描述研究对象的纳入和排除标准，清楚地显示研究对象的临床特征，包括年龄、性别、地区、疾病类型、病情程度以及有无并发症等。以便治疗性研究结果能被应用于相似的患者，而获得相似的临床效果。

四、是否注意研究结果统计学和临床意义的区别

在分析治疗性研究结果时，一定要衡量试验组和对照组间的统计学差异与临床疗效差异，这是评价治疗性研究价值的关键。

统计学意义是分析试验组与对照组间出现的差异是否来自被观察的干预措施本身的作用，其来自单纯机遇影响的可能性有多大。通常采用 $P<0.05$ 作为具有统计学意义或差异具有显著性，表示研究中发现的效果差异来自单纯机遇的可能性小于 5%，而由干预措施本身产生的真正效应大于 95%。统计学上的差异具有显著性意义并不涉及疗效差异的大小程度，也不能用于评价干预措施疗效有无临床意义，它唯一的意义只是评价这种差异存在的真实程度。

而治疗性研究中干预措施是否具有临床意义除直接考虑干预措施产生的临床疗效大小外，有时亦可从药物价格的高低、副作用出现的频率及其严重性等进行临床价值的评估。这就需要衡量研究的具体目的和具体指标，方能有效地进行临床意义的评价。

五、研究中干预措施内容是否明确

为了研究结果能正确应用和重复实践，研究分析报告中应尽可能详细地报告干预措施的内容和具体方法，如药物的剂型、剂量、给药途径、疗程以及其他的辅助方法等。在研究的实际观察中，是否严格执行以及是否依从性得到保证，同时是否严格地控制以防止沾染

和干扰的发生,都会影响到试验结果,应该在分析报告中详细地写明。

六、研究结果是否包括了全部的纳入对象

在治疗性研究的观察过程中,因为种种原因往往会中途丢失部分受观察患者,称为失访。因为失访的人群往往有不同的临床结局,在研究开始时建立的组间可比性会因为病例的失访而受到严重的影响,因而治疗性研究中通常要求病例失访率不应超出总观察数的10%。失访率若超出20%,则全部结果被视为失去真实性,而没有临床意义。因此,只有在研究实践中认真严格地观察、追踪,尽量减少病例的丢失,才能保证研究结果的真实性。

以上六条标准,依顺序代表治疗性研究中评价参考标准的重要性。它们可以帮助研究者以及临床医师在阅读文献时判断其科学性和实用性,从而作出正确的评价以提高自身的研究水平和指导临床干预措施的选择。

本 章 小 结

实施治疗措施相关的循证医学步骤包括:提出问题→查询证据→证据评价→证据应用→后效评价;治疗性研究设计遵循随机化、设立对照和盲法三大原则,确保研究结果真实可靠;其设计方案首选随机对照研究;治疗性研究评价的参考标准包括是否是真正的随机对照研究、是否观察和报告了全部的研究结果、被研究的对象是否明确、是否注意研究结果统计学和临床意义的区别、研究中干预措施内容是否明确、研究结果是否包括了全部的纳入对象。

(吴尚洁)

第十一章

预后研究证据评价

学习目标

1. **掌握** 预后研究的基本概念。
2. **熟悉** 预后研究的评价标准。
3. **了解** 预后研的究设计类型。

医生经常会被患者、同事等问及有关预后的问题。例如，一名 32 岁被诊断为"乳腺癌"行右乳改良根治术的年轻女性乳腺癌病例，患者及家属可能特别关心的问题包括：这个疾病是否会复发？日后能否怀孕及生育？怀孕会不会增加乳腺癌复发的概率？而作为临床医生，也会考虑：术后病理分期如何？是否需要术后辅助化疗、放疗、靶向或内分泌治疗？实际上，这些都是有关乳腺癌预后以及影响预后因素的问题，即乳腺癌复发率如何？妊娠对乳腺癌预后有无影响？

为了回答这些问题，需要了解预后研究的基本概念及研究类型，同时需要评估预后研究的真实性、重要性及研究结果的适用性。

第一节 预后研究的基本概念

预后（prognosis）是对疾病未来病程和结局（痊愈、复发、恶化、伤残、并发症和死亡等）的估计及对导致不同结局影响因素的研究，是疾病自然病程研究的一部分。疾病自然病程是指疾病的发生、发展及转归，而预后是指疾病诊断确立后的临床进程和影响这一过程的诸多因素。疾病预后研究（prognostic study）指对疾病各种结局发生概率及其影响因素的研究，至少包括率的估计和探究影响预后的因素这两个方面。其中，率的估计包括病死率、生存率、治愈率、复发率；对于病程短、可治愈的疾病，预后指标多用治愈率；对于病程长、不易治愈的疾病，多用复发率、缓解率；对于严重疾病，多用病死率（或存活率）、致残率等；慢性病预后研究常增加生活质量评价。而影响预后的因素主要包括可用来判断疾病预后的疾病亚型分类和一些临床指标。

第二节 预后研究常用的临床研究设计

很多种研究都能提供预后信息，常用的临床研究设计包括队列研究（前瞻性和回顾性）、病例对照研究、纵向描述性研究、系列病例分析、专家意见和个案报道。不同研究设计提供的预后研究证据质量水平完全不同。因此，在获取预后研究证据及应用证据前，掌握预后研究的不同设计方法及评估不同方法的优缺点对判断研究结果的真实性非常重要。

一、队列研究

队列研究是预后研究主要的研究方法，研究者对一组或多组患有特定疾病的群体进行随访，并追溯不同结局事件的发生。队列研究由病因（暴露、非暴露）推导结局（发病率、治愈率、缓解率、复发率和生存率等），可分为前瞻性队列研究和回顾性队列研究，是回答预后问题的最重要的研究设计方法。前瞻性队列研究指研究开始时，暴露因素已存在但疾病尚未发生（图 11-1），在随访过程之中，可获取暴露因素导致的不同结局。而回顾性队列研究指研究开始时，暴露与疾病均已发生（图 11-2），即研究结局在研究开始时已经发生，从而探讨过去的暴露因素与目前已发生某种疾病之间的因果关系，历史资料的完整性和真实性将影响研究的可行性和结果的可靠性。

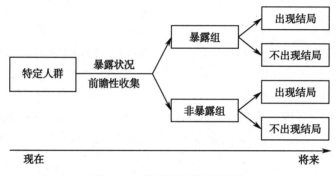

图 11-1　前瞻性队列研究设计

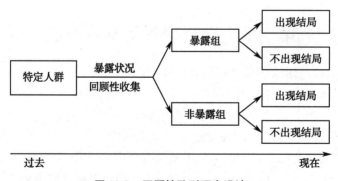

图 11-2　回顾性队列研究设计

运用队列研究进行疾病预后因素分析时，研究者根据是否存在某因素（暴露与否）将人群分组，然后随访一段时间，再确定患者是否出现阳性结局。因此，首先要确定研究因素和结局因素并记录随访的时间，这是队列研究的三大基本要素。

确定研究因素（暴露因素）是预后研究的主要内容，根据暴露因素的有无将人群划分为暴露组及非暴露组两组。根据暴露因素的不同水平或类型，分组可超过两组。暴露因素必须有明确规定，最好将暴露定量，明确划分暴露与非暴露人群的界限以及暴露因素分级标准。可影响疾病预后的因素很多，不同的疾病不尽相同，应结合专业知识尽可能将各种可能与预后有关的因素纳入研究因素，这样预后因素的分析才不会遗漏。临床预后因素的研究常比较复杂，可有多个预后因素互相作用，从而影响结局。应用单因素分析不能将多个预后因素对结局的影响分析清楚时，应采用多因素分析方法。

　　另一重要内容是确定研究的结局，即随访的终点（又称阳性结局）。阳性结局必须有一个明确和客观的定义，不能模棱两可，以免出现信息偏倚。对于某些结局，如死亡，是非常确定、没有疑问的。而其他的结局例如致残、疾病的缓解等，可明确定义，但确认发生的时间存在一定困难。结局包括研究终点和删失。

　　随访时间是指从研究起点至研究终点（出现阳性结局）或删失的时间。确定随访时间有以下注意点：预后研究需要一定的随访时间，才能观察到研究终点（或阳性结局）；随访时间必须足够长，使大部分患者有足够时间出现阳性结局、得出结论；需要根据疾病自然史或病程了解疾病结局发生的时间后确定随访时间。

　　生存分析是预后研究常用的统计学方法。在临床研究中，随访的起点往往不在同一个时间，因为不可能所有研究病例约好同一天起病，研究对象是逐渐入组的；同样随访终点（阳性结局）也不可能发生在同一时间，所以各个病例随访的时间长短不一。对于结束研究时尚未达到阳性结局者称为删失。研究随访时间较长时经常发生失访。如果研究的结局并非不可避免，受试者可能由于互竞风险而结束随访，例如研究终点为死亡时部分研究对象可能因为其他原因导致死亡而结束随访。大部分统计学方法认为研究对象失访或因互竞风险退出随访均归为删失。此时，预后分析是评估平均风险及发生时间较好的方法。生存分析围绕着这样一个精神，有多种计算方法，如寿命表法、Kaplan-Meier 法等，其中寿命表法为预后分析的基本方法。

　　队列研究的优点有：队列研究中研究因素和结局因素之间有一段连续的时间，两者间建立了清晰的因果关系，为临床的因果关系提供强有力的信息；可以直接测量某些暴露因素发展成疾病的危险性；在测量时尚不知结局因素可以避免暴露因素测量时的偏倚，也可以同时测量已知的混杂因素，以便在统计分析时加以控制。

　　队列研究的缺点有：需要花费很大的人力、物力和时间。阳性结局发生率较低者或从因至果的周期较长者，需要大样本及长时间的随访方能获得阳性结果。对于某些特殊暴露因素的群体，随访时间可能需要数十年，这样长时间的研究，代价自然也是不菲的。由于随访时间较长，研究初期确定的暴露因素经过一段时间后可能会发生变化，常常造成结局分析的偏倚。如有些吸烟者戒了烟，可能得出吸烟不导致肺癌发生的错误结论。

二、病例对照研究

　　病例对照研究也是预后研究的常用方法。相较于由暴露推导至结局的队列研究方法，病例对照研究是从疾病发生后开始，按照发病与否分为病例组和对照组，回顾性分析产生该种结局的有关因素，是由结果倒推至原因的研究方法（图 11-3）。例如，如果想研究吸烟与肺癌的关系，研究者需要比较肺癌患者与对照组吸烟的习惯。病例对照研究较为省时经济，更适合评估一些罕见病，也适用于一次性评估多种暴露因素与结局的关系。

　　通常认为病例对照研究不如队列研究真实有效。病例对照研究的对照组选择非常关键，若对照组选择不当，很容易造成选择偏倚。常见问题还有回忆偏倚等。病例对照研究不能提供生存率研究的证据，因此，在作疾病预后因素分析时，只能用于那些时间因素不重要的研究。常见的偏倚有以下三种。

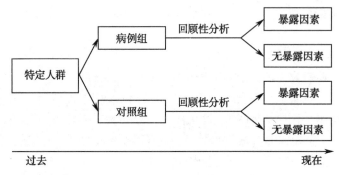

图 11-3　病例对照研究

1. 选择偏倚　选择进入研究的人群与未进入研究的人群之间存在的差别。例如在病例对照研究纳入对照组时，同意进入研究的人群可能比拒绝参与的人群更健康（体重更低、烟酒消耗更少、锻炼更多等），这会导致病例组与对照组之间存在差异，造成选择偏倚。

2. 回忆偏倚　回忆调查研究对象既往的暴露情况时，由于被调查者记忆失真或不完整造成病例组和对照组明确暴露与否所致的系统误差，多发生在病例对照研究。

3. 观察（者）偏倚　在实际观察中由于观察者的缘故而产生的系统误差，常发生在暴露组或病例组。例如，当观察者与病例组交谈时，会有意识地更加详细地询问是否存在暴露因素。例如临床医生对已知暴露于某特定因素者会倾向诊断相关疾病。

第三节　预后研究证据的评价

对于预后研究的证据，需评价其研究结果的真实性、重要性和适用性。

一、预后研究结果的真实性

研究对象的来源需作详细描述，并具有代表性。用公认的诊断标准准确定义研究对象。明确研究对象的纳入和排除标准，以便判断研究时有无选择偏倚。

预后队列研究在纳入研究对象时，起始点要十分明确，因为患者所处的病期和病程都将直接影响预后结局。只有保证研究对象纳入时处在大致相同的阶段，其预后结果才具有真实性。研究起始点最好在病程早期，至少应在相同病程阶段。

当研究对象因各种原因从原定的研究计划中退出，称为失访，这会影响研究的真实性。因为失访患者的结局是研究者不知道的。其影响程度取决于两方面，一是失访人群的质，即失访人群与未失访人群预后因素是否相似，如果失访和未失访者的人口学特征和临床特征较为相近，偏倚就会较小；二是失访人群的量，如果失访量小于观察人群总数的 5% 可认为产生的偏倚不大，而如果失访率大于 20% 则会严重影响结果的真实性。如失访在 5%～20% 之间，可根据情况而定，但需叙述失访原因。

研究时要根据疾病特点，对疾病终点进行准确定义，预后指标要明确，判断标准要客观，避免临床医师在判断预后结局时发生意见偏倚。研究终点必须有一个明确的定义或标准，不能模棱两可，以免出现测量偏倚。

如果预后结局是用"死亡"等硬指标，可不用盲法判断；但如果阳性结局的判断受主观因素影响，就必须采用盲法，以避免偏倚。避免研究者对结局进行直接判断，以避免疑诊偏倚和期望偏倚。

二、预后研究结果的重要性

预后研究结果是否报告了整个病程的预后结局，而不是某一时间点的结局，是其重要性的体现。计算生存率需要了解在某一段时间内发生的结果事件数，生存率常要求用 3 种方法表示：①某一时间点的生存百分率，即从疾病临床过程的某一点开始，一段时间后存活的病例数占总观察例数的百分比（比如 1 年生存率、5 年生存率）；②中位生存时间，即观察到 50% 的研究对象死亡的随访时间；③生存曲线，即在每个时间点，研究样本中没有发生该结果的比例。

置信区间代表了样本与真实人群的差异。预后结局概率的 95% 置信区间指按 95% 置信度估计的总体均数的所在范围。预后结局评估必须包括 95% 置信区间。从统计学角度判断预后研究结果估计的精确性，区间越窄，可信度越高。

三、预后研究结果的适用性

需考虑以下问题：该研究与患者是否差异过大？作者是否将研究对象情况介绍清楚？真实患者与研究对象比较，人口统计学、临床特征、诊断、纳入和排除标准是否相近？如果越接近，应用结果越有把握。

研究结果是否有助于作出临床治疗的决策和有助于对患者及其家属进行解释？根据预后的结果决定是否需要开始治疗：如证据显示不治疗预后也极佳，需讨论是否有必要开始治疗；证据显示不治疗预后不好，倾向对患者进行治疗；证据无法决定要不要治疗，这些研究证据也可以向患者及其家属提供预后信息。

第四节 循 证 案 例

一、提出临床问题

患者，女性，32 岁，因扪及右乳肿块就诊。患者已婚但是尚未生育。查体示右乳可扪及 1cm×1.5cm 质硬肿块。患者行右乳改良根治术，病理示：（右乳）浸润性导管癌；右腋窝下淋巴结 0/20（−）。免疫组化：ER（+）、PR（+）、HER2/neu（−）。

对于这样一个年轻尚未生育的早期乳腺癌病例，患者及家属可能特别关心的问题包括：这个疾病是否会复发？日后能否怀孕及生育？怀孕会不会增加乳腺癌复发的概率？首先研究者必须把患者提出的临床问题转化为可以检索（即包含关键词）并易于回答的问题。如：妊娠的乳腺癌患者复发率与不妊娠相比有无差别？妊娠是否为乳腺癌复发的危险因素？然后，通过在线检索工具检索比较乳腺癌诊断后妊娠和非妊娠患者人群的无病生存率的研究。最后，评价检索到的研究结果的真实性、重要性和适用性。

二、回顾性队列研究示例

雌激素受体状态已知的乳腺癌患者诊断后妊娠与预后关系：一项多中心回顾性队列研究。AMANT F，von MINCKWITZ G，Han S N，et al.Prognosis of women with primary breast cancer diagnosed during pregnancy：results from an international collaborative study［J］. Journal of clinical oncology：official journal of the American Society of Clinical Oncology，2013，31（20）.

1. 目的 此前有荟萃分析显示诊断为乳腺癌后妊娠的女性患者复发率低，但这一结论很可能是由选择偏倚造成的，因为患者往往在无复发后才选择妊娠。此外，尚无针对雌激素受体（ER）阳性的特殊患者人群探究妊娠效应的研究。本研究的目的是通过队列研究比较已知 ER 状态的乳腺癌诊断后妊娠和非妊娠患者人群的无病生存率（DFS）。

2. 方法 研究者开展了此项多中心队列研究，纳入了 2003—2011 年 45 岁以下的在乳腺癌诊断后任意时间发生妊娠（BCP）的患者，对照组为无妊娠的女性患者，排除了产后诊断的患者。分析主要采用 Cox 回归，在年龄、疾病分期分级、ER 状态、HER2 状态、病理、化疗放疗、曲妥珠单抗使用、激素治疗等相同或相近的基础上予以匹配，探究无病生存（DFS）和总生存（OS）与暴露因素（怀孕与否）的关系。

3. 结果 研究组共纳入 447 例怀孕患者，其中 311 人（69.6%）符合条件，和 865 例非怀孕患者被纳入对照组。怀孕患者的中位年龄为 33 岁，非怀孕患者的中位年龄为 41 岁，随访时间的中位数为 61 个月。怀孕对 DFS 的 HR 为 1.34（95%CI, 0.93~1.91; P=0.14），对 OS 的 HR 为 1.19（95%CI, 0.73~1.93; P=0.51）。Cox 回归显示，如果这些患者没有怀孕，其 5 年 DFS 率将从 65% 增加到 71%。同样，5 年的 OS 率也会从 78% 增加到 81%。

4. 结论 与非怀孕患者相比，BCP 患者的 OS 相似。在对患者进行咨询时需要注意这一结论，它支持在继续怀孕的情况下进行治疗。

本研究为多中心回顾性队列研究，纳入研究对象为 ER 状态已知的非转移性原发乳腺癌。主要结果为无病生存期，从明确病理诊断开始，至以下任一终点：局部复发、远处转移、发生第二原发肿瘤或任何原因所致死亡。为评估妊娠作为独立预后因素对结局的影响，将以下其他与预后相关因素进行分层分析：ER、淋巴结状态、辅助化疗、辅助激素治疗、年龄（<35 岁或≥35 岁）。本研究共有 311 例怀孕患者和与其搭配的 865 例非怀孕患者被纳入分析。总体中位随访时间（妊娠组和非妊娠组）为 61 个月。最终，两组复发率无差别（HR=1.34; 95%CI, 0.93~1.91; P=0.14）。本研究是在 ER 状态已知的患者人群中探讨妊娠与预后关系的最大样本量的研究，最终提供强大的数据进一步支持有生育意向的乳腺癌女性患者，妊娠不会给她们的预后带来不良影响。

本 章 小 结

预后研究是预测疾病病程及结局的研究。预后研究的结果有助于了解疾病的临床经过、提供临床决策。预后研究从确立疾病诊断开始，研究之后的临床过程和影响这一过程的诸多因素，至少包括率的估计和探讨影响预后的因素两方面。

预后研究设计包括队列研究、病例对照研究、横断面研究等。不同研究设计所提供的预后研究证据质量水平完全不同。因此，在获取预后研究证据及应用证据前，掌握预后研究的不同设计方法及不同方法的优缺点对后续判断研究结果的真实性非常重要。

预后研究评价原则包括评价其研究结果的真实性、重要性和适用性。

（刘天舒）

第十二章

预防和筛查性研究证据评价

学习目标

1. **掌握** 疾病筛查的基本概念。
2. **了解** 筛查性研究证据的评价原则。

现代预防医学在强调防止人群患病的同时，还要求达到早期诊断和早期治疗疾病的目标，旨在把疾病对人群的危害降到最低。目前，国内的筛查性研究多数是通过灵敏度、特异度、约登指数以及符合率等真实性和可重复性指标对筛查效果予以评价。然而，对于筛查方法的最佳间隔时间等筛查策略以及筛查方法和策略的健康效益和远期效果却未予以足够的重视。

在一定成本条件下如何选取具有较好社会效益的筛查方法和策略，或者在一定效用和效果的条件下如何选取花费较少成本的筛查方法和策略？与诊断性研究相比较，筛查性研究的评价原则有何不同之处？为此，本章节重点介绍有关疾病筛查的基本概念和评价原则。

第一节 基 本 概 念

疾病筛查是为已经处于患病危险或者已经被疾病影响，但尚未察觉疾病的一类人群提供的公共卫生服务。在此类目标人群中进行问卷调查或提供筛查检验测试，目的是确定是否进一步进行诊断试验或治疗，从而降低其患病的危险和危害。疾病筛查与疾病诊断的概念相近，但仍有不同之处。疾病诊断检测的目标人群是临床症状明显、需要确诊疾病的患病者，这些患者知道自身处于"病态"；而疾病筛查检测的目标人群主要是临床症状不明显的早期患者或具有高危因素的人群，此类人群尚不知自身处于"危境"。

疾病筛查的主要目的是将无症状或症状不显著的早期患者或具有高危因素者从正常的健康人群中区分出来，其主要的适用范围是普通人群或特定范围的人群，因而，其不同于针对某一特殊个体而直接进行的疾病诊断。

疾病筛查的意义在于运用简便、快捷的检验方法或检查手段筛检疾病，从而在疾病诊断之前能够提供有效的二级预防，以减少人群的死亡率和致残率，它是被大多数发达国家用于疾病防控的主要工具之一。当然，疾病筛查也可被用于确定高危人群，从而进行相应的干预，以达到疾病的一级预防，从而降低疾病的发病率。

因此，对于一篇有关疾病筛查的研究文献，除了要判别其筛查方法的有效性（能够辨别早期患者与非患者），还应了解人群通过筛查而被早期诊断疾病之后，是否能通过早期干预使阳性结果者今后的生活质量得以改善，以此来判断疾病筛查研究的正确性和意义。

第二节　研究设计和评价原则

一、实施疾病筛查的原则

实施疾病筛查有利亦有弊，它在发现早期患者和高危人群的同时，也有相对增加人群的"患病"时间、加重阳性结果人群心理负担等弊端。因此，在实施疾病筛查之初，应确定该筛查是否利大于弊，应同时考量筛查方法的准确性和治疗方法的有效性。如果在进行筛查并发现早期患者之后，却无有效的干预措施，那么，实施疾病筛查即无任何现实意义。

领先时间（lead time）指从筛检发现疾病到该患者因症状而去就诊的时间间隔。领先时间长的疾病，在筛检发现疾病后，有时间予以诊断和治疗，其健康结局优于症状明显后自动去就医的人群。例如，高血压及噪声性聋有较长的领先时间，而胰腺癌仅有一个短的领先时间。领先时间短的疾病进展很快，从筛检发现到因症状而去就诊仅有较短的时间，筛检发现后开始治疗与其自动就医后开始治疗相比，优点不明显。

目前，国内外筛查实施的原则被引用得最多的仍然是威尔逊（Wilson）和琼格尔（Jungner）在 1968 年为 WHO 疾病筛查工作所制定的《筛查实施原则》。这一原则在不同国家被具体应用时亦有所调整，但其核心的内容仍没有发生改变。我国"十二五"普通高等教育本科国家级规划教材的《流行病学》中所编写的筛查实施原则，即以威尔逊和琼格尔的 10 项实施原则为基础并进行了一定的调整。与威尔逊和琼格尔的 10 项实施原则相比，我国的原则对于被筛查人群、被筛查的疾病、被筛查的公共健康问题、筛查时应考虑的社会效益因素等均做了明确的限制及说明，此外，还考虑到了筛查计划中的伦理问题。表 12-1 对于威尔逊和琼格尔的 10 项原则和我国教材中引用的 10 项原则进行了对比。疾病筛查在符合以下前提原则时，才具有实施的价值和意义。

表 12-1　实施疾病筛查的原则

对比		威尔逊和琼格尔	我国
相同	1.	被筛查的内容应该是当地重要的健康问题	
	2.	对于被筛查的疾病或缺陷有可用于进一步诊断的条件	
	3.	对发现并确诊的患者及高危人群有条件进行有效的且可接受的治疗和干预	
	4.	被筛查的疾病或缺陷或某种危险因素有供识别的早期症状和体征或测量的标志	
	5.	需要清楚了解被筛查疾病的自然史，包括从潜伏期到临床期的全部发展过程	
	6.	要考虑整个筛查、诊断和治疗的成本和收益问题	
相似	1.	有合适的检查或试验	筛查试验必须快速、简便、经济、可靠、安全、有效且易被受检查者接受
	2.	试验是可以被人群接受的	有保证筛查计划顺利完成的人力、物力、财力和良好的社会环境条件
	3.	对于筛查人群，病例发现必须是一个持续的过程，而不是只进行一次筛查试验	发现病例的计划应该是一个持续的过程，要有连续并完整的筛查计划，能按照计划定期进行
	4.	提供被一致认可的政策	筛查计划应该能够被目标人群接受，有益无害，尊重个人隐私，制定保密措施；公正、公平、合理地对待被检对象

随机对照的研究方案也可用于探讨实施疾病筛查及早期治疗的意义。按照不同的筛查和治疗对象，以及随机分配实施的不同时机，可有两种随机对照的研究策略用于探讨实施筛查项目是否有意义，如图 12-1 所示，差别在筛查后干预时间不同。例如，在纽约用随机对照试验观察了约 6 万名 64 岁左右的妇女长达 23 年，比较经过筛检并干预的妇女与未经筛检的妇女患乳腺癌后的状况。随访 5 年时，筛检组乳腺癌死亡率比未经筛检组低 38.1%，10 年时低 28.6%，18年时低 22.7%。这一研究方案如图 12-1A 所示。图 12-1B 所示研究方案为妊娠妇女产前检查时筛查妊娠期亚临床性甲状腺功能减退症，评估筛查后早期干预与有症状干预的差异。

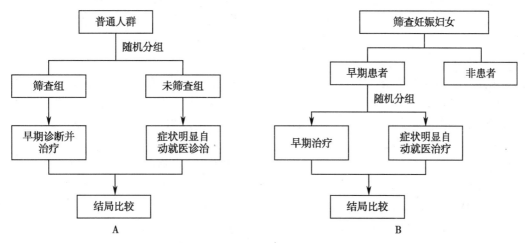

图 12-1　筛查疾病的随机对照研究方案

二、筛查的分类

筛查按照筛查对象的范围、筛查方法的数量可分为以下几类。

1. 人群筛查（population screening）　用一定的筛查方法对整体人群进行筛查，找出其中可能患病的高危人群，再进行确诊试验或治疗。例如，采用糖筛试验初检妊娠妇女，结果异常者再进行口服葡萄糖耐量试验进行确诊。

2. 选择性筛查（targeted screening）　对暴露在危险因素中的人群或高危人群进行定期健康检查，以达到早期发现疾病、及时提供干预的目的。例如，定期对矿工进行硅肺（肺尘埃沉着病）筛检；对石棉工进行石棉沉着病、肺癌的筛检；对接触铅作业职工及其他严重有毒、有害环境作业职工进行定期筛检。

3. 单项筛查（single screening）　用一种筛查试验筛查一种疾病，是目前应用最多的筛查类型。例如，采用乳腺 X 射线摄影常规筛查妇女乳腺疾病。

4. 多项筛查（multiple screening）　在筛查方案中，同时应用多种方法进行疾病的筛查，也可以同时针对多种疾病进行筛查。例如，我国通过采集足跟血进行检测和听力学测试的方法，对新生儿免费筛检苯丙酮尿症、先天性甲状腺功能减退症、葡萄糖 -6- 磷酸脱氢酶缺乏症、先天性听力缺陷等多种遗传或内分泌疾病。

5. 病例发现（case-finding）或机会性筛检（opportunistic screening）　筛检的对象是因其他原因而进行临床诊治或咨询，临床医生对就诊者加用其他筛检方法，以发现与主诉无关的疾病。

三、疾病筛查的流程

目前，疾病的基础筛查流程已经被国内外学者一致认可，并已应用于公共卫生领域。即对于健康人群，或是表面健康尚无症状或临床诊断的人群进行筛查性试验，将筛查人群按试验结果的阴性与阳性区分开；对于试验结果阳性者进一步实施疾病的诊断性试验；并根据诊断的结果区分为患者和非患者；对患者或高危人群实施治疗性或预防性干预。

然而，在实际操作过程中发现该筛查流程过于简单化，遗漏了部分结果不确定者，例如：结果未达到实施干预的标准，但也不满足阴性诊断结果者。所以对于策划、评估和实施筛查计划，建立明确且统一的筛查条件是至关重要的，其中筛查条件包括目标人群的年龄、性别等。

四、筛查模型

流行病学筛查模型是基于流行病学调查资料而采用的一种疾病筛查方法。通过建立恰当的筛查模型，可以使人群中大量尚未诊断的患者得到早期诊断和早期治疗，并且也可以使筛查的目标人群大大缩小，简化筛查的组织工作，节省大量的人力、物力和财力。

例如，对于糖尿病风险的筛查研究，常用方法是通过危险因素分析测定个体罹患糖尿病的风险大小。对于每位个体而言，所具有的危险因素越多，并且危险因素的等级越高，则罹患糖尿病的风险越大。利用危险因素记分法建立的社区糖耐量受损人群筛查模型则是一种简便、经济、有效的筛查工具。

此外，在流行病学调查资料的基础之上，数学模型也可以应用于疾病筛查模型的建立。例如，可利用人工神经网络建立筛查的预测模型。人工神经网络模型可以自动地从已知的数据或条件中总结出定量的规律，当研究者将未知样本的测量信息输入计算机后，待测信息经过人工神经网络的计算，可以预测出某种风险或事物的发生结果。采用人工神经网络作为疾病的初筛方法，可以避免传统的筛查方法存在的筛查效率低、费时、费力、费钱等问题，更适用于大规模的人群筛查。目前，人工神经网络已经成功地应用于疾病的流行病学筛查。高蔚等依据糖尿病及高危个体与正常人之间存在的特征差异，如体型肥胖、糖尿病家族史等，筛选糖尿病患者及高危个体，此时仅需给人工神经网络提供几个简单、易获取的指标，就可以使其正确地识别出 90% 的血糖异常者，减少了正常个体测定血糖所需的费用，其效益成本比率是普通筛查方案（口服葡萄糖耐量试验）的 1.6 倍。

五、筛查方案的评价原则

科克伦（Cochrane）和霍兰德（Holland）在 1971 年提出的 7 项评估标准仍是评估现代筛查方案的核心标准内容。这 7 项标准分别针对 7 个筛查要素，分别对简易性、可接受性、准确性、成本收益、可重复性、灵敏度以及特异度进行评估。

1. 简易性　该筛查方案所采用的检测方法应该是简单的，并且容易被理解。

2. 可接受性　筛查的参与者都是自愿参加的，所以检测方法必须是能够被参与者所接受的。

3. 准确性　检测所获得的测量值必须与实际值相符合。

4. 成本收益　综合考量检测的支出及检测应用后的获益。

5. 可重复性　将检测用于同一研究对象进行重复检测时，所得的结果应该保持一致。

6. 灵敏度　检测能够准确地发现研究对象是否患病。

7. 特异度　检测能够甄别出未患病的研究对象。

六、筛查结果的评估指标

评价任何一种筛查试验的优劣，必须先将试验结果与"金标准"检测结果（即应用公认的并且准确的诊断方法测得的结果）进行盲法比较。比较后会出现 4 种结果：真阳性（表示诊断结果和筛查结果都显示为阳性者）、假阳性（表示诊断结果显示为阴性而筛查结果显示为阳性者）、真阴性（表示诊断结果和筛查结果都显示为阴性者）、假阴性（表示诊断结果显示为阳性而筛查结果显示为阴性者）。

根据筛查试验与诊断试验的结果，通过计算公式将评价标准量化，用数字的形式直观地评价筛查试验的优劣。表 12-2 将评价指标按真实性、可重复性及收益三方面进行总结。

表 12-2　筛查结果的评价指标

分类	评价指标	定义和/或计算公式
真实性	灵敏度	灵敏度，即真阳性率，是评价筛查试验发现患病能力的指标
		灵敏度＝真阳性结果/临床诊断出的所有阳性结果×100%
		假阴性率，即漏诊率，是指实际患病但筛查试验为阴性的概率
		假阴性率＝假阴性结果/临床诊断出的所有阳性结果×100%
	特异度	特异度，即真阴性率，是评价筛查试验发现未患病能力的指标
		特异度＝真阴性结果/临床诊断出的所有阴性结果×100%
		假阳性率，即误诊率，是指实际未患病但筛查试验为阳性的概率
		假阳性率＝假阳性结果/临床诊断出的所有阴性结果×100%
	似然比	阳性似然比＝真阳性率/假阳性率，该比值越大，说明筛查试验的诊断价值越高
		阴性似然比＝假阴性率/真阴性率，该比值越小，说明筛查试验的诊断价值越高
	约登指数	约登指数＝（灵敏度＋特异度）−1，表示筛查试验正确鉴别患者和非患者的能力
可重复性	变异系数	当试验做定量测定时，可用变异系数表示可靠性
		变异系数＝标准差/均数×100%，该值越小，说明可靠性越好
	符合率	符合率，即准确度，指对同一批研究对象进行两次试验，检验结果均为阳性和均为阴性的人数之和占所有进行试验人数的比率
	一致性检验	Kappa 检验可用于检验不同地点或不同操作者对同一试验结果的一致性
收益	预测值	阳性预测值，即确诊的患病人数占所有筛查试验阳性结果的概率
		阳性预测值＝真阳性结果/筛查试验的阳性结果×100%
		阴性预测值，即明确未患病人数占所有筛查试验阴性结果的概率
		阴性预测值＝真阴性结果/筛查试验的阴性结果×100%
	卫生经济学指标	成本效益分析，用于分析试验的全部费用和取得的经济效益的关系
		常用效益成本比率表示，效益成本比率（benefit cost ratio，BCR）＝总效益/总成本，如 BCR>1，则筛查有实施价值
		成本-效果分析，用于比较两种干预措施，同时评价效果与消耗的成本
		常用增量成本-效果比率表示，增量成本-效果比率（incremental cost-effectiveness ratio，ICER）＝增加的成本/增加的效果，表示单位效果增加需要的成本增加，ICER 越小越好
		成本-效用分析，用于分析成本与生活质量的关系
		常用质量调整寿命年（quality-adjusted life year，QALY）、伤残调整寿命年（disability-adjusted life year，DALY）表示

　　一项筛查应当能从人群中发现一些过去未被识别的患者，发现率越高说明这项筛检的效果越好。当然，评估发现率时，还应同时考虑此种疾病的患病率高低，距上次同样筛查的时间间隔长短等影响因素。筛查还应当能够改善疾病预后，降低发病率、死亡率、合并症发生率，提高生存率。改善越大，则筛查的效果越好。

　　理论上，理想的筛查试验应同时具有高灵敏度和高特异度，但是在实际情况中，这二者是不可能截然分开的。研究者会发现对于某一筛查试验，通过调节其检测的临界点值以提高灵敏度时，其特异度值就会降低，反之亦然。故而，比较不同筛查方法的灵敏度和特异度时，有时很难判断哪一个应该优化。此外，对于多项筛查，仅仅比较它们的灵敏度和特异度，可能会发现其筛查效果并无太大差异。

　　当灵敏度和特异度无法帮助筛查人员选择适宜的筛查方法时，对于该筛查方法的收益评估就显得尤为重要。收益评估包括：预测值的评估、查出新病例及其预后情况以及卫生经济学的评价。其中，常被临床医生忽视的是筛查方法所带来的经济学效益，即社会效益。评价筛查方法和策略所产生的社会效益，不仅仅是计算其对于降低发病率和死亡率的贡献，还应该考虑质量调整寿命年（QALY）和伤残调整寿命年（DALY）的变化。DALY 是指从发病到死亡所损失的全部健康寿命年，它定量地评价了由于疾病造成的早死、残疾或失能而损失的健康寿命年数。计算 QALY 不仅需要考虑患者主观感受到的生命质量的改变，还需客观地反映疾病对健康和社会资源的危害程度。评价筛查方法的社会效益可通过分析计算不同筛查方法所损失的 QALY 和增加的 DALY，并结合成本费用及最佳筛查时间间隔得到，最后计算出增加一个 QALY 和减少一个 DALY 所需的费用，该分析结果可以为卫生部门提供良好的卫生决策依据。

　　当前，临床医生在制订筛查计划时，多数选用了真实性好且可靠性高的筛查方法，因此，多数的筛查评估均是围绕筛查方法的灵敏度和特异度进行的，却忽视了有效筛查模型的建立以及对于筛查效果的综合评估，特别是对筛查方法及策略的卫生经济学评价没有得到临床医生的广泛重视。筛查的最根本含义是采用理论模型支持的从大样本中筛选出最小的有代表性的样本。如果一味地追求理想的灵敏度和特异度，则忽略了筛查的根本含义。

　　目前，多数的筛查决策是针对单方法 - 单疾病，或是多方法 - 单疾病的。刘力松等应用多学科的优势建立了包括神经内科、心血管内科、内分泌内科等多学科联合的筛查模式，以进行脑卒中高危人群的筛查。相较于单方法或单学科筛查模式，多方法多学科联合筛查模式的优势在于能够确保目标人群可以得到更全面、更客观的综合性评估。然而，目前并未发现关于多学科联合针对多疾病的筛查模式的报道，针对此类筛查模式的实施和评估有待今后进一步的研究。

七、筛查性研究的偏倚

　　筛查性试验既是一种试验，它同样可能存在选择偏倚、信息偏倚、混杂偏倚（参见本书第七章的相关内容）。而在筛检试验中可能出现的特殊偏倚如下。

　　1. 领先时间偏倚（lead time bias）　筛检试验提前发现了那些尚未发展到明显疾病而来主动就医的患者，如果忽略这一点，在比较筛检出的患者及来医院就诊患者的存活期、病死率、治愈率等时，就可能因为领先时间偏倚而使结果偏离真实情况。

　　2. 病程长短引起的偏倚　病程短的疾病被筛检出的可能性低于病程长的疾病。在评价筛查性研究时应考虑病程长短可能带来的偏倚。

第三节　循证应用实践

李国荣等采用 Markov 模型对大规模的宫颈癌现场干预或临床试验进行预测分析、提供决策信息，从成本 - 效果、成本 - 效用的角度评价了宫颈癌的筛查方法和筛查策略。其研究方法和步骤如下。

1. 确定筛查方法　筛查方法采用醋酸染色观察（visual inspection with acetic acid，VIA）或者碘液染色观察（visual inspection with Lugol's iodine，VILI），任何一种检查结果为阳性者，则再进行阴道镜检查，并在阴道镜下取活检，以病理组织学检查结果作为筛查宫颈病变的金标准（以 CIN2 作为阳性结果）。据文献报道，以上 3 种筛查方法的灵敏度和特异度分别为：VIA（0.414，0.945）、VILI（0.4，0.847）、阴道镜检查（0.814，0.765）。

2. 确定筛查策略　研究分为 5 种筛查策略：终身筛查一次、每 1 年筛查一次、每 3 年筛查一次、每 5 年筛查一次、每 10 年筛查一次。

3. 确定筛查评价模型　利用 Markov 评价模型模拟了 10 万名妇女，预测其 20 年内的变化情况，与无干预队列相比较，评价不同筛查策略的费用和效果、减少的患病人数、死亡人数等指标。由 HPV 感染到宫颈癌的自然病程设立 6 个 Markov 状态，即：正常、HPV 感染、CIN1、CIN2、CIN3、宫颈癌。无干预队列只计算癌症的治疗费用，以及随访费用，而干预队列的费用包括整个人群的筛查费，CIN2、CIN3、宫颈癌的治疗费和随访费，以及对不同筛查策略如每 3 年筛查一次筛查出的 CIN1 患者每年筛查的费用。

筛查队列的效果和效用见表 12-3。

表 12-3　筛查队列的效果和效用

评价指标	每 1 年	每 3 年	每 5 年	每 10 年	终身
减少的宫颈癌患病率/(10 万)$^{-1}$	616.66	569.99	501.73	319.13	54.6
减少的宫颈癌死亡率/(10 万)$^{-1}$	2 826	2 368	1 934	1 129	379
每增加 1 个 QALY 的费用/元	532	223	221	324	232
每减少 1 个 DALY 的费用/元	490	208	208	309	213

（1）评价筛查收益

1）成本 - 效果：如表 12-3 所示，上述 VIA/VILI 联合阴道镜检查的筛查方法，以终身筛查 1 次或每 1 年筛查 1 次等 5 种筛查策略均可以降低宫颈癌的患病率和死亡率，在 20 年内可以降低宫颈癌的患病率 54.6/10 万～616.66/10 万，可以减少死亡率 379/10 万～2 826/10 万。筛查间隔的时间越短，减少的患病人数和死亡人数也越多，但是，增加的 QALY 和减少的 DALY 也越多。每 10 年筛查 1 次此种筛查策略，每增加 1 个 QALY 的花费比每 3 或 5 年筛查 1 次的费用高，这可能是由于治疗癌症的费用远远高于筛查的费用。此外，终身筛查 1 次减少的宫颈癌患病率和死亡率较少，并且增加的 QALY 也少，因此，筛查的间隔时间不宜过长。

2）成本 - 效用：如上表所示，每 1 年筛查 1 次，增加 1 个 QALY 的费用仅为 532 元，减少 1 个 DALY 的费用为 490 元。每 3 年和每 5 年筛查 1 次增加 1 个 QALY 的费用分别为 223 元和 221 元，减少 1 个 DALY 的费用均为 208 元。每 10 年筛查 1 次，增加 1 个 QALY 的费用为 324 元，减少 1 个 DALY 的费用为 309 元。

因此，醋酸染色观察/碘液染色观察联合阴道镜检查的方法筛查宫颈癌具有较好的成本-效果和成本-效用，在经济不发达地区建议每3～5年筛查一次。

（2）敏感性分析：上述研究所采用的 VIA 的灵敏度为 0.414，与文献报道相比偏低，可能与检查者的临床经验有关。鉴于此种情形，当 VIA 的灵敏度在 40%～75% 之间变化时，进行敏感性分析。每 3 年筛查 1 次与每 5 年、每 10 年、终身筛查 1 次相比，不同的灵敏度费用波动不大，当 VIA 灵敏度等于 0.7 时，每 3 年和每 5 年筛查 1 次增加 1 个 QALY 的费用相同，但每 3 年筛查 1 次减少的宫颈癌死亡人数和患病人数均较每 5 年筛查 1 次多，筛查效果比每 5 年筛查 1 次好。故而，3 年是最佳的筛查间隔。

本 章 小 结

疾病筛查是将正常健康人群与患者或高危人群分开的一种初筛方法。在评价一项筛查性研究时，应先评判其是否符合实施疾病筛查的 10 项前提原则，评估研究是否有实施的价值。对于研究的筛查方案，可分别从简易性、可接受性、准确性、成本收益、可重复性、灵敏度以及特异度进行评估。而对于筛查结果则可以从真实性、可重复性、收益这三个方面进行评价。

（许良智）

第十三章

不良反应研究证据评价

学习目标

1. **掌握** 不良反应评价方法。
2. **了解** 不良反应的概念和分类；网状 meta 分析。

1956—1961 期间，沙利度胺（反应停）被用于治疗妊娠期呕吐，在 17 个国家和地区广泛应用。随后出现了畸胎事件，表现为婴儿四肢短小、形似海豹，称之为"海豹婴"。其中受害人数达 10 000 多人，死亡人数达 5 000 多人。反应停事件是历史上比较严重的药物不良反应导致的重大公共卫生事件。

第一节 不良反应的概念

药物在治疗疾病的同时也可能会对机体产生不良反应（adverse effect），因此客观、科学地评价药物的安全性和有效性十分重要。

WHO 国际药物监测中心关于药物不良反应的定义为正常剂量的药物用于预防、治疗、诊断疾病时出现的有害的、与治疗目的无关的反应。我国《药品不良反应报告与监测管理办法》第六十三条关于药物不良反应的定义为：合格药品在正常用量用法下出现的与用药目的无关的有害反应。

不良反应全面、系统的概念应定义为：使用各种措施、手段、方法进行预防、治疗、诊断疾病时，出现的有害的，与预防、治疗、诊断目的无关的反应。

一、药物不良反应分类

任何药物都会产生不良反应，但是由于人的个体差异，导致表现结果相差很大。药物不良反应可以根据其发生机制、发生频率、严重程度进行分类。

根据发生机制，药物不良反应可以分为：与剂量相关的不良反应以及与剂量无关的不良反应。二者的区别在于药物剂量与不良反应情况是否在剂量曲线上体现为正相关，后者一般由个体差异引起。

根据发生频率，国际医学科学组委会（CIOMS）将其分为：十分常见（频率≥10%）；常见（频率 1%～10%）；偶见（频率≥0.1%，<1%）；罕见；十分罕见。

按照药物对人体的伤害程度，可将其分为 6 级。1 级为轻度：停药后很快好转，无需治疗。2 级为中度：需要治疗或者干预，但是无需住院，容易恢复。3 级以上为重度。3 级：需要住院，住院时间>7d。4 级：造成永久性损伤（如器官损伤或者残疾）。5 级：对生命有危险，需急救（如休克、窒息）。6 级：死亡。

二、药物安全性研究

任何药物进入临床试验前必须进行一系列的基础研究，如通过药物化学研究确定其化学结构；通过药理与毒理学研究确定其药理、毒理机制等。而评价药物有效性和安全性的临床试验主要分为 4 期（表 13-1）。

表 13-1　评价药物有效性和安全性的临床试验主要分期

分类	目的
Ⅰ期临床试验	初步人体药物试验，观察人体耐药程度和药物代谢动力学
Ⅱ期临床试验	随机双盲对照试验，初步评价药物有效性和安全性
Ⅲ期临床试验	多中心临床随机对照试验，进一步评价药物有效性和安全性
Ⅳ期临床试验	新药上市后进行的长期临床监测。对广泛使用的药物研究其疗效和不良反应（包括常见不良反应、少见不良反应、长效不良反应）

所以新药上市后的安全性监测是很重要的，上市后若发现严重不良反应，应按规定停用、召回。

第二节　不良反应的评价

目前，涌现出较多关于治疗方式有效性、安全性的传统循证研究和网络 meta 分析，其中关于安全性的研究多涉及不良反应。本节重点介绍不良反应的纳入研究类型、检索、评价等相关知识。

一、不良反应的评价指标和纳入研究类型

部分原始文献在报道治疗措施有效性（疗效）的同时也报道了其安全性或者不良反应。但是有些治疗措施或治疗手段出现的不良反应为远期不良反应、罕见不良反应、未识别的不良反应。因此，为更规范评估药物的不良反应，研究者应该选择最常见、医生和患者都认为很严重的症状或体征作为不良反应的研究指标，同时考虑远期反应和近期反应。

大部分纳入的研究类型为随机对照试验，且多为药物治疗时的不良反应。为了全面系统评价药物不良反应，对远期不良反应、罕见不良反应、未识别的不良反应等还需要纳入队列研究、病例对照研究、个案报道等进行系统分析和研究，这样才能使不良反应的系统评价更加全面。

二、不良反应研究的检索

1. 不良反应的数据资源

1）参考书：*Meyler's Side Effects of Drugs*；*The Side Effects of Drugs*（SEDA）。

2）杂志：*The Complete Drugs Reference*。

2. 检索策略　使用主题词、副主题词以及自由词进行检索，适当变更检索策略，尽量不

漏掉相关研究。下面以 MEDLINE 为例，列举常见的主题词和副主题词和具体疾病针对性自由词。

主题词：drug toxicity；adverse drug reaction。

副主题词：adverse effects；poisoning；toxicity；chemically induced；complication。

检索自由词时应该选择一些高敏感性或者某种疾病特有的不良反应。除常见的毒性、副作用、有害作用以外，还有比如疲倦、乏力、恶心、呕吐等临床表现。

三、不良反应研究的质量评价

1. 不良反应的诊断　判断不良反应与治疗措施之间是否存在因果联系是治疗措施安全性评价中非常重要而烦琐的工作。以药物治疗为例，目前国际上判断药物治疗与过程中出现的不良反应的因果联系评定方法有 Karch 法和 Lasagna 法等。

（1）可以从以下几个方面判断药物与不良反应之间的因果关系

1）用药与不良反应出现的时间顺序是否合理。

2）反应是否属于该药已知的不良反应类型。

3）停药或者减轻剂量，不良反应是否减轻或者消失。

4）症状消失后再次给药是否再次出现相同不良反应症状。

5）充分考虑其他混杂因素：比如病理状况、联合用药、治疗方式改变等。

（2）治疗药物与不良反应之间的因果关系判断结论

1）肯定：用药和出现反应的时间顺序很合理；该反应与已知的药物不良反应相符合；停药后不良反应停止；重新给药，不良反应再次出现；其他原因不能解释。

2）很可能：时间顺序合理；该反应与已知的药物不良反应相符合；停药后不良反应停止；无法用患者疾病合理解释。

3）可能：时间顺序合理；该反应与已知的药物不良反应相符合；患者疾病或者其他治疗也可能造成此种不良反应。

4）有条件：时间顺序合理；该反应与已知的药物不良反应不相符合；无法用患者疾病合理解释。

5）可疑：不符合上述各项标准。

除上述主要方法以外，还有计分推算法：APS（adverse drug reaction probability scale），又称 Naranjo 计分法，是国际上比较常用的方法。总分 12 分，其中 ≥9 分判断为肯定有关；5～8 分判断为很可能有关；1～4 分判断为可能有关；≤0 分判断为可疑。

2. 不良反应证据的评价　证据的评价主要从真实性、重要性、实用性三个方面进行评价。其中真实性主要从以下 4 个方面进行判断：①除治疗措施和其他相关因素，资料中所涉及的各组患者，其主要临床特点和基线状况是否界定清楚，是否组间相似；②不良反应证据是否为盲法观测结果；③对不良反应的观测追踪时间是否足够长，资料是否完整；④不良反应证据是否满足病因或危险因素判断标准。

对不良反应重要性评价目的是确定其对患者的危害程度以及精确程度，主要通过因果关联强度的大小以及 95%CI 来体现。

如果不良反应的真实性好、重要性强，需要进一步考虑其实用性。实用性要求：需要权衡治疗措施的有效性和安全性两方面的利弊关系；准备备选的治疗方案；与患者沟通，结合患者意见，综合考虑。

3. 不良反应各种类型研究的质量评价 不良反应各种类型研究的质量评价主要有临床试验的 RCT 试验、病例对照以及队列研究、病例报告等。

影响临床试验不良反应质量评价的因素主要有以下四个：①监测不良反应的方法、时间、频率；②选择性地报告结果；③盲法；④利益冲突。其中，评价临床试验不良反应证据的质量标准主要包括实施阶段和报告阶段的评估（表13-2）。

表 13-2　评价临床试验不良反应证据的质量标准

阶段	内容
实施阶段	是否给出不良反应具体定义
	是否报告监测不良反应的方法
	（常规方法还是自发报告；问卷或患者日记或系统跟踪）
报告阶段	是否提供对照组数据
	属于哪类不良反应
	是否有患者在统计不良反应时被排除

疗效评价的最佳研究设计为 RCT 试验。但受客观限制，一个样本量小且随访时间短的 RCT 试验，其提供信息的可靠性不如一个大样本、实施好、随访长的队列研究。设计类型为病例对照或队列研究的不良反应质量评价参照本书相关章节。

评价病例报告研究的不良反应数据真实性，应该考虑以下 4 个方面：①病例报告是否有良好的预测价值。因病例报告无对照组，出现不良反应可能仅是巧合，故易形成假警报；②干预措施与不良反应之间，是否存在可以解释的生物学机制；③病例报告是否提供了足够的信息以便评估；④不可靠信息是否会造成假警报，对社会产生负面影响。

四、不良反应的网状 meta 分析

网状 meta 分析是指将传统直接头对头比较（direct head to head comparison）和间接比较同时合并起来进行 meta 分析，构成了一个网的形状。其主要功能是对处于同一个证据的所有干预措施进行综合评价并排序。网状 meta 分析能实现找出相对安全性最高、不良反应最小的药物和治疗方式。网状 meta 分析操作软件有 R、Stata。除网络图以外，网状 meta 分析的输出结果一般还有 loop 图、阶梯图和 rank 排序。值得注意的是最后结果的解读还应结合实际。

本 章 小 结

不良反应是使用各种措施、手段、方法预防、治疗、诊断疾病时，出现的有害的，与预防、治疗、诊断目的无关的反应。不良反应的评价指标、纳入研究类型、质量评价是需要重点关注的内容。网状 meta 分析的方法可以帮助实现找出相对安全性最高、不良反应最小的药物和治疗方式。

（让蔚清）

第十四章

证据的应用

学习目标

> **掌握** 循证决策的概念；循证决策的5个步骤。

医师每天面对不同临床症状和体征的患者，针对患者的具体情况应用不同的诊断方法，提出适当的治疗措施，采取相应的护理手段，分析疾病发生可能的危险因素，并对其预后进行判断，上述过程即为临床决策。可以说临床决策贯穿于医疗活动的各个环节。不言而喻，临床决策的准确性极大影响着医疗的质量和安全。

传统的临床决策往往来自医师自己的临床经验与直觉，以及专家意见和权威书籍中的观点。但随着循证医学的发展，传统的决策思维和越来越多的经典医疗决策受到质疑。究其原因，一是由于很多临床经验的积累和专家意见的形成并非源自科学严谨的研究设计与实施，其所得到的结论难免会有偏倚；二是权威书籍中的观点存在时间滞后性，新技术、新进展很难从书籍中获得，致使一些有效的疗法得不到推广，一些无效甚至有害的疗法却被广泛使用；三是不同医疗机构和不同地域医师的许多临床决策不能达到一致，某些决策甚至相互矛盾，经不起时间或空间的检验。此外，许多临床医师所作的临床决策是武断的或是多变的。即使就同一个患者而言，让同一位医师间隔一段时间先后判断两次，决策的结果也往往不一致。四是随着患者获取最新医学信息能力的不断增强，以及患者对医疗质量的要求越来越高，传统的临床决策不仅不易被患者接受，更可能使患者失去对医师的信任。

那么在这个倡导5P医学模式的时代，即预防性（preventive）、预测性（predictive）、个性化（personalized）、参与性（participatory）和精准医疗（precision medicine），如何科学有效地进行临床决策，实现"以患者为中心"的个体化、微创化的精准诊治，从而更好地为患者服务呢？循证决策无疑是解决上述问题的新模式，本章将重点解决这个问题。

第一节　循证决策的概念

循证决策是指遵循证据的临床实践，即在临床实践中应用循证医学的原理，根据最佳研究证据、临床经验和患者的选择进行临床决策。循证决策包括三大要素：第一是患者，第二是医师，第三是最佳证据。患者生病找医师诊治，医师要正确诊疗患者，除了自己的临床经验及已掌握的医学理论知识外，医师还应更新、丰富自己的知识，掌握新技能，寻找当前研究的最佳证据，客观评价患者的具体情况，结合患者自己意愿，将三大要素有机结合，制订最佳方案,从而卓有成效地解决患者问题。

循证决策不是一个简单的科学问题,在资源有限的情况下,它又是一个经济和伦理问题。在临床中运用循证决策常常会遇到诸多困难。首先,医师所面临的情况具体而且复杂,有人文的、社会的、政治的、经济的多方面问题。其次,21 世纪科学技术知识的累计可能比过去几千年的总和还要多,要在医学信息的汪洋大海里找到相关的最佳证据,困难是不言而喻的。有些证据相互矛盾,有些证据本身有缺陷或者根本没有好的证据支持决策。再者,患者的期望过高,或新技术的不成熟可能带来风险,等等。由于诸多的因素影响这个过程,因此学习并掌握循证决策的步骤尤其重要。

第二节 循证决策的步骤

循证决策的过程即是实践循证医学的过程,具体可以分 5 个步骤:①针对具体患者提出并构建临床问题;②全面收集有关证据;③严格评价证据;④临床应用证据;⑤后效评价。如何提出并构建问题、如何进行证据查询、如何评价证据在前面的章节都有描述,在此不一一赘述。本章重点讲述在决策过程中如何科学地分析证据,结合临床医师的经验和患者的价值观进行最佳决策,正确、合理地应用证据,并进行后效评价。

一、证据的分析

仅凭经过评价的最佳证据绝不可能做出正确的临床决策。每例患者除了有很多与同类患者相似的共性外,还有其各自的特性。使用证据为具体患者做临床决策时需对证据进行分析,权衡各种方案的利与弊,再与医师的临床经验及患者的价值观结合起来综合考虑,并让患者理解权衡诊疗利弊的重要性,在通过沟通和解释后,与患者共同做出最佳决策。因此,在找到相关证据后要从以下方面分析证据(表 14-1)。

表 14-1 证据分析时应考虑的因素

分析要点	具体内容
适用性分析	患者与研究证据中纳入的患者特征相似吗?
	患者和研究标准存在怎样的差异的情况下,使结果不能适用于患者?
利弊分析	利大于害吗?
	有替代方案吗?
	不使用有关疗法有什么后果?
	证据影响你现在的处理吗?
	患者的价值观及对疗效和副作用有什么看法?
可行性分析	检查或治疗技术在你所在的医院是否开展?技术是否成熟?
	患者的依从性如何?
	患者是否能够承担或接受费用?

1. 患者与研究证据中纳入的患者特征相似吗? 因为患者并没有真正参与到试验研究当中,所以在进行临床决策前,首先要将证据中的 PICO 与患者的 PICO 进行比较,只有证据中 PICO 的每一项与现实患者中 PICO 相似或一致,证据才有可能应用于患者,才能进行决策。要考虑证据中研究对象的基本特征(如年龄、性别、病情的轻重缓急、疾病的

不同类型等)、诊断标准、纳入和排除标准是否符合。如证据中研究的患者主要是轻型患者而你面对的是一个重症患者,证据等级即使再高也仍然不适合。许多研究排除了老年人群,而在老年人群中,许多药物毒副作用的发生率和发生程度均会提高,这就可能导致在相同的治疗方案下,老年患者与研究证据中的患者相比产生毒副作用的风险不同。在进行适用性分析时,可以从研究中的纳入和排除标准开始。当然,患者很难和研究中的标准完全匹配;萨克特(Sackett)等人建议,可以反方向回答这个问题,你的患者和研究标准存在怎样的差异?证据中这些差异是否影响结果,而使证据中的结果不能适用于当前的患者?

2. 患者可以得到的利益和风险是什么? 决定循证决策时医师不仅要评估患者能从证据中获得怎样的利益,还要评估这项结果可能给患者带来哪些风险,权衡利弊。因此,你需要通过相应的临床评价,在考虑患者个体临床特征的情况下,判断个体患者的风险程度。有些干预措施能够带来明显的治疗效果,但副作用明显,或不良事件发生的可能性增加,患者有可能更倾向于选择疗效欠佳但是不良反应更少的治疗方案。此外,许多患者往往有多种合并症,而这可能会影响药物之间的相互作用。利弊平衡差距越大,越容易作出临床决策。差别越小,越不容易作出临床决策,这主要取决于患者的价值取向甚至费用。

3. 证据中的干预措施在当地可行性如何? 证据中的诊断试验在当地可及性如何?干预措施可行性怎样?是否受到条件限制(包括经济上、技术上以及患者接受程度上)?尤其在有创性治疗试验中,临床医师的技能是衡量其是否能使用证据的一个重要条件。当普通医师的技能达不到参与试验的医师的技能时,就必须慎重考虑该试验结果的适用性。其次,还要考虑患者的依从性。当干预方式是药物时,如果患者同时在服用其他药物,或者某种治疗方案需要患者一天服用多次药物,患者的依从性就会明显降低。药物的剂量和给药途径也可能影响患者的依从性。总之,在临床实践中并非所有高质量的、利远远大于弊的证据都能顺利地应用于临床。例如,一项治疗措施很容易操作,效果也很好,但花费很高,那么它应用于临床的障碍也可能会很大。

二、临床医师经验在循证决策中的作用

临床经验有三个不同层面,一是进行医学实践活动的基本能力,如问诊、查体及与患者沟通的能力;二是综合判断各种因素,进行决策的能力;三是关于干预效果的经验累积。

前二者是利用证据进行循证实践不可缺少的基本技能,最后一种关于效果的临床经验也是证据,但它是原始的、未经严谨科学研究证实的证据,其质量低于科学研究证据。因此,当高质量研究存在时,循证决策应基于研究证据,当研究证据不存在时,则需要由临床医师经验补充。另外,研究证据往往是有限的、局部的,而临床医师的经验是大量的、广泛的,所以在很多情况下,临床经验是唯一的也是最好的证据。

由此可见,临床经验是循证实践的基础,研究证据与临床经验相互补充,缺一不可。但是,在强调经验重要性的同时,必须谨防经验至上的情况。在重要证据缺乏时,循证医学提倡医师积极地开展相关科学研究。

三、患者及其家人的价值观以及医患沟通在循证决策中的作用

循证决策非常强调并确保决策符合患者及其家人的价值观和意愿。因为患者和临床医

师的价值观可能存在本质的区别,不同患者间价值观的差异也很大。为了确保临床决策符合患者的价值观和意愿,让患者参与决策显得十分必要。这一过程有赖于有效且良好的医患沟通。

在进行医患沟通时,医师经常面临很复杂的情形。一方面,随着社会的发展、生活水平的提高,患者对预期结果的要求越来越高,而对风险的承受能力越来越低。另一方面,由于现代通信发达,患者的信息来源丰富,有些患者对相关知识的掌握有时比医师还多;而有些患者又因受教育水平较低、理解能力差,虽经反复沟通,对病情仍不能理解,不愿做决策,并要求医师代为决策;有些患者受亲朋好友的影响或不正确的商业广告宣传的影响,坚持拒绝最佳证据或盲目要求某种技术;有时患者与家人意见不统一,患者的经济承受能力有限等也为决策带来困难。

除了以上众多的原因,在充分了解患者的价值观及意愿后,如何将这些复杂的信息有效地传达给患者,正确引导患者及其家人进行最恰当的临床决策,对于临床医师同样是一个巨大的挑战。第一,分析证据后,医师需清楚地罗列诊断或治疗方案,包括替代方案,指出证据来源和对证据的分析。第二,提供有效、实用、与患者疾病相关的信息,并要权衡利弊。临床医师尽可能用通俗的语言为患者提供有关治疗费用、每种治疗方案会产生什么效果和不良反应、并发症及可能出现的风险等情况,让患者了解疾病发生发展过程中可能出现的特殊情况,了解每个人可能存在的特殊体质,了解现有医疗技术的局限,不能过高、过分地期望治疗方案的效果。第三,与患者共同分析、充分交流,医患双方共同参与治疗决策的制订。每位患者有不同的经历和文化背景,对疾病的认识大相径庭,临床医师需分析患者心理,引导患者做出正确决策;对于明显违背医疗原则的患者要求,应当坚决拒绝。事实证明:患者参与循证决策的程度越高,越能理解所获得的证据,所做出的选择也更能体现患者的意愿和价值观。经充分的医患沟通和患者参与的决策,不仅能增强患者对医师的信任,提高患者治疗依从性和疗效,还为构建和谐的医患关系奠定了基础。

四、随访患者,并对结果进行评价

最后一步需了解应用证据进行临床实践后的效果,进一步指导今后的实践。临床医师需随诊患者,进行效果评价,好则推而广之,不好则分析原因,找出问题,并针对问题进行新的循证和实践。

第三节　循证决策的基础

一、高素质的临床医师

医师是实践循证医学的主体,高素质的临床医师是循证医学实践的有力保证。首先,要求医师具有崇高医德和较强的医患沟通能力,在循证决策过程中要以患者而非疾病为中心,深入了解患者的期望和价值取向,并设身处地地站在患者的角度,充分沟通,共同作出最佳决策。其次,医师在问诊、查体、诊断等方面,要对患者进行无偏倚观察,准确收集第一手信息。患者的第一手信息不正确可能导致错误的诊断,在错误诊断引导下的最佳治疗证据没有任何价值。此外,缺乏临床实践经验的医师即使得到了最好的证据,也可能不会准确地使用,所以医师应不断更新、丰富自己的新知识、新技能。循证医学并不提倡患者就诊后才去寻找有关的治疗方案,医师平时就应该经常学习、掌握相关领域最新医学动态,而不仅仅在遇到临床问题时才开始收集证据,否则有时会错过最佳的治疗时机。另外,很重要的一点,医师需掌握临床流行病学的基本理论和临床研究方法,掌握寻找、评价、分析和应用证据的能力,才能进行循证决策。

二、最佳证据

最佳临床研究证据是指应用临床流行病学原则、方法以及有关质量评价的标准,对临床研究的文献经过认真分析与评价而获得的最新、最真实可靠且有临床重要应用价值的研究成果。最佳证据主要来源于设计合理、方法严谨的临床随机对照试验研究,及对这些研究所做的 meta 分析及系统评价。经专家严格筛选和评价的最佳证据可以从 *ACPJC* 副刊发表的《内科学年鉴》、《循证医学杂志》、Cochrane Library、Clinical Evidence 等途径获得,以指导临床医疗实践。

三、患者的参与

患者是医疗实践的主要参与者之一,是医疗活动的中心。医师的诊治决策,必须通过与患者共同分析、充分交流,医患双方共同参与,才能取得相应疗效,医师和患者平等友好的合作关系及医患双方共同参与的诊治决策是实践循证医学的关键。

第四节　进行循证决策需注意的问题

一、专家临床经验和意见的价值

过去人们过于迷信个别专家的所谓"经验"而忽略了知识的更新,认为他们的经验是金科玉律。假如这些专家的经验来源于缺乏严谨科学方法保证的临床研究、动物试验、实验室研究以及过时的教科书或是主观臆断的经验,轻信这类权威专家意见就容易导致临床决策的严重错误。但是,如果是建立在循证医学基础上的经验就值得推崇,因此循证医学并不排斥科学的经验积累。这就提醒研究者在听取专家意见时要注意他们经验的来源。

二、Cochrane 系统评价作为最高质量证据的依据

Cochrane Library 由六个数据库组成,包含不同类别高质量、相互独立的证据文献来指导医疗决策的制订。Cochrane 系统评价编委会由权威的统计学、流行病学和方法学专家组成,并且在系统评价过程中参考的研究结果必须满足一定的质量评价标准,有不断更新的统一工作指南。在对文献进行评价的过程中,Cochrane 系统评价的作者会针对不同步骤采用不同的方法来减少偏倚。当新的证据产生后,Cochrane 系统评价也会及时进行更新。所以 Cochrane 系统评价不仅可以为医学研究和决策人员提供了高质量的证据资源,也能为患者提供有效的医疗信息。

三、没有最佳证据存在时的临床决策

没有最佳证据不等于没有证据,若当前尚无随机对照试验等高质量证据,可依次参考

级别较低的证据或依据经验处理患者(如少见病),总之要应用当前可获得的最佳证据。一旦高级别证据发表,就应及时使用新证据。可能有效但尚无可靠证据时,要考虑副作用、经济承受能力以及患者的选择等问题。此时,作为临床医务工作者应该积极开展或参加临床研究,积极提供证据。

四、研究证据之外的影响因素

研究证据只是影响临床循证决策的因素之一,它只回答了一个方面的问题,即一项治疗在最理想的医疗条件下是否有效及效果的大小,但是一项有效的干预措施,从经济上讲可能并不划算,可能患者不愿意接受,也可能太复杂,在本地实际条件下难以重复;此外,即使是同一高质量的证据,在不同的地区或国家,或是应用于不同的患者,也可能由于经济水平、付费方式、临床医师经验、患者的伦理观念和价值取向、相关疾病所致的负担大小、患者对治疗措施的接受程度等方面的不同,而作出不同的选择和运用。

五、循证医学的不足——证据的缺乏

据估计,一个临床医师平均每周会遇到约 60 个待回答的问题,每一患者会同时存在多个问题。期待每一个临床问题都有现成答案在当前是不现实的。比如 RCT 是 EBM 的重要方法,但高质量的 RCT 需要大样本量,需要长时间随访,成本极高。许多少见病、罕见病难以进行 RCT 研究。不确定性是临床医学的基本特征,即使 EBM 得到充分发展,一定程度的不确定性仍然不可避免。在科学性和不确定性之间寻求最佳平衡点,是临床医学艺术性的体现,也是医师综合素质的反映。

第五节　循证决策临床实例

【案例 14-1】

患者,男,67 岁,以"间断心悸、气短 1 年,伴头晕半月"为主诉入院。1 年前患者无明显诱因出现心悸、气短,就诊于当地医院,行心电图检查,结果示:"心房颤动";行冠脉造影:"前降支中段约 30% 狭窄"。给予药物治疗(具体不详),上诉症状进行性加重;半月前患者出现头晕、乏力,不易缓解。既往患"肾小球肾炎"病史 5 年,否认高血压、糖尿病、脑血管疾病病史;否认吸烟饮酒史;否认家族性遗传性疾病病史。

体格检查:端坐卧位,口唇发绀,双肺呼吸音粗,双肺底可闻及少量湿啰音;心浊音界向左下侧扩大,心率 92 次 /min,心律绝对不齐,第一心音强弱不等,胸骨左缘 3~4 肋间可闻及舒张期奔马律;双下肢轻度凹陷性水肿。

辅助检查:心电图示"快心室率型心房颤动";BNP 为 165pg/ml;心脏超声示"EF35%,左室大,室壁运动幅度弥漫性减弱";肺静脉成像示"心房内无血栓形成"。

诊断:1. 心动过速性心肌病、心律失常、持续性心房颤动、心功能不全、心功能Ⅲ级;2. 冠状动脉粥样硬化;3. 慢性肾小球肾炎。

1. 提出并构建临床问题　临床问题主要分为 4 类:诊断问题、治疗问题、病因和不良反应问题、预后问题。在处理临床问题时,医师常根据 PICO 原则将问题翻译成可检索、可回

答的问题。P：患者的临床特征，I：关注的干预措施或者暴露因素；C：对照措施，如果是诊断研究，通常为"金标准"；O：关注的结局指标。

从本例出发，根据 PICO 原则可以提出的临床问题举例如下（表 14-2）。

表 14-2　根据 PICO 原则针对案例 14-1 提出的临床问题

问题类型	临床问题	PICO	可回答的问题
诊断	肺静脉成像对诊断心房内血栓的意义	P：持续性心房颤动患者 I：肺静脉成像 C：经食道超声心动图 O：确诊心房内血栓形成	肺静脉成像对于诊断心房内血栓的敏感性和特异性有多大？
治疗	心房颤动合并心力衰竭的患者能否应用屈奈达隆？	P：心房颤动合并心力衰竭的患者 I：屈奈达隆 C：安慰剂 O：死亡率	屈奈达隆能否降低心房颤动合并心力衰竭患者的死亡率？
病因和不良反应	肾小球肾炎是否增加心动过速患者心肌病的患病风险？	P：心动过速的患者 I：患有肾小球肾炎 C：不患有肾小球肾炎 O：心肌病的患病率	肾小球肾炎是否增加心动过速患者心肌病的患病风险？
预后	心动过速性心肌病患者心动过速终止后心肌病能否治愈？	P：心动过速性心肌病患者 I：终止心动过速 C：未终止心动过速 O：心肌病治愈率	心动过速性心肌病患者心动过速终止后心肌病治愈的概率有多大？

2. 全面收集有关证据　获得最佳证据的快捷途径是从循证医学证据等级资源的最高层开始，没有找到相关证据，则转向下一层。目前临床医生常用的数据库大致可以分为两大类：一类是传统型数据库，即原始文献数据库，如 PubMed、Embase 等。使用这类数据库要求临床医生自己检索相关文献、评价文献的质量、分析整合得出结论。它的优点为时效性强、免费检索、能获得最新最前沿的临床研究证据，缺点是需要医生有较强的临床流行病学知识对证据进行评价分析的能力、比较费时费力。另一类是现代模式的数据库，也称为二次分析数据库，如 UpToDate、Best Evidence、EBM guidelines、MD consult、Cochrane Library 等。它的优点是由专家进行原始文献的筛选、评价和分析，临床医生检索到证据后可直接应用，方便省时。缺点是其往往不是免费的，且为保证时效性需要定时更新。

以"屈奈达隆能否降低心房颤动合并心力衰竭患者的死亡率？"为例检索相关文献。具体检索策略制订步骤请参考本教材相关章节，本章仅以"心房颤动"（atrial fibrillation）和"屈奈达隆"（dronedarone）作为关键词检索 Embase 数据库，得到 Tarapués M 等人的 1 篇系统评价和 Xia Y 等和 Hohnloser S 等发表的 2 篇 meta 分析。在检索 UpToDate 后，得到 Connolly SJ 等人和 Køber L 等人的两篇 RCT 研究。检索 Cochrane Library，共得到 Dagres N 发表的 1 篇系统评价和 Chatterjee S. 发表的 1 篇 meta 分析。检索 PubMed，得到 323 篇原始文献。

3. 严格评价证据　循证医学强调证据，要求研究者尽可能地选择高质量的研究。证据的等级水平是影响证据可靠性的重要因素之一，在分析证据的可靠性时可参照表 14-3 所列的项目,结合自己研究的目的,对证据的等级进行评级,以对证据的真实性做出评价。

表 14-3　不同研究问题的证据水平分级标准

分级	诊断	治疗	病因和不良反应	预后
Ⅰ级	系统评价(包括meta分析等)			
Ⅱ级	横断面研究(随机患者或包括疾病各阶段的患者)	随机对照试验(RCT)	前瞻性队列研究	起始队列研究
Ⅲ级	非随机患者的横断面研究或病例对照研究	非随机对照试验或队列研究及病例对照研究	回顾性队列研究或病例对照研究	回顾性队列研究或病例对照研究
Ⅳ级	病例系列报告	病例系列报告	横断面研究	病例系列报告

　　根据临床研究的证据水平分级标准,本文检索到系统评价(包括 meta 分析)为Ⅰ级证据;Connolly SJ 等和 Køber L 等发表的两篇 RCT 研究为Ⅱ级证据。Køber L 等发表的题为"Increased Mortality after Dronedarone Therapy for Severe Heart Failure"的论文中的实验为随机、双盲、安慰剂对照的平行试验,研究方案设计合理,研究过程遵循严格的纳入标准和排除标准,研究终点明确,该研究因考虑安全问题而提前终止了试验。Connolly SJ 等于 2012 年发表在 *NEJM* 上的"Dronedarone in High Risk Permanent Atrial Fibrillation"同样因考虑安全问题提前终止了试验,该研究的纳入标准、干预方案、数据的处理和分析、质量控制方法均设计合理,实施严格。这两篇 RCT 研究的真实性和重要性均较好,均能为临床决策提供最佳的证据。

　　对于本例提出的问题,Køber L 等的 RCT 研究表明,对于重度心力衰竭及左心室功能下降的患者,屈奈达隆由于使心力衰竭恶化而增加了患者早期死亡的风险;该研究在中位数为 2 个月的随访中发现,接受屈奈达隆治疗的患者死亡率较对照组明显增高(8.1% 与 3.8%)。Connolly SJ 等人的 RCT 研究同样表明屈奈达隆增加了心血管不良事件的发生风险,比如持续性心房颤动患者的心力衰竭、卒中和死亡等,因此该类患者不应给予屈奈达隆治疗。Chatterjee S 等人的 meta 分析结果提示,在人群中广泛应用屈奈达隆增加了全因死亡率和心血管疾病的死亡率,并导致心力衰竭恶化。Hohnloser S. 等人基于 9 664 例心房颤动患者的 meta 分析结果表明,屈奈达隆对于不同类型心房颤动患者的治疗效果具有异质性:对于非持续性心房颤动患者,应用屈奈达隆将获益;而对于持续性心房颤动患者,心血管疾病死亡率明显增加(HR=2.32;95%CI,1.13~4.75),因心力衰竭而住院的概率也增加(HR=1.674;95%CI,1.05~2.67)。

　　4. 临床应用证据　Connolly SJ 等人的 RCT 研究的主要纳入标准为:持续性心房颤动或心房扑动、年龄 65 岁以上,并至少包括以下危险因素之一:冠心病、卒中或短暂脑缺血发作史、症状性心力衰竭(NYHA 分级Ⅱ~Ⅲ级)、EF≤40%、外周动脉疾病、年龄在 75 岁以上的高血压或糖尿病患者。主要排除标准包括阵发性心房颤动或持续性心房颤动应用植入型心律转复除颤器(ICD)、白天心率在 50 次 /min 以下、QTc>500ms(对于加速性室性自主心律患者 QTc>530ms);Køber L 等的 RCT 研究中要求受试者年龄在 18 岁以上,因新发或加重的心力衰竭而住院,心功能(NYHA 分级)Ⅲ级或Ⅳ级。这些证据中受试者的临床基本特征与本例患者基本符合,证据适用于该患者。

　　与患者及家属沟通病情,针对该患者,除了抗凝、抗心力衰竭治疗外,对于其快速心室率的心房颤动，可行转复窦性心律或控制心室率治疗。转复窦性心律的方法有：①口服抗心律失常药物胺碘酮。其优点是适用于心力衰竭合并心房颤动的患者，另外价格便宜，患者的经济负担小；其缺点是容易产生多器官毒副作用，较常见的不良反应有皮肤光过敏反应、角膜微沉淀、甲状腺功能异常、肺间质纤维化、肝功能损伤等。②房颤射频消融术：其优点是可在短时间内根治心房颤动，明显改善患者的症状并提高生活质量；缺点是手术成功率仅在 70% 左右，另手术存在风险（如血管穿刺导致的血肿、气胸；导管操作导致的心肌穿孔、心脏压塞等），且手术费用较贵。③控制心室率可通过口服抗心律失常药物实现，简单易行。但缺点是心房颤动持续存在，患者的心力衰竭可能会进行性加重。

患者与家属详细了解了所有可能的治疗措施后，为避免让患者的心力衰竭进行性加重，决定接受转复窦性心律治疗。但是了解到胺碘酮的多器官毒副作用后拒绝使用胺碘酮治疗；并咨询能否应用新型抗心律失常药物屈奈达隆。经过以上循证决策的步骤，根据 PICO 原则提出临床问题，收集、评价、分析证据，告知患者及家属新型抗心律失常药物屈奈达隆虽然不含有碘基，避免了胺碘酮的上述毒副作用，但根据目前的证据，屈奈达隆会加重心力衰竭的进展，增加患者全因死亡率和心血管疾病死亡率，而该患者心功能低下，故医师和患者及家属不考虑应用屈奈达隆治疗。最终考虑三维标测下进行房颤射频消融术，医师与患者及家属反复沟通手术的风险，患者及家属表示愿意接受风险，签署知情同意书后行手术治疗。

5. 后效评价　该患者房颤射频消融术后心房颤动节律终止并转为窦性节律，其心悸、气短症状明显好转。出院后随访 1 年，胸片示心脏缩小，心脏超声示 EF 为 51%。在治疗期间并未出现严重不良反应或心血管不良事件。

【案例 14-2】

患者，女，35 岁，因"右下腹隐痛 15d，发现右侧卵巢囊肿 10d"入院。15d 前患者于夜间休息时出现右下腹针扎样疼痛，持续 2h 后减轻。后间断出现右下腹憋胀样隐痛。10 日前超声检查发现：右侧卵巢有约 7.5cm×8.0cm 大小囊性回声。既往 3 年前曾因"多囊卵巢综合征"服用枸橼酸氯米芬 3 个周期诱导排卵，2 年前行子宫下段剖宫产术。月经婚育史：平素月经不规律，初潮 14 岁，周期 30～65d，经期 3～5d，月经量少，无痛经。28 岁结婚，孕 1 产 1，育有 1 女。

体检检查：生命体征稳定，心肺查体无异常。腹部查体：平坦，触诊无压痛及反跳痛，无腹肌紧张，听诊无异常。

妇科检查：外阴阴道无异常，宫颈柱状上皮中度外移，子宫无异常，子宫右后方可触及 8cm×7cm 大小囊实性肿物，边界清楚，表面光滑，活动可，无压痛。左附件区未及异常。

辅助检查：经阴道超声示子宫右后方可见 8.0cm×7.5cm 囊实性回声区，囊性区呈分隔样，囊性部分透声尚可，实性区可见丰富血流信号，血流阻力指数为（RI）0.4。超声诊断为右侧卵巢囊实性肿瘤（不排除恶性肿瘤）。肿瘤标记物系列均在正常范围内。余辅助检查无异常。

初步诊断：卵巢肿瘤。

1. 提出并构建临床问题 根据 PICO 原则可以提出的临床问题举例如下（表 14-4）。

表 14-4 根据 PICO 原则针对案例 14-2 提出的临床问题

问题类型	临床问题	PICO	可回答的问题
诊断	MRI 对鉴别良、恶性卵巢肿瘤的意义	P：诊断不明确的卵巢肿瘤患者 I：MRI 检查 C：超声检查 O：术后病理确诊	MRI 与超声相比对鉴别卵巢肿瘤良性、恶性的敏感性和特异性的差别
治疗	卵巢良性肿瘤合并局灶癌变术后是否需要行化疗	P：术后病理提示卵巢良性肿瘤、局灶癌变患者 I：手术 + 术后化疗 C：单纯手术治疗 O：死亡	对卵巢良性肿瘤伴局灶癌变患者术后行化疗是否可以降低患者死亡风险？
病因和不良反应	应用促排卵药物是否会增加卵巢癌患病风险？	P：不孕症患者 I：应用促排卵药物诱导排卵 C：未使用促排卵药物 O：卵巢肿瘤发生	应用促排卵药物是否会增加卵巢肿瘤发病风险？
预后	单侧卵巢良性肿瘤伴局灶癌变仅行单侧卵巢切除术，术后复发率是多少？	P：术中病理结果示单侧卵巢良性肿瘤伴局灶癌变患者 I：仅行单侧卵巢切除术 C：双侧卵巢切除术 O：卵巢肿瘤复发	单侧卵巢肿瘤伴局灶癌变仅行单侧卵巢切除术，是否增加术后卵巢肿瘤复发率？

2. 全面收集有关证据 以"应用促排卵药物是否会增加不孕症患者卵巢肿瘤患病风险？"检索相关文献。具体检索策略制订步骤请参考本教材相关章节，本章仅以 ovarian cancer/ ovarian neoplasm/ ovarian carcinoma 和 ovulation induction/ stimulate/ promote/ clomiphene（中文数据库以"卵巢恶性肿瘤"和"促排卵"）为检索词进行检索，检索日期限定为 2016 年 6 月。检索结果如表 14-5 所示。

表 14-5 检索结果汇总表

数据库	检索结果 / 篇	与本例临床问题相关 / 篇
PubMed	114	18
The Cochrane Library	4	1
UpToDate	14	14
Embase	75	48
Springerlink	2 537	8
万方数据知识服务平台	20	2

3. 严格评价证据 在检索完成获得相应的证据后，需要从中找出论证强度最高的文献。本例经去重、并经进一步评价筛选，选取 1 篇 Ivana Rizzuto 发表的系统评价"The system to evaluate the risk of ovarian cancer in women treated with ovarian stimulating drugs for infertility"、Modan B 等的前瞻性队列研究"Cancer incidence in a cohort of infertile women"和 Venn A 等的前瞻性队列研究"Risk of cancer after use of fertility drugs with in-vitro fertilisation"作为本例的证据。

获得相关文献后，就该开始对所获得的证据进行评价。不同类别的研究其评价标准并不完全一致，具体请参考该教材的相应章节或表 14-2。就本病例而言，通过文献检索选取了三篇文献，其中 Ivana Rizzuto 发表的系统评价总结了 11 篇病例对照分析和 14 篇队列研究，对文章的纳入标准、干预方案、文献检索和获取途径、数据的处理和分析、质量控制方法均有很好的描述，根据证据等级进行划分，将其列入 I 级证据。在 Venn A 的研究中，采用了证据等级较高的前瞻性队列研究，同时给出了研究的纳入标准，并均衡混杂因素，给出了随访时间和随访结局、统计学方法和指标，总体来说研究方法合理，统计学方法准确，结果可信度高。Modan B 等人的研究，虽然采用了证据等级高的前瞻性队列研究，陈述了研究的招募时间范围和暴露数据，给出了参与者的来源和选择方法，同时给出了统计学方法和统计学指标，但是本文中并没有明确指出研究排除标准，没有指出随访的具体方法和随访结局，同时没有采用盲法，没有质量控制方法，总体来说，证据质量并不高，不建议采纳。

4. 临床应用证据 在对证据进行评价后，得到了两篇高质量的相关文献。Ivana Rizzuto 在系统评价中指出，与未服用促怀孕相关药物的不孕症女性以及与普通女性人群相比，目前尚没有有效的证据可以证明卵巢恶性肿瘤发病率的增加与促怀孕药物有关。Venn A 的前瞻性队列研究发现原发性不孕可使卵巢肿瘤发病率增加，但促排卵药物的应用并没有增加卵巢肿瘤的发病率。所以该证据是否适用于该个体患者，仍需要进一步分析。

分析研究纳入标准及排除标准与个体患者之间的差异。在 Ivana Rizzuto 的系统评价中，给出的纳入标准为年龄大于 18 岁的女性，至少有一侧卵巢，与该患者情况相符。在 Venn A 的研究中，纳入标准为澳大利亚境内因不孕症就诊的女性，并且将至少应用了一个周期的促排卵治疗的女性归为暴露组，同时排除了非澳大利亚居民，和女性的年龄未知。该患者并不符合其地区设定，因此将该结果应用于该患者时便需要更加谨慎。

综上，根据目前证据，尚不能认为服用促排卵药物会增加卵巢肿瘤发生的风险。就促排卵药物与卵巢肿瘤发生的相关性而言，在不孕症患者中应用促排卵药物是基本安全的。但因不孕症本身就是卵巢肿瘤发生的危险因素，所以仍建议患有不孕症的女性能够按时体检。

5. 后效评价 可以对服用促排卵药物的不孕症患者进行追踪，对促排卵药物影响卵巢肿瘤发病风险进行评估，并对结果进行统计学分析，然后将所得结果与原始文献进行比较，将相关数据总结整理成文献发表，产生证据。

本 章 小 结

虽然循证医学带来了一场医学革命，但正像任何新生事物一样，循证医学不是完美无缺的，更不是万能的。在临床决策中不能夸大其作用，更不能生搬硬套。应该认识到随着医学科学的不断发展，证据也在发展变化，在应用证据时多分析、多思考，认真评价其质量，不能把目前的证据看成至高无上的教条，应随着新证据的出现不断更新自己的医疗行为。

（刘广芝）

第十五章

循证实践指南

学习目标

1. **掌握** 循证实践指南的定义；循证实践指南的评价。
2. **熟悉** 循证实践指南制定的方法。
3. **了解** 循证实践指南的临床应用。

临床实践指南（clinical practice guideline，CPG）是人们根据特定的临床情况，系统制定出的帮助临床医生和患者做出恰当处理的指导意见。临床实践指南能帮助临床医生将最好的证据转化为最好的临床实践。随着循证医学的发展，体现循证医学精髓的指南成为现代医学临床实践不可分割的一部分。制定和推广循证实践指南，成为当前规范医疗卫生服务的重要举措。然而，目前发表的很多实践指南并不总是以循证医学为基础的。一个好的临床实践指南应该以当前最佳的科学证据为依据，降低临床实践的不一致性，减少不同医疗机构和不同临床医师间医疗水平的差异，避免不必要的诊断检查，防止采用无效甚至有害的治疗手段，给患者以最经济有效的治疗。

第一节 基 本 概 念

1990年美国医学研究所对CPG的定义为：系统开发的多组临床指导意见，帮助医生和患者针对特定的临床问题做出恰当处理，选择、决策适宜的卫生保健服务。20年来，循证医学的快速发展也导致临床实践指南制定的方法发生了巨大的转变，基于循证医学的临床实践指南已逐渐成为制定指南的趋势。因此，2011年美国医学研究所对临床实践指南的定义更新为：通过系统评价相关科学证据，并对各种备选干预方式的利弊进行评价后，提出的最优指导性文件。这一更新后的定义更符合循证医学的要求。

循证实践指南是被系统地开发出来的，其内容要经过严格的评价，用以在特定的临床环境中帮助医务工作者对医疗活动进行决策。一个可靠的指南必须做到以下几点：①基于对现有证据的系统评价；②由来自专业团队、各学科的专家和主要相关团体的代表共同制定；③适当地考虑患者重要的亚群体和偏好；④过程透明，使干扰、偏倚和利益冲突最小化；⑤对各备选干预措施及相应的结局之间的关系提供合理的解释，并对证据质量和推荐意见进行分级；⑥当有重要的新证据时，要对原有指南进行合理的重新审议和修订。

第二节 循证实践指南的制定方法

开发高质量临床实践指南是国际上近年来规范医疗服务、加强医疗质量管理、控制医疗费用行之有效的方法。临床实践指南一般分为"专家共识指南"和"循证实践指南"两大类。专家共识指南的制定较为简单,通常由一组专家开会讨论,将多次讨论后达成的共识形成推荐意见作为指南,这种指南大多数缺乏证据基础,推荐意见易受参会专家的各方面因素的影响,因此其可靠性和质量有待评价。

随着指南制定程序的不断规范,越来越多的指南都是在系统检索和评价了相关证据之后制定出来的。循证实践指南的制定过程包括:成立指南开发小组,提出相关临床问题,系统检索文献,使用正确的方法对证据进行严格评价,并结合实践经验、根据证据的级别和强度提出推荐意见。此外,还包括系统评估、推广普及、修订更新等指南推出后的工作计划,使指南能与时俱进。制定循证临床实践指南的方法学基于证据的方法学,其结论或推荐意见须有可靠的证据支持,将推荐意见与相关的证据质量明确地联系在一起是循证临床指南的明显特征。

苏格兰校际指南网络(Scottish Intercollegiate Guidelines Network,SIGN)建于 1993 年,SIGN 推荐的循证指南制定的方法较为全面,其主要步骤和方法如下。

1. 组建指南开发小组 开发小组由来自不同地区的多学科人员(15~20 人)组成。开发小组的成员应该能够代表所有相关的专业团队,还要有患者、其他相关从业者及合适的志愿者组织参与,其有利于指南的制定和最终的推荐。

2. 确定指南拟解决的主要问题 制定一个循证实践指南往往耗费大量的时间和资源。为了确保充分利用这些资源,应该针对解决一个特定的医疗保健需求制定指南。而且确保应用该指南能够提升医疗质量并改善患者预后,且指南制定后可以被有效地推广和实践。

3. 文献的系统评价 SIGN 推荐的指南制定方法必须基于循证医学的系统评价,指南中的每一个关键问题都要进行证据的系统评价,必须提供证据列表作为支撑文件。系统评价中文献必须满足以下几点:①运用清晰的检索策略全面检索文献;②根据明确的纳入和排除标准筛选文献;③采用公认的方法学原则评估纳入的文献。

4. 证据的质量评估 指南开发小组还需要对纳入的所有文献的整体质量进行评估。

(1)证据总体质量的评价,包括:①可靠性,即相关证据的偏见风险的评估;②一致性,即研究间结果是否一致;③针对性,即证据是否直接针对指南的目标人群或者人群特征的不同将会影响最终结果;④全面性,即是否获得了所有相关的证据。

(2)证据的解释,包括:①患者意愿,即是否权衡利弊,以患者结局指标的最大改善为目标;②临床实践,即是否与现有的医疗实践有较大的差距;③资源分配,即是否会导致大规模的资源重新分配,卫生系统是否支持改进的措施。

5. 依据对证据客观评价的结果提出推荐意见 经过严格的证据评价达成共识后,可参照证据水平和推荐意见强度对照表对推荐意见强度进行标注。有充分证据时,根据证据提出推荐意见;没有证据或证据很弱时,根据讨论达成的共识(或一致)性意见提出推荐意见。有时候高质量证据的推荐级别并不一定较高,需要同时考虑目标人群的花费和可接受度。

循证实践指南一般都标注推荐意见级别和证据等级,但不同的国家和学术机构采用的标准不同。为了建立评价证据和推荐意见分级的国际标准体系,2004 年由 GRADE

（Grading of Recommendations Assessment，Development and Evaluation）工作组制定了 GRADE 证据质量和推荐分级。GRADE 评级系统突破了只从研究设计角度考虑证据质量的局限性，它依据未来的研究是否改变研究者对目前疗效评价的信心以及改变可能性的大小将证据质量分为高、中、低、极低四个等级（见表 4-2），将推荐意见分为强、弱两个级别。当明确显示干预措施利大于弊或弊大于利时，应评为强推荐；当利弊不确定或无论质量高低的证据均显示利弊相当时，则视为弱推荐。基于随机对照临床试验的证据在 GRADE 证据质量分级系统中，被评为高质量。但并非所有随机对照临床试验的质量都一致，下述五种情况将降低其证据质量：研究的局限性、研究结果不一致、间接证据、结果不精确、报告有偏倚。GRADE 涵盖所有医学专业和临床护理领域的各种临床推荐意见，简单明了，易于掌握。Cochrane 协作网、世界卫生组织（WHO）等多个国际组织已经广泛使用该评级系统。

　　在 GRADE 系统出现之前，应用较多的是 2001 年 5 月牛津循证医学中心制定的证据水平评价标准，基于研究设计、论证因果关系的力度不同将证据水平分为五级。推荐建议则根据证据的质量、一致性、临床意义、普遍性、适用性等将推荐意见分为 A（优秀）、B（良好）、C（满意）和 D（差）四个等级。以治疗性研究证据为例，表 15-1 列出了牛津循证医学中心的临床证据水平分级和推荐级别。

表 15-1　牛津循证医学中心临床证据水平分级和推荐级别（2001 年）

推荐级别	证据水平	证据来源（治疗性研究证据）
A	1a	同质性 RCT 的系统评价
	1b	单个 RCT（置信区间窄）
	1c	全或无病案系列（治疗前所有患者均死亡或部分死亡，治疗后仅部分死亡或全部存活）
B	2a	同质性队列研究的系统评价
	2b	单个队列研究（包括低质量 RCT，如随访率 <80%）
	2c	结局性研究（指描述、解释和预测干预措施对临床最终结局的作用和影响的一类研究，最终结局不同于中间指标，主要包括生存、生命质量、疾病负担等）
	3a	同质性病例对照研究的系统评价
	3b	单个病例对照研究
C	4	病例系列研究（包括低质量队列和病例对照研究）
D	5	基于经验，未经严格论证的专家意见

　　6. 咨询和同行评价　召开会议，同行专家向指南小组提出疑问及对指南初稿做出评价。指南小组根据建议进一步修订指南。修订版再送同行专家进行评价，也需要发给至少两名外行审稿人，以便从患者的角度进行评定。最后，SIGN 编辑组对指南进行审查并做出评价。

　　7. 指南的制定和发表　清晰的定义、语言和格式对于一个好的指南至关重要，因此指南的内容要用明确的语言表述，并且准确地定义所有的条款。在指南的书写格式方面，可以根据不同的对象、不同的问题以及不同的目的做出适当的选择。

　　8. 指南的执行　确保循证实践指南的实施至关重要。在指南的执行过程中会遇到两大类障碍：指南本身的内部障碍和临床实践过程中相关的外部障碍。SIGN 处理内部障碍的方法：①根据公认的方法开发指南；②确保指南中的定义、语言和格式清晰明确；③提供指南的方式与目标群体、主题和预期用途相适应。SIGN 处理外部障碍的四种策略：改进指南执行进程；提高认知和教育；合作；实施资源支持。

9. 患者参与　在医疗过程、医疗重点关注内容以及预后预期方面，患者可能和专业的医护工作者持有不同的观点，因此患者参与指南的制定更能反映患者的需求。患者、护理者和研究者一起工作，确保从患者或护理者的角度参与指南的制定。

第三节　循证实践指南的评价标准

临床实践指南的质量取决于在制订指南的过程中是否能够合理地控制可能存在的偏倚因素，从而确保推荐建议内部和外部的真实性，以及临床应用的可行性。低质量的临床实践指南不仅不能起到临床指导作用，反而会误导临床医师。因此，对已发表的指南，读者应具备评价和鉴别其质量高低的能力，以便选择性地应用。

一、评价临床实践指南的基本原则

对临床实践指南的评价主要分为真实性、重要性和适用性评价三个方面。

1. 真实性评价　好的指南必须遵循循证医学的原则和方法，强调临床实践指南应建立在证据的基础上，并根据证据的可信程度对建议进行分级。评价的要点包括：①指南编写者是否做了全面、可重复的文献检索？检索是在最近一年内进行？②是否对每项建议均标明了其相关证据的等级，并提供了原始证据的链接或文献？评价主要集中在对证据的收集、评估和合成，以及如何将推荐意见与相关的证据紧密结合方面。

2. 重要性评价　经过对实践指南真实性评价后，还要明确指南是否回答了临床需要解决的重要问题，这些问题是临床医生必须面对的。但要注意的是临床所面临的问题相当复杂，指南不可能囊括所有的临床问题。

3. 适用性评价　适用性评价应考虑在本地区疾病负担（burden of disease）是否很低而无需参考指南？患者对治疗价值观和愿望的利弊的评价是否与指南一致？执行该指南所需的成本有多大，即同样的资源用于其他的措施是否有更大的收益？对于患者，是否有实施该指南不可克服的困难？因此，一个指南的成功实施依赖四个因素，即疾病负担（burden）、价值取向（belief）、费用（bargain）和障碍（barrier），需要综合考虑，根据个体化的原则运用指南。

二、评价临床实践指南的常用工具

为了科学客观地评价循证实践指南，不同的国家和学术团体制定了许多专门的指南评价工具。迄今，大约有 20 多个评价工具。目前有 3 个评价工具比较全面系统，分别是 Cluzeau 量表（包含 37 个评价条目）、美国 COGS 评价标准（包含 18 个条目）和欧洲 AGREE 评价标准（23 个条目）。下面将主要介绍欧洲 AGREE 量表。AGREE（appraisal of guidelines research and evaluation，AGREE）是由 13 个国家的研究者制定的一种指南研究和评价的评估工具。AGREE 量表的作用是为临床实践指南的质量审查提供一个框架。AGREE 量表通过 6 个领域（包括指南的范围和目的、参与人员、指南开发的严格性、指南的清晰性与可读性、指南的适用性和指南撰写的独立性）及 23 个条目来对指南进行评价（表 15-2）。

表 15-2　AGREE Ⅱ评价工具

Ⅰ 指南的范围和目的（涉及指南的总目的、具体的临床问题和适用的患者）

  1. 明确说明指南的撰写目的

  2. 详细描述了指南所涵盖的临床问题

  3. 明确了指南针对的目标人群，并对其特征（年龄、性别、临床类型等）进行了描述

Ⅱ 参与人员

  4. 指南制定小组的成员包括所有相关方面的专家

  5. 指南考虑了目标患者的意愿和喜好

  6. 指南的使用者已明确

  7. 指南发表前在目标使用者中进行了预测试

Ⅲ 指南开发的严格性

  8. 采用严格系统的方法检索证据，应提供检索证据的详细策略，包括使用的检索词、信息来源和文献涵盖的时间

  9. 清晰描述了证据的纳入和排除标准

  10. 详细描述了形成推荐建议的方法

  11. 形成推荐建议时充分考虑了干预措施的获益、风险和副作用

  12. 推荐建议与支持证据之间有明确的联系

  13. 指南发表前接受了制定小组以外专家的同行评议

  14. 提供了更新指南的程序

Ⅳ 指南的清晰性和可读性

  15. 推荐建议明确而无歧义

  16. 针对不同临床状况提供了不同的治疗选择

  17. 关键的推荐建议可以很容易找到

  18. 提供了指南方便应用的工具（如概要、教育工具、针对患者的宣传单等）

Ⅴ 指南的适用性

  19. 讨论了应用该指南的过程中可能遇到的困难

  20. 讨论了应用该指南过程中可能的费用

  21. 提供监督和审查指南执行情况的评估指标

Ⅵ 指南编撰的独立性

  22. 赞助单位的观点不影响指南的制定

  23. 指南制定小组成员的利益冲突在指南中有所说明

在具体使用 AGREE Ⅱ评价工具时，可以对表中每个条目进行评分（7 分制），以衡量该条目标准的执行程度。如果质量较高，完全符合条目要求的为 7 分；如果质量非常差，或没有条目要求的相关信息的为 1 分；介于二者之间的根据测评人员的判断给予 2～6 分，分值的高低取决于报告的完整性和质量。由于评价不可避免地存在一定的主观性，所以每一篇指南应由 2～4 名参评人员进行评价。然后根据公式将所有参评人员的评分进行综合，得到该领域的标准化总分。标准化总分 =（实际总分 - 最低可能分数）/（最高可能分数 - 最低可能分数）（表 15-3）。

表 15-3　AGREE 各领域得分的计算方法举例

参评人员	条目1/分	条目2/分	条目3/分	总分/分
评估员1/分	5	6	6	17
评估员2/分	6	6	7	19
评估员3/分	2	4	3	9
评估员4/分	3	3	2	8
总分	16	19	18	53

最高可能分数 =7（完全符合）×3（条目数）×4（评估员人数）=84。

最低可能分数 =1（完全不符合）×3（条目数）×4（评估员人数）=12。

该领域的标准化总分 =（实际总分 − 最低可能分数）÷（最高可能分数 − 最低可能分数）=（53−12）÷（84−12）= 0.57×100% =57%。

AGREE 评价原则中 6 个领域的得分是独立的，不能被合计为一个总的质量得分。尽管这些领域的分数可以用来比较指南，帮助决定是否使用或者推荐一个指南，但是，不能对得分设立一个阈值评价一个指南的好坏。最后应根据评价结果综合判断该指南的质量以及是否值得推荐应用该指南。

第四节　循证实践指南的临床应用

临床实践指南是为帮助临床医师处理临床问题而制定的技术指导性意见，并非法规文件，是推荐应用而非强制应用。允许临床医生根据具体情况更改或决定是否采用，应避免不分患者具体情况强制性、盲目教条应用临床实践指南。循证实践指南和具体的临床实践不可避免地存在着差距，因此临床医生在应用循证实践指南的过程中应充分考虑以下问题。

一、该实践指南是否真实有效

1. 该指南是否考虑了所有重要的临床决策和预后？必须从患者以及医生的角度综合考虑可以采取的临床决策以及可能的临床预后。

2. 该指南鉴别、筛选、综合证据的流程是否合理、明确？循证实践指南所参考的证据必须合理、明确，并且应对证据的类型进行分级。

3. 该指南是否针对不同的预后进行了合理、明确的描述？该指南必须对所有可能出现的预后以及出现该预后的原因进行清晰描述。

4. 该指南是否考虑了最近重要的进展？指南的参考证据应该包含最新的证据。

5. 该指南是否经过了同行评议以及同行测试？理想的情况下，指南应该经过不同情况下的测试，以确定临床医生是否愿意应用该指南以及该指南是否能达到预期的效果。

二、该实践指南的建议是什么

1. 该指南的适用性以及临床重要性如何？指南中的决策是否简单易行，适合大多数临床医生应用？

2. 该指南的推荐等级如何？该指南所依据的证据应明确罗列出来，并且根据常用的评级标准确定推荐等级，研究结果的效应应该较明显，以支持证据的使用。

3. 指南中有多少不确定的证据？指南中所依据的证据有多少是不确定的也需要知晓。应该有敏感性分析的结果。

三、该实践指南是否有益于患者

1. 指南的主要目的是否具有临床重要性，是否能够提高医疗质量，与患者的目标是否一致？

2. 指南是否适用于患者？患者的实际情况必须符合指南的适用标准。

本 章 小 结

在循证实践指南的临床应用中，提倡既要以科学证据为基础进行医疗决策，又要结合临床经验和患者利益，在诊疗中遵循个体化的诊治原则。临床医学既是科学也是艺术，在重视循证实践指南的同时，不应忽视个人临床技能的重要性，如与患者良好的沟通和交流等临床技能，只有科学灵活地运用循证实践指南，才会使患者得到最佳的结果。

（李亚斐）

第十六章

系统评价与 meta 分析

学习目标

1. **掌握** meta 分析的基本步骤、文献评价原则、结果应用解释。
2. **熟悉** 循特殊类型 meta 分析。
3. **了解** 系统评价与 meta 分析的基本概念。

第一节　系统评价的概念

循证医学的核心理念是临床实践应基于证据，因此"证据"的形成及其质量是实践循证医学的关键，所有已完成的和正在进行的医学研究都可以成为证据。在循证医学中，系统评价和 meta 分析方法是产生高质量证据的重要方法。对于某种疗法有效性和安全性评价问题，基于大样本随机对照试验和其他相关随机对照研究进行系统评价（systematic review）后所得出的结果常常是最佳证据之一，被临床指南广泛引用。

系统评价是指按照严格的纳入标准广泛收集关于某一医疗卫生问题的研究，并对纳入的研究进行全面的质量评价和分析，必要时进行定量合并的统计学处理，以得出综合结论的一种研究方法。该方法旨在整理、汇总多项研究结果，提供可靠的证据，促进决策。系统评价的研究问题不仅局限于对干预措施的疗效评价，目前已拓展到病因、诊断、预后和动物实验等多个领域。

Cochrane 协作网是一个国际性组织，旨在通过制作、维护和提高决策所需的系统评价证据可及性，帮助人们制定遵循证据的（知证）卫生决策。Cochrane 系统评价是指在 Cochrane 协作网统一工作手册指导下，在相应 Cochrane 专业评价组编辑部指导和帮助下完成并发表在 Cochrane Library 的系统评价。Cochrane 系统评价实施全程都有严格的质量控制措施，同时开发了专业的系统评价软件作为辅助，故其被公认是目前相对最成熟、质量最高的系统评价方法。

第二节　系统评价的基本步骤

系统评价是通过收集、评价和合成原始临床研究结果，得出综合性结论的一种研究方法。系统评价是一种科学研究方法，也是一项系统工程，其中有诸多研究步骤。本节将基于 Cochrane 系统评价工作手册简述系统评价的一般步骤。

一、明确研究问题

正确的选题是系统评价的第一步。这一步骤需要花费一些时间,也需要系统评价者的积极参与和专业知识的积累。可以通过明确研究对象(participants)、干预(intervention)、对照(comparisons)和结局(outcome)来确定研究问题,即 PICO 原则。

二、确定文献的入选标准

入选标准一般基于研究问题(PICO)要素以及研究问题的相关内容考虑并设置。一般还应包括研究发表文献的语言、发表的年限、研究的类型等。

三、文献检索

主要过程是根据研究问题的 PICO 确定检索策略,包括明确检索数据库、确定检索词、编制检索策略、实施检索和文献管理。需要注意的是要全面查找所有相关的临床研究,不仅要检索常用的综合性文献数据库资源(如 MEDLINE、Embase、Cochrane 中心对照试验注册库等),还应尝试检索专题数据库、引文数据库、学位论文数据库和灰色文献数据库等。注意不要遗漏各类研究注册网站,以及监管机构和一些其他来源的临床研究报告。强烈建议系统评价人员应当与经验丰富的图书馆员或信息学专家密切合作。

四、临床研究的选择与纳入

Cochrane 协作组推荐了选择和纳入的过程。主要包括:合并不同来源的检索结果,删除同一报告的重复记录;阅读标题和摘要,删除明显不相关的报告;检索相关报告的全文;将同一研究的多个报告联系在一起;仔细阅读报告全文,确定是否符合合格标准;必要时联络研究者,确认研究的相关信息(要求研究者提供更多的信息,例如缺少的方法学或结果信息);对研究的纳入做出最终决定并收集数据;标记或记录尚未报告且正在进行的试验,以便将它们添加到正在进行的研究列表中。在选择研究的过程中,应详细记录排除的原因,同时绘制选择研究的流程图。

五、数据提取

应当保证系统评价数据的准确性、完整性,并保证系统评价的更新和共享。注意尽量减少偏见和人为错误。研究报告的来源多种多样,因此将同一研究的多个报告联系在一起是很重要的。最好是由两名研究人员独立提取数据,并且通过双人核对确保数据的准确。而且,从不同的研究报告中提取的结果常常需要将数据转换为可用于分析的样式。

六、对纳入的文献进行研究质量评估

需要对单个研究在设计、实施和分析过程中,防止或减少偏倚或系统误差的情况进行质量评估。针对随机对照试验开发的评估工具众多,常用的包括 Jadad 量表(Jadad scale)评分、Cochrane 风险偏倚评估工具和风险偏倚风险工具更新版(RoB 2)等方法。由于非随机研究的研究设计多样,目前尚无一种通用的研究质量评估工具。Newcastle-Ottawa Scale(NOS)是较为常用的工具之一,简单易操作,其中分别有针对队列研究和病例对照研究的条目。

七、分析数据

在必要时进行 meta 分析,meta 分析的核心计算是将多个研究的统计量汇总。在合并数据之前,需要对多个研究结果进行异质性检验,以判断多个研究是否具有同质性。如果确实存在异质性,下文将详细介绍有关的解决方法。meta 分析常使用森林图展示 meta 分析结果。此外,还需要通过绘制漏斗图或相关检验来判断是否存在发表偏倚或其他偏倚。

八、总结结果,得出研究结论

系统评价结果报告应当遵循 PRISMA 2020 报告规范。

第三节　文献质量评价工具

对纳入的研究进行质量评价是系统评价的核心步骤之一,评价原始研究的质量对客观判断系统评价结果和结论的真实性、可靠性至关重要。由于综述中得出的结论取决于纳入的研究结果,如果这些结果有偏倚,那么对这些研究的 meta 分析结果将产生误导的结论。评价文献质量和偏倚风险的方法较多,可采用清单、一览表或量表评分等。针对不同的研究设计类型,质量评价工具和方法也有明显差别。

针对随机对照试验,文献质量评价的工具有很多,目前被广泛使用的包括 Jadad 量表(Jadad scale)和 Cochrane 偏倚风险评估工具。前者强调的是研究报告的质量,简单易操作,但有些项目定义不够明确;后者则强调了试验设计和实施的方法学质量,条目定义清晰规范。因此,此处推荐使用 Cochrane 偏倚风险评估工具。

Jadad 量表由 Alejandro R.Jadad 和他的团队成员在 1996 年开发并发表,最初的版本包括三个条目(随机化、盲法和退出),得分为 0～5 分,后续改良 Jadad 量表有八个条目(表 16-1)。

表 16-1　改良 Jadad 量表评分标准

条目	回答	得分 / 分
1. 研究是否随机	是	+1
	否	0
2. 随机化方法是否恰当	是	+1
	否	0
	未描述	−1
3. 研究是否使用盲法	是	+1
	否	0
4. 盲法的使用是否恰当	是	+1
	否	0
	未描述	−1
5. 受试者是否退出或脱落	是	+1
	否	0
6. 是否对入选 / 排除标准有清晰的描述	是	+1
	否	0

续表

条目	回答	得分 / 分
7. 是否对评估不良反应的方法有描述	是	+1
	否	0
8. 是否对统计分析方法有描述	是	+1
	否	0

2008 年，Cochrane 协作组发布了 Cochrane 偏倚风险（risk-of-bias，RoB）评估工具，该工具在 2011 年进行了修订，发布了更新版（RoB 2）。这个工具是由众多方法学家、编辑和评价者组成的工作小组共同开发的。该工具侧重于评估研究中各类偏倚的风险。它是一项基于"维度评估"的工具，即需要对研究的质量从不同"偏倚风险"维度进行严格独立评估。该工具涵盖六个维度：选择偏倚、实施偏倚、信息偏倚、随访偏倚、报告偏倚及其他偏倚。该工具中没有评分系统。对偏倚风险的评估需要系统综述的研究者进行判断，该过程应当完全透明。系统综述的研究者需要对每个维度做评价，判断为"低风险""高风险""风险不清楚"，同时需要提供支持该评价的理由。

这一工具自发布以来已经得到了广泛的应用。2019 年，Cochrane 偏倚风险评估工具的更新版本发布。在最新的版本中有几个值得注意的变化：引入了信号问题及相关的算法；对偏倚的评估是在单一结果水平上；某些偏倚的名称描述更清楚；增加了整体风险偏倚评估，并且对于总体风险偏倚的判断过程更加明确清晰。Cochrane 偏倚风险评估工具 2 的详细条目列于表 16-2。更多关于 Cochrane 偏倚风险评估工具 2 的信息可以通过偏倚风险工具网站获取。

表 16-2　Cochrane 偏倚风险评估工具 2

偏倚领域和信号问题 *	回答		
	低风险偏倚	高风险偏倚	其他
随机化过程中的偏倚			
1.1　分配序列是否随机？	Y/PY	N/PN	NI
1.2　受试者分配干预措施前，是否保持分配序列隐藏？	Y/PY	N/PN	NI
1.3　组间基线差异是否提示随机化过程存在问题？	N/PN	Y/PY	NI
偏倚风险评估（低 / 高 / 有一定风险）			
可选：如果存在偏倚，可能的方向是什么？			
偏离既定干预的偏倚			
2.1　研究过程中研究对象是否知道他们接受哪种干预？	N/PN	Y/PY	NI
2.2　研究过程中医护人员是否知道受试者接受哪种干预？	N/PN	Y/PY	NI
2.3　如果以上两个问题回答是 / 可能是 / 不清楚则回答：是否存在由于试验环境引起的偏离既定干预？	N/PN	Y/PY	NA/NI
2.4　如果上一个问题回答是 / 可能是 / 不清楚则回答：与既定干预的偏离是否可能对研究结局造成影响？	N/PN	Y/PY	NA/NI
2.5　如果上一个问题回答是 / 可能是则回答：与既定干预的偏离是否在组间均衡？	Y/PY	N/PN	NA/NI
2.6　是否使用恰当的分析方法来评估干预的效果？	Y/PY	N/PN	NI

偏倚领域和信号问题 *	回答		
	低风险偏倚	高风险偏倚	其他
2.7　如果上一个问题回答不是 / 可能不是 / 不清楚则回答：未能分析随机分配的受试者数据是否（对结果）有潜在的重大影响？	N/PN	Y/PY	NA/NI
偏倚风险评估(低 / 高 / 有一定风险)			
可选：如果存在偏倚，可能的方向是什么？			
结局数据缺失的偏倚			
3.1　是否可以获得全部，或几乎全部的随机化受试者的数据？	Y/PY	N/PN	NI
3.2　如果上一个问题回答不是 / 可能不是 / 不清楚则回答：是否有证据证明结局数据的缺失没有对结果造成偏倚？	Y/PY	N/PN	NA
3.3　如果上一个问题回答不是 / 可能不是则回答：结局数据的缺失是否与其真值有关？	N/PN	Y/PY	NA/NI
3.4　如果上一个问题回答是 / 可能是 / 不清楚则回答：结局数据的缺失是否很可能与其真值有关？	N/PN	Y/PY	NA/NI
偏倚风险评估(低 / 高 / 有一定风险)			
可选：如果存在偏倚，可能的方向是什么？			
结局测量的偏倚			
4.1　结局测量的方法是否不恰当？	N/PN	Y/PY	NI
4.2　组间结局测量或确定是否存在差异？	N/PN	Y/PY	NI
4.3　如果以上两个问题回答不是 / 可能不是 / 不清楚则回答：结局评估者是否知道研究受试者所接受的干预措施？	N/PN	Y/PY	NI
4.4　如果上一个问题回答是 / 可能是 / 不清楚则回答：如果知道接受了何种干预措施，结局的测量是否会受到影响？	N/PN	Y/PY	NA/NI
4.5　如果上一个问题回答是 / 可能是 / 不清楚则回答：如果知道接受了何种干预措施，结局的测量是否很可能会受到影响？	N/PN	Y/PY	NA/NI
偏倚风险评估(低 / 高 / 有一定风险)			
可选：如果存在偏倚，可能的方向是什么？			
结果选择性报告的偏倚			
5.1　结果的数据分析是否与在获取揭盲结局数据之前就已预先确定的统计分析计划一致？	Y/PY	N/PN	NI
正在评价的结果数据可能是基于以下结果选择性报告的：			
5.2　从多个合格的结局测量（例如尺度、定义、时间点）的结果中选择性报告？	N/PN	Y/PY	NI
5.3　从多个合格数据分析的结果中选择性报告？	N/PN	Y/PY	NI
偏倚风险评估(低 / 高 / 有一定风险)			
可选：如果存在偏倚，可能的方向是什么？			
整体偏倚			
偏倚风险评估(低 / 高 / 有一定风险)			
可选：结果的总体偏倚的方向可能是什么？			

　　Y= 是；PY= 可能是；PN= 可能不是；N= 不是；NA= 不适用；NI= 不清楚。

　　*：偏离预期干预引起的偏倚的信号问题与分配干预的效果有关。

　　与随机对照研究相比,非随机对照研究更容易受到偏倚风险的影响。由于非随机对照研究的设计多样,例如非随机对照试验、队列研究和病例对照研究等,目前尚无一种通用的偏倚评价工具。目前最常用的是"纽卡斯尔 - 渥太华量表(Newcastle-Ottawa Scale,NOS)",该量表包括 3 大块(人群选择、可比性、结果测量),共计 8 个条目,分别开发了针对队列研究和病例对照研究的 NOS 评价标准,采用星级评分系统,队列研究满分为 13 颗星,病例对照研究满分 9 为颗星(表 16-3、表 16-4)。

表 16-3　队列研究的 NOS 条目

栏目	条目	评价标准
研究人群选择	暴露组的代表性如何(1星)	①真正代表人群中暴露组的特征 *;②一定程度上代表了人群中暴露组的特征 *;③选择某类人群,如护士、志愿者;④未描述暴露组来源情况
	非暴露组的选择方法(1星)	①与暴露组来自同一人群 *;②与暴露组来自不同人群;③未描述非暴露组来源情况
	暴露因素的确定方法(1星)	①固定的档案记录(如外科手术记录)*;②采用结构式访谈 *;③研究对象自己写的报告;④未描述
	研究起始时尚无要观察的结局指标(1星)	①是 *;②否
组间可比性	设计和统计分析时考虑暴露组和未暴露组的可比性(最高2星)	①研究控制了最重要的混杂因素 *;②研究控制了任何其他的混杂因素 *(此条可以进行修改用以说明特定控制第二重要因素)
结果测量	研究对于结果的评价是否充分(1星)	①盲法独立评价 *;②有档案记录 *;③自我报告;④未描述
	结果发生后随访是否足够长(1星)	①是(评价前规定恰当的随访时间)*;②否
	暴露组和非暴露组的随访是否充分(1星)	①随访完整 *;②有少量研究对象失访但不至于引入偏倚(规定失访率或描述失访情况)*;③有失访(规定失访率)但未行描述;④未描述随访情况

*:给星点。在"研究人群选择"和"结果的测量"模块中,每个条目最多一颗星;"组间可比性"模块最多可给出两颗星。

表 16-4　病例对照研究的 NOS 条目

栏目	条目	评价标准
研究人群选择	病例确定是否恰当(1星)	①恰当,有独立的确定方法或人员 *;②恰当,如基于档案记录或自我报告;③未描述
	病例的代表性(1星)	①连续或有代表性的系列病例 *;②有潜在选择偏倚或未描述
	对照的选择(1星)	①与病例同一人群为对照 *;②与病例同一人群的住院人员为对照;③未描述
	对照的确定(1星)	①无目标疾病史(端点)*;②未描述来源
组间可比性	设计和统计分析时考虑病例和对照的可比性(最高2星)	①研究控制了最重要的混杂因素 *;②研究控制了任何其他的混杂因素 *(此条可以进行修改用以说明特定控制第二重要因素)

栏目	条目	评价标准
暴露因素的测量	暴露因素的确定（1 星）	①固定的档案记录（如外科手术记录）*；②采用结构式访谈且不知访谈者是病例或对照 *；③采用未实施盲法的访谈（即知道病例或对照的情况）；④未描述
	采用相同的方法确定病例和对照的暴露因素（1 星）	①是 *；②否
	无应答率（1 星）	①病例组和对照组无应答率相同 *；②描述了无应答者的情况；③病例组和对照组无应答率不同且未描述

*：给星点。在"研究人群选择"和"暴露因素的测量"模块中，每个条目最多一颗星；"组间可比性"模块最多可给出两颗星。

第四节　meta 分析

1976 年，吉恩·格拉斯（Gene Glass）首次提出了对多个同类研究统计量的整合的方法，他将该方法称作是 meta 分析（meta-analysis）。meta 分析是对一系列个体研究的统计分析。随后，该方法广泛应用于医疗健康领域。20 世纪 80 年代末，meta 分析被引入我国，中文常翻译为荟萃分析。

Cochrane Handbook 中将 meta 分析定义为对来自两个或多个独立研究结果的统计学合并，它是一种最常用的统计学方法。meta 分析是为循证医学提供临床证据的重要技术和工具，该方法的突出优势包括增加检验效能、提高准确性、回答单个研究无法回答的问题和解决相互矛盾的观点引发的争论等。然而，值得注意的是，meta 分析也可能会带来潜在的误导，尤其是在未仔细考虑特定的研究设计、研究本身存在严重的偏倚，或研究间的异质性太大等情况下。

因此，只有当系统评价中纳入的研究资料适合使用 meta 分析时才建议使用，这样可以大大提高分析结果的可靠性和精确性；但当资料出现上述不适合 meta 分析的情形时，建议仅汇总描述各研究，对分析结论应慎重。

一、异质性检验

系统评价中研究过程中任何种类的变异都被称为异质性（heterogeneity）。meta 分析的核心是将多个研究的统计量合并，按照统计学原理，只有同质的资料才能进行统计量的合并，反之则不能。如果个体研究结果的置信区间重叠较少，这通常表明存在统计学异质性。更正规的是对异质性进行统计学检验，该检验主要评价了所观察结果间的差异是否仅由机遇所致。较小的 P 值（异质性检验的 α 水平一般取 0.10，即 $P<0.10$）提供了干预效应存在异质性的证据。纳入研究的异质性大小还可以用 I^2 来评价，I^2 的计算公式如下所示。

$$I^2 = \left(\frac{Q - \mathrm{d}f}{Q}\right) \times 100\%$$

其中，Q 是异质性检验的卡方统计量，$\mathrm{d}f$ 是自由度。该公式描述了由异质性而不是抽样误差（机遇）所致的干预估计值变异（异质性）占总变异的百分比。一般认为，$I^2<50\%$ 时，异质性可以接受；$I^2 \geqslant 50\%$ 时，可能存在实质的异质性。

如果异质性变异检验结果 $P>0.10$ 时,可认为多个同类研究具有同质性,可使用固定效应模型(fixed effect model)。当异质性检验 $P<0.10$ 或者 $I^2>50\%$ 时,首先应探索分析并寻找引起异质性的原因,并进行亚组分析或 meta 回归。也可采用随机效应模型(random effect model)合并结果,但要注意的是该模型针对的是不能解释的异质性的统计处理方法,并不能替代对异质性的原因分析。当不存在异质性时,随机效应模型和固定效应模型的结果相同;当存在异质性时,随机效应模型估计的置信区间会比固定效应模型的更宽。

二、合并统计量

meta 分析的核心内容是将多个同类研究的结果合并成某个单一效应量。对于不同类型的指标,结果合并的方法不同,因此 meta 分析首先要确定合并统计量,并计算每个研究的结果。如果需要分析的指标是连续性变量,可以选择平均差(mean difference,MD)或标准化均差(standardized mean difference,SMD)为合并统计量。如果需要分析的指标是二分类指标,可以选择比值比(odds ratio,OR)、相对危险度(RR)或危险差(risk difference,RD)为合并统计量。

对于二分类结局资料,常用的固定效应模型可以根据资料类型选择 Peto 法、Mantel-Haenszel 法或倒方差法(inverse variance)。随机效应模型多采用 D-L 法(DerSimonian 和 Laird 倒方差法)。Peto 法仅能合并 OR,其他三种方法能合并统计量 OR、RR 和 RD。连续性资料的固定效应模型可以选择倒方差法。

倒方差法得名于每个研究所赋权重来自效应估计方差的倒数(如标准误平方分之一)。因此,较大样本的研究(其标准误较小)比较小样本的研究(其标准误较大)所赋权重大。但当数据稀少时(不管是事件发生率低还是样本量小),倒方差所用的效应估计值的标准误可能欠佳。而 Mantel-Haenszel 法根据使用的效应指标(如 RR、OR、RD),采用了不同的加权方式,当研究内容为小概率事件时,其表现出较好的统计性能。D-L 法是最简单,也是最常用的随机效应模型方法。更多的统计学相关公式在此处不做展示,读者可查阅相关文献进行学习。

三、森林图

meta 分析常用森林图(forest plot)展示其统计分析结果,可以参考下文示例中的森林图(图 16-1)。森林图展示了个体研究和 meta 分析的结果估计和置信区间。森林图中,中间一条数值为 0 或 1 的中心垂线为无效线(效应量为组间均数差异时,无效线在 0 处;效应量为 RR、OR 或 HR 时,无效线在 1 处)。每一横线代表每个研究效应值的 95% 置信区间范围,中央的小方块为该研究效应指标(如均值差 MD、RR 或 OR)所处的位置,方块大小代表研究权重。当该横线触及或跨越中线,则表示试验组与对照组的结局效应差异不具有统计学意义,反之,若该横线完全落在无效线的左侧或右侧,与无效线不相交时,则表示差异有统计学意义。最下方的菱形的中心所在位置表示合并效应值的估计,该菱形的宽度表示合并效应的置信区间范围。

四、漏斗图

漏斗图(funnel plot)是最常用的考察纳入的研究是否存在发表偏倚的方法之一,漏斗图的横坐标为单个研究的效应值,纵坐标常用样本量大小表示,或者使用效应量的标准误或是标准误的倒数。该方法的假设是小型研究比大型研究更容易受到发表偏倚的影响。如果研究人员完成了一项大型随机试验，即使结果是阴性的，它也更可能被发表。然而，对于小型试验来说，情况可能有所不同。如果发表偏倚确实存在，很可能是由于小型阴性结果的试验未发表造成的。

小样本研究的数量远多于大样本研究，其结果广泛分布在图形底部，随着试验规模的增加，试验结果会趋近于真实效应，但数量相对较少，图形顶部分布密集、狭窄，因此呈现为类似于一个倒置的漏斗。当发表偏倚发生时，常常小规模研究的分布是不对称的，更多的研究显示出阳性的结果，而那些阴性的结果则未发表。所以会出现不对称的漏斗图，不对称越明显，偏倚程度也就越大。

漏斗图法是一种定性的方法，主要通过研究者考察散点图情况做判断，存在很大的主观性。目前，有几种定量方法用于评价是否存在发表偏倚，常用的有 Egger's 检验和 Begg's 检验。Egger's 检验是用标准化效应量对效应估计值的精度（标准误的倒数）做回归分析，截距大小来表示漏斗图的不对称程度，如果存在发表偏倚，回归线的截距将偏离起点。Begg's 检验通过秩相关分析来检验效应量大小与标准误之间的相关性。Egger's 检验比 Begg's 检验的检验效能稍高，但当纳入文献数量较少时（少于 10 篇），这两种方法的检验效能均较低。

五、亚组分析

亚组分析（subgroup analysis）指根据某些因素将所有受试者数据分成不同的亚组，通常比较不同亚组的结果是否一致。例如，可以对不同受试者特征（如性别、年龄或病情严重程度）或不同的研究（如在不同地点实施）进行。亚组分析也可作为分析异质性结果的方法，或用于回答有关特定患者、干预类型或研究类型的问题，对临床指导个体化处理有重要意义。

需要注意的是，亚组结果可能有误导性。由于各亚组的样本量通常较小，所以容易因偶然性而得出错误的结果。并且，亚组分析进行越多，出现假阴性和假阳性显著性检验的可能性越多。因此，对于亚组的分析的结果要谨慎解读。Cochrane 系统评价建议作者应说明是否亚组分析是事先确定的或在知晓研究结果后才实施的（事后分析）。如果一个亚组分析是事先确定的分析之一，则其可靠性更高。否则，进行大量的事后亚组分析以解释异质性是数据捕捞，其可靠性较低。

六、敏感性分析

敏感性分析（sensitivity analysis）是通过改变不确定的值或标准对原始分析或 meta 分析进行重复分析。meta 分析过程中的不确定性常常会影响结果的稳健性。因此，需要借助大量的敏感性分析充分评估结果的稳健性和可靠性，并发现或确定研究过程中哪些不确定因素带来了影响。在进行敏感性分析时，总是可以问这样一个问题：基于这些结果所做的决策是否可靠？

在实践中，系统评价的作者可以通过改变一些不确定的条件对某一类研究或人群进行分析。例如，探讨随机对照设计的试验或非随机对照试验的治疗效果，以评估研究设计的影响；排除一些低质量或高偏差的研究，以评估研究质量对结果的影响。注意不要将敏感性分析与亚组分析混淆。虽然敏感性分析常常会重点分析所有研究中的一个子集，但不会分析那些排除掉的研究。在敏感性分析中，常常是从不同的角度估计同一件事情。

敏感性分析通常可以从以下角度考虑：①研究设计，包括受试者特征、干预措施特征、对照特征、终点指标以及研究类型；②数据，包括数据分析集、样本量大小、缺失数据的处理；③分析方法，包括使用不同的统计模型，例如固定效应模型或随机效应模型。敏感性分析不仅限于以上提到的这些内容。

敏感性分析的因素最好研究方案中事先确定，但其常常是在系统评价过程中确定的。如果通过敏感性分析找到了可能影响系统评价结果的某一重要因素或决策时，应尝试获取更多的信息或资源来解决，比如可以尝试联系研究者获取数据。但如果无法获取更多的信息时，就必须注意对结果的解释要慎重。*Cochrane Handbook* 建议系统评价中敏感性分析的最佳报告方式是制作敏感性分析结果汇总表。

七、实例分析

关于二甲双胍与罗格列酮治疗 2 型糖尿病的疗效差异一直存在争议，故需要进行 meta 分析，评估和比较二甲双胍与罗格列酮治疗 2 型糖尿病的有效性和安全性。用关键词"（metformin AND rosiglitazone AND diabetes AND HbA1c）OR（二甲双胍 AND 罗格列酮 and 2 型糖尿病 AND 糖化血红蛋白）"进行检索，得到满足文献入选标准且可以提取数据的文献共 12 篇，有关治疗 6 个月后的糖化血红蛋白的数据整理如下（表 16-5）所示。

表 16-5　12 篇文献的治疗 6 个月后的糖化血红蛋白数据整理

纳入研究	发表年份	二甲双胍组			罗格列酮组			两组均数差值	标准误
		n1	mean1	s1	n2	mean2	s2		
Viljanen AP 等	2005	12	−0.60	0.82	14	−0.30	0.90	−0.30	0.337 5
Stocker DJ 等	2007	38	−1.19	0.13	37	−1.08	0.14	−0.11	0.031 2
Bilezikian JP 等	2013	84	−0.49	0.75	73	−0.49	0.70	0.00	0.115 8
Yoon KH 等	2011	114	−0.92	0.96	117	−0.82	0.79	−0.10	0.115 8
Natali A 等	2004	28	−0.33	1.10	24	0.09	12.00	−0.42	2.458 3
Yener S 等	2008	16	−1.00	1.11	23	−1.10	1.57	0.10	0.429 2
Iliadis F 等	2007	15	−1.70	1.10	14	−1.00	0.70	−0.70	0.340 1
Kiyici S 等	2009	16	−0.30	0.79	19	−0.70	0.79	0.40	0.268 1
Jung HS 等	2005	13	−1.00	0.98	14	−1.50	1.01	0.50	0.383 1
Skov V 等	2014	90	−1.31	0.15	93	−1.26	0.19	−0.05	0.025 3
Fidan E 等	2011	20	−1.20	0.95	20	−1.00	0.92	−0.20	0.295 7
Rosenstock J 等	2006	150	−1.80	1.00	155	−1.60	1.00	−0.20	0.114 5

该研究的主要终点为连续性资料（糖化血红蛋白），合并效应量为均数差（WMD），考虑基于异质性检验结果选择使用倒方差法的固定效应模型或 D-L 法的随机效应模型。借助 Stata 软件完成 meta 分析的统计部分及绘图部分，操作方法如下。

1. 数据按如下格式输入 Stata 软件（表 16-6）。

表 16-6 Stata 数据格式

name	year	Studylabel	n1	m1	s1	n2	m2	s2
Viljanen AP	2005	ViljanenAP（2005）	12	−0.60	0.82	14	−0.30	0.90
Stocker DJ	2007	StockerDJ（2007）	38	−1.19	0.13	37	−1.08	0.14
Bilezikian JP	2013	BilezikianJP（2013）	84	−0.49	0.75	73	−0.49	0.70
Yoon KH	2011	YoonKH（2011）	114	−0.92	0.96	117	−0.82	0.79
Natali A	2004	NataliA（2004）	28	−0.33	1.10	24	0.09	12.00
Yener S	2008	YenerS（2008）	16	−1.00	1.11	23	−1.10	1.57
Iliadis F	2007	IliadisF（2007）	15	−1.70	1.10	14	−1.00	0.70
Kiyici S	2009	KiyiciS（2009）	16	−0.30	0.79	19	−0.70	0.79
Jung HS	2005	JungHS（2005）	13	−1.00	0.98	14	−1.50	1.01
Skov V	2014	SkovV（2014）	90	−1.31	0.15	93	−1.26	0.19
Fidan E	2011	FidanE（2011）	20	−1.20	0.95	20	−1.00	0.92
Rosenstock J	2006	RosenstockJ（2006）	150	−1.80	1.00	155	−1.60	1.00

2. 在 Stata（Version 16 或以上版本）输入下列命令，系统评价的基本信息罗列如下。

meta esize n1 m1 s1 n2 m2 s2, esize（mdiff, unequal）fixed studylabel（studylabel）

```
meta-analysis setting information
 Study information
  No. of studies：12
   Study label：studylabel
   Study size：_meta_studysize
  Summary data: n1 m1 s1 n2 m2 s2
  Effect size
    Type：mdiff
    Label：Mean Diff.
    Variable：_meta_es
    Precision
    Std. Err.：meta_se
 Std. Err. adj.：Unequal
    CI：[_meta_cil，_meta_ciu]
    CI level：95%
Model and method
    Model：Fixed-effects
    Method：Inverse-variance
```

3. 继续输入"meta summarize"的命令后，会输出 meta 分析的结果。

```
Effect-size label：Mean Diff.
 Effect size：meta_es
 Std. Err.：meta_se
```

Study label: studylabel

meta-analysis summary　　　　　　　Number of studies = 12

Fixed-effects model　　　　　　　　Heterogeneity：

Method：Inverse-variance　　　　　 I2（%）= 18.36

　　　　　　　　　　　　　　　　　 H2 = 1.22

Study	Mean Diff.	[95% Conf. Interval]		% Weight
Viljanen AP（2005）	−0.300	−0.961	0.361	0.31
Stocker DJ（2007）	−0.110	−0.171	−0.049	35.71
Bilezikian JP（2013）	0.000	−0.227	0.227	2.60
Yoon KH（2011）	−0.100	−0.327	0.127	2.59
Natali A（2004）	−0.420	−5.238	4.398	0.01
Yener S（2008）	0.100	−0.741	0.941	0.19
Iliadis F（2007）	−0.700	−1.367	−0.033	0.30
Kiyici S（2009）	0.400	−0.125	0.925	0.48
Jung HS（2005）	0.500	−0.251	1.251	0.24
Skov V（2014）	−0.050	−0.100	−0.000	54.53
Fidan E（2011）	−0.200	−0.780	0.380	0.40
Rosenstock J（2006）	−0.200	−0.424	0.024	2.65
theta	−0.075	−0.112	−0.038	

Test of theta = 0：z = −4.02　　　　　　　Prob > |z| = 0.000 1

Test of homogeneity：Q = chi2（11）= 13.47　　Prob > Q = 0.263 5

在 Stata 输出结果中，异质性变异的检验统计量 Q 为 13.47（自由度 d.f.=11），对应的 P=0.264>0.10，故不能认为 12 个研究的两组均数差值存在异质性变异（异质性检验的 α 一般取 0.10）。本例异质性评估统计量［I-squared（variation in WMD attributable to heterogeneity）］I^2=18.4，可以认为异质性变异不明显（<50%），可以认为异质性变异不明显，因此采用固定效应模型是合适的。

固定效应模型的平均效应估计值 $\hat{\theta}$ 为 −0.075，有关该效应的检验结果 P=0.000 1，95% 置信区间为（−0.112，−0.038）。由于 95% 置信区间的上限为 −0.038<0，故可以推断 $\mu_1<\mu_2$，即：服用二甲双胍的糖尿病人群的糖化血红蛋白平均水平低于服用罗格列酮的糖尿病人群，故可以推断二甲双胍降糖效果优于罗格列酮。

4. 输入"meta forestplot, nullref"的命令，即可输出森林图（图 16-1）。

本例中输出的森林图显示，各研究效应分布在无效线两侧，合并效应值落在无效线 0 左侧，置信区间上限<0，提示两组差异有统计学差异，服用二甲双胍的糖尿病人群的糖化血红蛋白平均水平低于服用罗格列酮的糖尿病人群。

Study	二甲双胍组			罗格列酮组				Mean Diff. with 95% CI	Weight（%）
	N	Mean	SD	N	Mean	SD			
Viljanen AP(2005)	12	−.6	.82	14	−.3	.9		−0.30 [−0.96, 0.36]	0.31
Stocker DJ(2007)	38	−1.19	.13	37	−1.08	.14		−0.11 [−0.17, −0.05]	35.71
Bilezikian JP(2013)	84	−.49	.75	73	−.49	.7		0.00 [−0.23, 0.23]	2.60
Yoon KH(2011)	114	−.92	.96	117	−.82	.79		−0.10 [−0.33, 0.13]	2.59
Natali A(2004)	28	−.33	1.1	24	.09	12		−0.42 [−5.24, 4.40]	0.01
Yener S(2008)	16	−1	1.11	23	−1.1	1.57		0.10 [−0.74, 0.94]	0.19
Iliadis F(2007)	15	−1.7	1.1	14	−1	.7		−0.70 [−1.37, −0.03]	0.30
Kiyici S(2009)	16	−.3	.79	19	−.7	.79		0.40 [−0.13, 0.93]	0.48
Jung HS(2005)	13	−1	.98	14	−1.5	1.01		0.50 [−0.25, 1.25]	0.24
Skov V(2014)	90	−1.31	.15	93	−1.26	.19		−0.05 [−0.10, −0.00]	54.53
Fidan E(2011)	20	−1.2	.95	20	−1	.92		−0.20 [−0.78, 0.38]	0.40
Rosenstock J(2006)	150	−1.8	1	155	−1.6	1		−0.20 [−0.42, 0.02]	2.65
Overall								−0.07 [−0.11, −0.04]	

Heterogeneity: $I^2 = 18.36\%$, $H^2 = 1.22$
Test of $\theta_i = \theta_j$: $Q(11) = 13.47$, $p = 0.26$
Test of $\theta = 0$: $z = −4.02$, $p = 0.00$

−5　　　0　　　5

Fixed-effects inverse-variance model

图 16-1　二甲双胍与罗格列酮疗效比较分析的森林图

5. 继续输入"meta funnel plot"可输出该分析的漏斗图。输入"meta bias，begg"或"meta bias，egger"命令，可输出 Begg's 检验和 Egger's 检验结果。漏斗图（图 16-2）显示所收集的各个研究的效应指标的散点全部落在漏斗虚线范围内，说明没有明显发表偏倚的迹象。

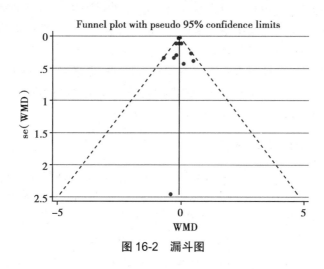

图 16-2　漏斗图

第五节　系统评价与meta分析的特别主题

一、网状meta分析

系统评价和 meta 分析常用来评估干预措施的有效性和安全性，可为临床医生、决策者和患者提供可靠的医疗信息。现实情况是,针对某一特定疾病有多种干预措施,但传统的 meta 分析一次只能比较两种干预措施。由于缺乏"头对头"试验数据,因此无法获得比较两种干预措施的直接证据。为了解决这个问题,出现了同时比较多种干预措施的方法,称为网状 meta 分析(NMA),或混合疗效比较 meta 分析。

网状 meta 分析是一种利用网络,综合所有干预措施间的直接和间接证据,同时比较三种或三种以上干预措施的技术。有了所有可获得的直接和间接证据,网状 meta 分析可以对网络中任何一对干预措施之间的相对效应做出估计,通常比单一直接或间接比较的结果更精确。该方法还可针对给定的研究终点对不同的干预效应进行排序。

三种或三种以上干预措施间的直接比较可以联系起来形成一个干预网络。网状图是对干预措施间的网状结构的一种可视化描述。网状图由结点和连线组成,每一个结点代表一种干预措施,其大小代表干预措施纳入的患者数量;结点之间的连线表示纳入分析的研究中两种干预措施进行了直接比较,其粗细代表直接比较的干预措施的研究数量。

如图 16-3 所示,干预措施 A 分别与 B、C、D 之间都进行了直接比较,纳入 meta 分析含有 A 和 B 直接比较的研究最多。从图 16-3 中可以发现,干预措施 C 和 D 之间没有进行直接比较,但可以通过公共比较组如干预措施 A 作为中间媒介,间接计算干预措施 C 与 D 在疗效和完全性方面是否存在"真正"的差异,称为间接干预比较(indirect treatment comparison,ITC)。间接比较能估计在试验中没有直接比较的两种干预措施间的相对效应。间接比较的基本假设是,通过结合"A vs. C"和"A vs. D"的相对效应来估计"C vs. D"的相对真实效应。间接比较不是随机比较,可能存在观察性研究中的常见偏倚,如混杂偏倚。

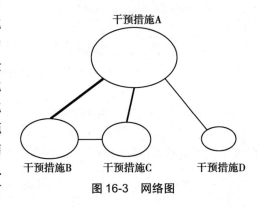

图 16-3　网络图

网状 meta 分析有很多种分析方法。所有方法的核心要求是,分析中包括的所有干预措施可以形成一个相互连接的网络。一种最直接的网状 meta 分析方法是 meta 回归,另一种常用的网状 meta 分析方法是贝叶斯框架下的层次模型。

二、个体患者资料系统评价

个体患者资料(individual patient data,IPD)系统评价是一种特殊的系统评价,它与常规的系统评价不同,它不是直接利用已发表的研究结果的总结数据进行合并,而是从原始研究的负责人、数据共享库或平台获取每个受试者的原始数据,重新进行数据核对,并以统一方法重新分析汇总结果。IPD 通常包含每个受试者的人口统计信息,如年龄、性别、健康状况的性质,以及关于所接受的治疗或检测结果。该方法比其他形式的系统评价需要更多的时间、资源和专业知识,但质量更高。因此,大部分 IPD 系统评价由协作组实施并发表,协作组通常由以下部分构成:项目管理组或秘书组、顾问小组成员(若有)、提供数据的研究者。

IPD 系统评价有着传统系统评价无法超越的优势:IPD 方法可以大大改善现有数据的质量,并弥补个别研究报告的不足。IPD 综述常常包括未发表的试验或灰色数据。在发表的研究中,常常可能没有报道期望的数据,或者有很多受试者没有纳入分析,那么如果原始研究提供每一个受试者的原始资料，将极大地避免发表偏倚。当有每个受试者的原始数据和必要的额外数据时，就可以更彻底地评估偏倚风险，也能够更详细和灵活地进行统计分析。研究者可以在患者层面处理缺失的数据，分析所有感兴趣和重要的结果，检查分析的假设，更加方便地进行亚组分析，或进行更复杂的分析。例如，可以深入分析患者的特征，开发复杂的预测或预后模型。研究者也可以更新随访的生存结局，报道超出研究报告的数据结果。当解释研究结果时，系统评价的作者还可以与包括提供数据的研究者在内的多学科团队共同探讨研究结果的临床实践意义。

IPD 系统评价通常比常规的系统评价要花费更长的时间和更多的费用，并且要求一定的技能用以获取、管理和分析数据。一般来说，当目前已发表的系统综述或其他汇总结果质量不高时，会考虑开展一项 IPD 系统评价。另一个重要的考虑是要能收集到足够多的患者个体数据进行可靠的分析。在开始 IPD 系统综述之前，作者需要仔细考虑研究成功需要的技能和资源。

需要注意的是，虽然 IPD 方法有助于避免研究中分析报告相关的偏倚，但通常它不能避免与研究设计或实施相关的偏倚。如有此类问题，该研究应从 meta 分析中排除。此外，在 IPD 系统评价中获得所需的所有数据常常是不可能的，因此需要警惕那些不能获得的研究数据带来的偏倚。如原始研究的研究者不回应或拒绝参加，一些阴性或不利的研究数据就可能无法获取，那么会导致 IPD 系统评价出现偏倚。因此，在不能获得所有研究个体患者数据的 IPD 系统评价报告中应说明无法获得个体患者数据的原因以及由此导致的偏倚的可能性，并且谨慎下结论。

三、前瞻性 meta 分析

前瞻性 meta 分析（prospective meta-analysis，PMA）是一项有计划的、主动的 meta 分析方法，是指单中心随机试验与主动的同期开展的 meta 分析相结合的一种方法。这有别于传统的方法，即研究者设计、实施并发表一项临床试验，但没有更远期的研究计划，他们常常会被动地等待其他研究者将该研究与类似的随机试验进行结果合并，即完成一项系统综述研究中的传统回顾性 meta 分析。或者，他们也可能会计划开展一项包含该研究的传统 meta 分析。但在前瞻性 meta 分析中，研究者会在计划、实施一项临床试验的同时设计一项包含该试验结果的 meta 分析。

前瞻性 meta 分析避开了传统回顾性 meta 分析中存在的一些问题和挑战。在 PMA 中，随机试验的研究结果产生之前就被识别并确定将其纳入 meta 分析。在单个研究结果产生之前，研究者就事先明确假设并建立前瞻性研究的选择标准。而且，在任一研究结果产生之前，PMA 允许事先确定分析计划，包括亚组分析。因此，PMA 避免了传统 meta 分析中依赖事后数据分析结果的潜在问题。

此外，一项 PMA 中的所有中心必须有统一的干预和结局。这样就可以避免回顾性 meta 分析中不同干预之间的差异和不同结局测量的差异。如果没有 PMA 研究者的共同规定，某些单个中心可能会产生冲突的数据，这些数据在一项科学的 meta 分析中是无法进行合并的。

如果启动得足够早，PMA 将为正在进行中的试验提供更为标准的试验设计、数据收集和其他试验流程。PMA 中的所有中心可能都会同意使用相同的仪器来测量特定的结果，并在相同时间点测量结果。因此，那些传统回顾性 meta 分析中因缺乏标准而引起的一些问题将可以得到解决。如果没有 PMA 研究人员的共同决策和标准化规则，一些中心可能会产生相互矛盾的数据，从而无法进行合理的 meta 分析。

基于患者个体数据的 PMA 类似于多中心临床试验，具有类似的优势，包括增加样本量、增加治疗和人群的多样性以及提升识别异质性的能力。传统的多中心试验在所有中心必须统一实施某一特定方案以减少各中心间干预的差异，而 PMA 使研究人员在试验实施方面具有更大的灵活性。各中心可以根据当地实际情况设计相应的方案，该方案只需要与 PMA 方案中的一些特定关键要素一致即可。

PMA 往往由某一协作组织开展实施，他们可以采集并分析个体患者数据。不像传统的多中心试验，当事先设计的 meta 分析发挥最大化效能时，他们允许纳入研究的方案有差异。对于培养研究人员而言，一项 PMA 常常比一项多中心随机试验需要更少的资源。因此，PMA 项目可以通过合作增加研究的能力。

第六节　系统评价的注册与报告规范

为了提高系统综述和 meta 分析报告的质量，1999 年和 2009 年有关组织分别提出了 QUOROM 指南和 PRISMA 声明。为了解决系统综述与 meta 分析报告质量不佳的问题，一个国际组织于 1999 年制定并发表了 meta 分析报告质量（quality of reporting of meta-analyses，QUOROM）指南。2009 年，该指南进行了更新，并更名为系统评论和 meta 分析报告规范（preferred reporting items for systematic reviews and meta-analyses，PRISMA）。随着这两份声明的广泛使用，系统综述报告的质量已经有所提高。近年来，PRISMA 也被改编和修订，衍生出许多不同的版本，以适应不同类型系统评价的报告。过去十多年中，系统评价出现了许多创新，在方法和术语方面取得很大进展。为了适应新的需求，Page 等对 PRIMSA 2009 进行了更新和修订，并于 2021 年 3 月在 *BMJ*、*PLOS Medicine* 等 5 家期刊同期在线发表。

PRISMA 2020 声明为系统评价提供了最新的报告指南，它重点对过去十年在系统评价方法和术语方面取得的进展进行了更新。PRISMA 2020 声明由 27 项条目组成的清单、详细说明的扩展清单、PRISMA 2020 摘要清单和流程图组成。

为保证系统评价的真实性和透明性，与其他类型研究一样，系统评价研究也被要求注册，主要的注册平台是 PROSPERO 网站，注册时需要填写系统评价研究方案的简要内容，网站将永久保存简要内容。待审核后即可获得 PROSPERO 注册号。

本 章 小 结

循证医学的核心理念是临床实践应基于证据，"证据"的形成及其质量是实践循证医学的关键，所有已完成的和正在进行的医学研究都可以成为证据。系统评价和 meta 分析方法在循证医学中是产生高质量证据的重要方法。

（吕敏之　李春波）

第十七章

生命质量评价

学习目标

1. **掌握** 健康相关生命质量的定义和评价。
2. **熟悉** 健康相关生命质量量表的建立和评估；患者报告结果在健康相关生命质量评价中的应用。
3. **了解** 健康相关生命质量评价的临床应用。

慢性疾病对患者造成的危害远不止躯体症状和生理功能的变化，患者的情绪、社会活动、人际交往、家庭角色等均会受到不同程度的影响。1948年世界卫生组织（WHO）指出"健康不仅是没有病和不虚弱，而是使生理、心理、社会功能三方面都处于完满的良好状态"。但是，目前临床常规的疾病评估方法主要关注患者的生物学改变，回答的是有病或者没病，而不是完整意义上的健康。例如，同样是恶性肿瘤患者，一例接受了手术切除，且属于预后较好的病例，但对肿瘤的恐慌使其频繁就诊，情绪低落，惶惶不可终日；另一例晚期患者，非常乐观，尽可能地参与家庭和社会活动。这两例患者的健康状态如何评价？

第一节 健康相关生命质量的概念

一、生命质量的定义

1993年世界卫生组织生命质量评估组定义生命质量（quality of life，QOL）为"个体在不同的文化背景和价值体系下，与个体目标、期望、标准以及所关心的事物有关的生存状况的体验"。生命质量的内涵强调依从于每一个体独特的生活体验，具有明显的主观特性，尊重个体的价值观，尊重个体的社会价值。

二、健康相关生命质量的定义

应用生命质量的理论与方法来评价健康，即"健康相关生命质量"（health-related quality of life，HRQOL），是在疾病、医疗干预、个体经济收入、年龄老化、社会环境变化等影响下，与经济、文化背景和价值取向相联系的主观满意度。这一定义体现了HRQOL具备综合反映健康状态的能力，符合生物-心理-社会的医学模式，并确立了评价HRQOL所需要的领域和维度。各个领域不仅与疾病有关，彼此之间构成因果关系，而且与社会、经济以及其他因素有着错综复杂的关联。尽管疾病往往造成损伤和残疾，伤残进一步导致较差的 HRQOL，然而疾病与 HRQOL 的关系并非线性或单向关系。例如，脑梗死后肢体瘫痪的患者，随着对疾病认知度的加深、健侧肢体代偿能力的提高、家庭的支持、社会活动的恢复等，可在患侧肢体功能永久丧失的情况下，HRQOL 得到改善。

三、健康相关生命质量的评估内容

《国际功能、残疾和健康分类》(ICF)、WHO 的生命质量测定等界定 HRQOL 构成的多种体系陆续建立，这些体系将客观标准、疾病相关参数与患者自我报告的症状和感受结合起来，主要包括 5 个方面的评估。

1. **躯体症状** 疾病症状等。
2. **生理功能** 脏器功能水平、认知状态、角色状态、性功能等。
3. **心理功能** 情绪良好、压抑、抑郁、焦虑等。
4. **社会功能** 社会关系、工作角色、业余爱好、财政状况等。
5. **精神状态** 宗教信仰、个人价值观等。

这些领域充分体现了 HRQOL 的评估以患者为中心，并以主观评价为主要内容。但是，目前 HRQOL 的评估是否应该包括客观指标如收入、生态环境等存在较大的争议。

四、健康相关生命质量的评估方法

由于生命质量的大多数内容为受试者的主观体验，因此，目前最常用的评估形式是量表和患者报告结果。

第二节 健康相关生命质量量表的建立与评估

一、量表的分类

根据使用对象，主要分为两种，一类是测量患者一般健康状态的普适量表（generic QOL instrument），另一类是疾病特异性的专用量表（disease-specific QOL instrument）。

普适量表包含常规生活活动和心理状况，其评估内容适用于不同类型的疾病、不同种族、不同语言人群。普适量表的优势在于不受疾病诊断影响，能够直接比较不同疾病的严重性、采取不同干预措施的利弊，比如系统性红斑狼疮与消化道溃疡的治疗比较，有利于决策者权衡不同疾病的损害或治疗对患者的影响，从而对有限的资源作出有效的决策。然而，这类量表常常未包含与研究疾病特征有关的条目，忽视了研究疾病所受影响的重要功能方面，因而该类量表用于特殊疾病评估时信度往往不高，可能存在对某些条目应答率低的情况。例如，欧洲五维度表（EQ-5D）包括行动状况、自我照顾、日常活动、疼痛 / 不舒服、焦虑 / 抑郁等维度，选择没有疼痛，通常代表较好的 HRQOL，但对于痛觉丧失的患者来说，实际情况恰恰相反。

疾病专用量表是为某一类疾病或疾病的某一亚型制定的量表，能有效地反映该类疾病对患者 HRQOL 的影响，适用于该类疾病不同干预措施的比较。但是，疾病专用量表也有它的局限性，受地区特征、文化传统、信仰、风俗、生活方式等影响，有时需建立不同的量表，常常难于对不同的疾病进行同等的评价。例如，类风湿关节炎的健康评估问卷（HAQ）、肿瘤的欧洲癌症治疗研究组织（EORTC）量表等均是被广泛应用的疾病专用量表。

二、量表的构成

量表通常构架为生理功能、心理功能、社会功能、总体状况、角色功能等不同的维度（domain）或称为亚量表（subscale）；每一维度又可以包含不同方面（facet），如生理功能可以分为日常生理功能、认知水平、角色功能等三个方面；每一个方面又可以由多少不等的条目（item）构成。

三、量表的建立

量表的设计过程中需考虑的要素包括应用的临床背景、研究目的、应用的对象、量表的概念框架、条目池的建立与条目选择、反应项的选择、数据收集方式、监管模式、应答时间范围、评分标准、条目或亚量表的权重、格式、填表负担、翻译和文化调适等。

量表的建立必须经过一系列严谨规范的步骤。首先，形成量表的概念框架，根据疾病背景和研究目的，明确研究对象和内容；其次，建立研究议题小组和核心小组；第三，通过总结疾病特征、搜索文献、组织医护人员和患者访谈等，形成条目池，经过研究小组讨论确定进入量表的条目；第四，预试验观察量表的准确性、合理性以及完成和应答情况，修正或删除表述歧义、无法理解、重复出现的条目，并采用专家或患者重要性评分、变异系数、主成分分析等传统方法或者等级反应模型、分部评分模型等深入分析和筛选条目，形成量表的初级版本；第五，扩大样本量，完成量表的效度、信度和可行性的检验，根据结果调整量表的内容和结构；第六，重复量表质量的评价。

四、量表的评价

无论在量表的建立过程中，还是量表的适用对象、语言等发生改变时，均需要对量表的信度、效度、可行性和反应性进行评价（表17-1），从而保证量表的调查结果真实、可靠。

表 17-1　HRQOL 量表的评价

评价维度	指标	检验参数或考察内容举例
信度	重测信度或评定者内信度	组内相关系数
	评定者间信度	组间相关系数
	内部一致性信度	Cronbach's α 系数
效度	内容效度	所有条目对量表构成方面的适用性
		所有条目与研究人群特征相关性
		所有条目与量表测定目的相关性
		患者对量表内容的理解能力
	结构效度	区分和聚合效度
	效标效度	ROC 曲线（连续性变量）
		灵敏度和特异度（二分类变量）
	文化调适效度	概念等价性
		条目等价性
		语义等价性
		操作等价性
		测量等价性

评价维度	指标	检验参数或考察内容举例
反应性		最小显著差异
		患者随时间的变化
可行性		完成率
		完成时间
		条目应答率

1. 信度（reliability） 信度即可靠性，是对量表所得结果的稳定性和同一领域所有条目一致性的评价。影响量表信度的三大因素包括测定内容、测定时间和评定者。对这三大因素常用的检验方法有重测信度、评定者间信度、内部一致性信度、折半信度等。

（1）重测信度（test-retest reliability）：在相同条件下，间隔一定时间，同一患者前后两次完成量表所能达到的一致性程度，是体现量表稳定性的重要指标。间隔时间的长短对重测信度有较大的影响，过短造成患者的主观体验受记忆影响，过长则患者的 HRQOL 已发生变化，原则上应在 HRQOL 无变化的期间内进行。常应用 Kappa 值来检验两次测量结果一致性程度，若是连续变量可采用组内相关系数（intra-class correlation coefficient，ICC）进行统计。一般来说，Kappa 在 0.40～0.75 或 ICC>0.6，说明重测信度较好；若 Kappa 或 ICC>0.75，则极好。

（2）评定者间信度（inter-reviewer reliability）：能反映不同测定者间的一致性，测定工具管理的标准化和对测定者进行该标准的培训是提高评定者间信度的前提。多采用 Kappa 值或组内相关系数进行检验。

（3）内部一致性信度（internal consistency reliability）：如 α 系数（Cronbach's alpha）是检验亚量表内部条目之间一致性水平的指标。理想情况是每一个亚量表 α 系数均≥0.70，达到这一水平说明量表各条目所测内容具有同源性。需注意的是，在临床研究中，在缺乏重测信度的前提下，内部一致性信度将受到质疑。

2. 效度（validity） 效度即有效性，检验量表测定内容与真实情况的吻合程度，也就是检验量表的真实性和准确性。但患者主观体验的真实性很难明确，因此，需多方面效度评价，包括内容效度、结构效度、效标效度、文化调适效度等。

（1）内容效度（content validity）：表明测定的内容能否真实反映或真正代表所要测定现象，是首要关注的量表特性之一，但内容效度涉及的方面非常广泛，且无法应用定量方法进行检验，故对内容效度优劣的评价存在困难，仅能观察文献中有关内容效度的描述，评估其是否准确、全面和详细。内容效度包括条目生成（如条目生成方法，条目来源、选择、编辑和删减，条目评估的定量工具，研究对象等）、数据收集方式和工具监管模式、回忆周期、反应选择项、测定工具标准化和培训、患者理解能力、条目和亚量表的评分系统、应答者和管理者责任等。

（2）结构效度（construct validity）：是指测定工具测到所要测量理论结构和特质的程度，表明研究结果与假设之间的一致性，即测定工具是否真正测量到假设检验。结构效度又可分为区分效度（discriminant validity）和聚合效度（convergent validity）。区分效度应用于测定工具能识别出具有或不具有某种特征的检测对象；聚合效度是指不同测量方法测定同一特征时测量结果的相似程度。

（3）效标效度（criteria-related validity）：指所建量表和已有的标准测定结果（"金标准"）

的一致程度。标准测定结果可以是成熟的量表、临床指标或长期临床随访结果。效标效度分为两种：一种为同时效度（concurrent validity），即用所评定量表和标准测定工具同时测定一组研究对象，评价两者测定结果的一致性；另一种是预测量表（predictive validity），即量表能否预测未来事件（如疾病复发、治疗反应等）。然而，大多数生命质量研究很难找到"金标准"，如在研究中使用了标准测定工具，则需提供它的基本原理、灵敏度、特异度和预测值等信息。

（4）文化调适效度（cross-cultural validity）：由于社会、经济、信仰、文化背景等诸多方面的差异，同一量表在应用于不同国家、不同民族、不同语言人群过程中，需要对量表进行翻译和文化调适。此类文献报道应注明源语言版本的发展情况和目标语言版本的翻译过程、进行翻译和回译的专家信息、翻译者间是否独立、文化差异的调整内容、检验患者理解难易程度的预试验等。

3. 反应性（reactivity） 随时间变化或干预措施后，患者的情况发生改变，相应生命质量也发生变化，量表反映这种变化的能力称之为反应性。临床研究常以"统计学显著"来判定疗效差异，但只是数值上有显著差异不代表一定具有临床意义。患者需改善多少，患者或医护人员才认为此改变具有重要性或有意义，该阈值即为最小显著差异（minimal important difference，MID）。MID 作为定量的反应性指标经常被用于治疗疗效评估和比较的研究。

4. 可行性（feasibility） 量表的实施需不费时、易操作、不繁重，对患者具有低风险，尽可能控制在 20min 内完成，这样才能获得完整的、有效的真实信息。量表的完成率和条目的应答率是常用的量表可行性评价指标。

第三节 患者报告结果在 HRQOL 评价中的应用

HRQOL 的核心内容是患者对健康的主观满意度，往往需要患者通过自我报告的形式提供关于他们的自我感受、正在从事的活动以及对自身健康和生活满意程度的信息。该评价手段即为患者报告结果（patient reported outcome，PRO），已被证实具有较好的有效性和实用性。有效的患者报告结果通常要求与年龄、性别、诊断无关且适用范围广泛，并对能发现微小而重要的临床差异足够敏感。PRO 受到越来越多临床工作者的青睐，其中部分原因是它们从患者的角度出发，补充了客观检查无法获取的重要症状信息，已成为临床研究必需的评价指标。例如在类风湿关节炎的新药疗效评价研究中通常纳入患者对疾病状态的整体自我评估、关节疼痛程度的感受、HAQ（疾病专用量表）以及 SF-36（普适量表）等评价指标，用于明确新药对类风湿关节炎患者 HRQOL 的影响。

PRO 包括了来自患者的一切报告。通过在医院诊室、患者记录日记或其他可能的方式获取患者对疾病或治疗的反应，可以是单项指标的测量、事件记录、症状主诉或有关健康相关生命质量量表填写等。PRO 从患者角度了解其疾病状况和身体的总体感觉，有利于患者参与治疗决策，有助于了解疾病负担，为健康资源分配决策提供指南。

第四节 健康相关生命质量评价的临床应用

近十年来，健康相关生命质量量表的临床应用越来越广泛，并持续受到重视，卫生保健领域及其制定的方针都需考虑健康相关生命质量结果的影响。

　　大量的健康相关生命质量量表为临床医师以及研究者们提供了重要的信息，这些信息有助于评估疾病对患者生存的总体影响。生命质量的研究开拓了临床医学研究的一个新领域，而在该领域应用科学方法建立和评价生命质量可以帮助临床医师进一步全面评估患者病情、指导临床医师正确和合理地选用药物，同时还有助于医疗管理部门比较不同疾病间的医疗成本，进行成本 - 效用、成本 - 效益分析，优化医疗资源的分配和医疗政策的制定。

本 章 小 结

　　健康相关生命质量的概念强调通过生命质量的理论与方法来评价健康，关注个体的价值观和社会价值。健康相关生命质量量表为临床决策以及临床研究的制定开展提供了重要的支持和参考。

（马莉莉）

第十八章

成本 - 效果分析

学习目标

1. **掌握** 临床经济学评价的基本元素和类型。
2. **了解** 成本 - 效果分析的文献评价标准。

第一节 基 本 概 念

在临床实践中,医生和患者不仅需要考虑不同诊疗方式的临床结局,同样需要关注医疗本身及相关成本。我国是一个发展中国家,卫生投入不足,卫生总费用只占国内生产总值(GDP)的 5% 左右。同时我国目前面临严重的人口老龄化问题,以及服务可及性增加、技术进步等因素,我的卫生费用及需求迅速上涨。因此,将经济学的原理和方法应用于医药卫生领域研究具有十分重要的理论及实践意义。政府制定卫生政策需要考虑卫生资源的分配,临床医师起着医疗保健资源利用这扇大门守门人的作用,临床医师面临如何更好地使用这笔钱,每一项检查、每一个治疗方案都需要考虑是否值得、是否具有成本 - 效果。因此,临床医生的医疗实践要有经济学观点,需要从临床结果和资源消耗两方面综合考虑医疗服务,开展相关研究和临床实践,为政府制定相关政策提供循证医学证据。

临床经济学(clinical economics)是指临床医生及相关人员应用经济学的原理和方法评价临床诊断、预防和治疗技术与措施的经济学效果,找出影响合理利用有限资源的因素,为临床医生在临床实践中进行决策提供科学依据。

临床经济学研究的目的是在临床实践中对不断出现的新的诊疗措施进行科学的评价,从对社会是否有利的角度作出经济分析,提出经济学上的依据,达到以最合理有效的方式分配和利用有限的卫生资源的目的。临床医师应熟悉临床经济学评价中的基本概念、掌握临床经济学评价方法,并应用于临床实践。

一、临床经济学评价的基本元素

1. 成本(cost) 指在临床医疗或者卫生服务过程中的投入或资源消耗。一般而言,在临床经济学中,成本包括直接医疗成本、直接非医疗成本、间接成本和隐性成本四类。

(1)直接医疗成本(direct medical cost):指卫生服务过程中用于治疗、预防、保健的成本,包括住院费、药费、诊疗费、实验室检查费、影像检查费、手术费、病房费、康复费等费用。

（2）直接非医疗成本（direct non-medical cost）：指患者因寻求医疗服务而直接消耗的医疗资源以外的资源，如交通费、食宿费、营养食品费等。一般情况下，直接非医疗成本因条件差异大，难以准确计算。因此如果所占比例较小，在研究中可将其忽略。

（3）间接成本（indirect cost）：为社会成本，指由于疾病而丧失的资源。包括与发病率（morbidity）有关的成本、与死亡率（mortality）有关的成本。间接成本的计算有一定的困难，常用的方法包括人力资本法和意愿支付法。人力资本法是用工资率、失业率、期望寿命、退休年龄等计算由于病残或死亡引起的收入的减少。但缺点是不同的人群的收入并不相同，同时对没有收入的老人、儿童、失业者很难测定。意愿支付法，即直接测定由于减少疾病的病残和死亡个人自愿支付的费用。缺点是穷人和富人有不同的支付意愿，个人主观预期结果的大小影响支付意愿。

（4）隐性成本（hidden cost）：指因疾病或实施预防、诊断等医疗服务所引起的疼痛、忧虑、紧张等生理上和精神上的痛苦及不适，如精神损失等。隐性成本也叫无形成本，隐性成本通常不单独测量，因为：①隐性成本难以用货币准确测量，且计量隐性成本本身通常要付出较多的成本；②在测量效用时，隐性成本已被包含在产出的测量中，无需重复测算。

2. 效果（effectiveness）　就是产出测量，指临床医疗或者卫生服务过程中的产出，即医疗结果。广义地讲，效果指医疗或卫生服务方案实施后所取得的结果，可能是好的结果，也可能是不好的结果。狭义地讲，效果指的是好的、有用的结果，也就是能满足人群需要、给人们带来好处或满足感的结果，比如发病率的下降、并发症的减少、死亡率的下降。常用的效果如疗效、生存或者死亡率等。广义的效果包括效用（utility）、效益（benefit）。为便于比较，在评估不同卫生措施的投入产出时，效果转为效益，常用货币单位进行衡量。评估生存或者死亡结果时，如果校正了生命质量，效果转为效用。

二、临床经济学评价的基本类型

1. 最小成本分析（cost minimization analysis，CMA）　也可称为成本最小化分析或成本确定分析（cost identification analysis）。最小成本分析是指测定不同医疗措施的成本并进行成本比较，假定这些措施的效果是相同的，选择最经济、效果最好的措施。例如，围手术期预防应激性溃疡，预防措施为应用抑酸药物，一种措施为静脉应用质子泵抑制剂（PPI），另外一种措施为口服应用。对于可以口服药物的患者，两种方案的疗效相同。但前者成本较高，后者成本很低，所以，口服方案花费最少，但是有同样的效果，应选择口服药物预防围手术期的应激性溃疡。但是这种方法有一定的局限性，只能比较同一种疾病相同效果时的成本，故使用范围较窄。

2. 成本 - 效果分析（cost-effectiveness analysis，CEA）　是分析成本消耗后得到的效果。其表示方法为每一效果单位所耗费的成本（成本 - 效果比）或每一个增加的效果所需要耗费的增量成本（增量成本 - 效果比）等。这就使两种不同的医疗措施，在进行比较选择时，有了相同的评价单位，从而为临床决策提供科学的依据。

（1）成本 - 效果比（cost/effectiveness，C/E）：成本 - 效果比是 CEA 的一种表示方式，即每延长 1 个生命年、挽回 1 例死亡、诊断出 1 个新病例或提高 1 个结果单位所花的成本。通常 C/E 值越小，就越有经济效率，单一的 C/E 值是没有意义的，主要用于两个或两个以上项目的比较，并且是比较有相同结果单位的两个项目。临床上，两项措施的比较常常关注新的措施疗效增加的同时成本的变化。如果新的措施不仅疗效增加，成本也减少，在其他条件相同（如适应证）的情况下，肯定会选择新的措施。如果新的措施疗效增加的同时，成本也增加了，比较两种措施的成本-效果比，即单位效果所付出的成本，选择成本-效果比更低的方案。如果新的措施疗效增加的同时，成本也增加了，并且成本-效果比也高于传统的措施，又如何选择呢？无论从群体或者个体角度看，临床疗效是需要首先考虑的，而成本-效果比只适用于有限的资源用于可以无限放大的群体中。如果希望增加投入来获得更高的产出，如何评判成本-效果分析的结果呢？增量分析可以帮助权衡。

（2）增量成本-效果分析（incremental cost-effectiveness analysis）：由于成本-效果分析包含着对两种或两种以上的措施进行比较，因此成本-效果比还不能充分显示两者的相互关系，故常用增量成本-效果分析表示。通过计算研究组和对照组的成本差值与健康产出差值之比，即增量成本-效果比（incremental cost-effectiveness ratio，ICER），判断研究物相比对照物的经济性优劣，能充分说明由于附加措施导致成本增加时，其相应增加的效果是多少以及是否值得推荐。增量成本-效果比是对卫生干预方案进行经济学评价中最常用的分析指标。在经济学理论中，通常采用边际分析来指导经济决策。在临床经济学评价中，必须报告边际分析的结果，即增量成本-效果分析的结果。

$$\frac{新成本-旧成本}{新效果-旧效果}=\frac{增加的成本}{每一个增加的效果单位}$$

$$\frac{\Delta C}{\Delta E}=\frac{C_N-C_0}{E_N-E_0}$$

ΔC 表示两个方案成本之差，ΔE 为两个方案效果之差，$\Delta C/\Delta E$ 为增量比 C_N 为新成本，C_0 为旧成本，E_N 为新效果，E_0 为旧效果。

ICER 是两组之间成本和产出两个维度的比较，表示研究组相比对照组获得单位健康产出增量所需要支付的成本增量。目前世界贸易组织（WTO）关于成本-效果阈值分析的推荐意见为：当 ICER<人均国内生产总值（GDP）时，可认为增加的成本完全值得，具有成本-效果优势；当人均 GDP<ICER<3 倍人均 GDP 时，认为增加的成本可以接受，具有成本-效果优势；当 ICER>3 倍人均 GDP 时，则认为增加的成本不值得，不具有成本-效果优势。ICER 指标中也体现了对卫生干预方案的净收益的考量。通过 ICER 和阈值进行比较的决策方式，等同于将健康产出通过阈值货币化，然后比较不同方案的净收益。

3. 成本-效用分析（cost-utility analysis，CUA）　成本-效用分析是成本-效果分析的一种特殊形式，其结果的测定是将各个不同方案的不同结果都转化为效用指标，效用值（utility）是根据生理或心理功能对每一种疾病或不同的健康水平进行量化得到的数值，范围为 0~1，完全健康为 1，死亡为 0。通常用质量调整寿命年（quality-adjusted life year，QALY）、伤残调整寿命年（disability-adjusted life year，DALY）来衡量。QALY 可以直接或间接进行测量。直接测量法中的标准博弈法（standard gamble，SG）、时间权衡法（time trade-off，TTO）、视觉模拟评分法（visual analogue scale，VAS）；间接测量法中的欧洲五维健康量表（EQ-5D）、六维健康测量量表（SF-6D）、健康效用指数（health utility index，HUI）和健康质量量表。

4. 成本-效益分析（cost-benefit analysis，CBA）　在比较不同的医疗措施时，除了上述用 QALY 为单位外，将某一项目及医疗服务的所有成本和效果均用货币量为单位表示，就是成本-效益分析。成本-效益分析作为一种经济决策方法，可将其用于政府部门的计划决策中,以寻求在投资决策上如何以最小的成本获得最大的效益。常用于评估需要量化社会效益的公共卫生事业项目的价值。

第二节　成本 - 效果分析的文献评价标准

一、临床经济学评价方法

临床经济学评价方法包括最小成本分析、成本 - 效果分析、成本 - 效用分析、成本 - 效益分析四种类型。表 18-1 回答了两个问题:①是否对两种以上的方案进行了比较;②是否同时检查了每一种方案的成本和效果两个方面。

表 18-1　临床经济学评价方法

维度		是否同时检查了各种方案的成本与效果		
		否		是
		仅检查效果	仅检查成本	
是否对两种或两种以上的方案进行比较	否	1A 部分评价 效果描述	1B 部分评价 成本描述	2 部分评价 成本 - 效果描述
	是	3A 部分评价 效力或效果分析	3B 部分评价 成本分析	4 完整的经济评价 最小成本分析;成本 - 效果分析; 成本 - 效用分析;成本 - 效益分析

二、成本 - 效果分析的文献评价标准

成本 - 效果分析的文献评价标准包括三方面内容,即经济分析的结果是否正确、结果是什么、结果是否适用于患者。

1. 结果是否正确

(1) 是否提供了完整的经济分析?

(2) 是站在何人的立场上进行评价?

(3) 是否比较了所有相关的临床措施?

(4) 成本和效果的测量是否正确?

(5) 成本和效果资料是否进行增量分析?

(6) 是否进行了敏感性分析?

(7) 估计的成本和效果是否来源于干预人群?

2. 结果是什么

(1) 增量成本和效果是多少?

(2) 各亚组增量成本和效果有无不同?

(3) 允许变化的不确定结果是多少?

3. 结果是否适用于患者

(1) 治疗的收益或益处是否超过成本或危害?

(2) 患者是否有相似的临床结果?

(3) 患者是否有相似的成本?

第三节 成本 - 效果分析的循证实践

一、临床案例

患者男性，12岁，以"口干、多饮、多尿3年伴恶心、呕吐2天"为主诉入院，入院后完善相关检查，诊断为1型糖尿病、糖尿病酮症酸中毒，经胰岛素给药、补液、补钾等治疗后好转，后续拟采取进一步措施控制血糖。每日多次注射（multiple daily injection，MDI）胰岛素和持续皮下胰岛素输注（continuous subcutaneous insulin infusion，CSII），采用何种方式？国际青少年糖尿病联盟推荐使用的胰岛素强化治疗方案主要包括MDI和CSII，强化治疗方案能有效控制血糖、改善微血管病变。与MDI相比，CSII能更好地控制血糖，降低糖尿病急性并发症的发生率。但CSII的治疗成本更高。在医疗资源有限且有多种有效治疗方案的情况下，采用哪种方式控制血糖？

二、临床问题

1型糖尿病患者控制血糖，选择每日多次注射胰岛素还是持续皮下胰岛素输注？

三、文献检索

通过输入关键词，可以检索到相应的文献：冷雪霏，杨洪秀，肖敦明，等.青岛地区儿童青少年1型糖尿病持续皮下胰岛素输注与每日多次注射胰岛素治疗的成本效果比较[J].中国卫生资源，2021，24（04）：397-404.DOI：10.13688/j.cnki.chr.2021.200644。

四、文献评价

1. 结果是否正确？ 这一问题强调临床经济学分析是否真实地反映了其中某一项临床措施可能提供更好的成本 - 效果。与其他类型的研究一样，临床经济评价的真实性取决于使用的方法是否正确。

（1）文献提供了完整的经济评价，同时比较了每日多次注射胰岛素和持续皮下胰岛素输注的临床结果和成本。

（2）站在为社会节约资源的角度考虑问题。

（3）对所要比较的方案作了详细的描述。

（4）成本和临床效果都采取了合适的测量和评价方法。临床结果来源于文献分析，包括单一的随机对照临床试验、一系列临床试验的系统复述、临床试验的合成资料（meta分析）等。结果考虑了置信区间，符合实际临床工作情况。

（5）研究进行了增量成本 - 效果分析。

（6）采用单因素和概率敏感性分析。

（7）估计了治疗人群的基线成本 - 效果。

2. 结果是什么？ 每种措施的增量成本和效果是多少？是否针对不同亚组人群中增量成本和效果进行分析？根据单因素敏感性分析及概率敏感性分析结果，判断不确定因素对结果的影响有多大？

通过研究可以得知，模拟60年，对于青岛地区患1型糖尿病的青少年：CSII组的直接医疗成本比 MDI 组高 67 137 元；CSII 组的预期寿命、质量调整寿命年均比 MDI 组高 0.41 年；CSII 组的增量成本 - 效果比为 163 749 元 / 质量调整寿命年，低于 2019 年青岛市地区的人均国内生产总值的 1.5 倍（186 423 元）；CSII 治疗具有性价比。敏感性分析显示，在胰岛素泵价格为 60 000 元、模拟 60 年的情况下，胰岛素泵升级价格降幅越大，ICER 越低。当胰岛素泵升级价格分别下降 10%、20%、30%、40% 和 50% 时，CSII 组的 ICER 均低于 2019 年青岛市人均 GDP 的 1.5 倍。因此，CSII 具有性价比。当以 2019 年青岛市人均 GDP 的 1.5 倍和 3.0 倍为阈值时，CSII 组具有成本 - 效果的概率分别为 62.8% 和 93.7%。

3. 结果是否能用于临床实践？ 在得到了两种措施的经济分析结果以及经济分析的精确性评价之后，需要回答的是，患者是否适用这一结果？给患者选择何种治疗更合理？有两点可以帮助作出选择：一是成本 - 效果分析的增量比，二是患者在多大程度上与经济分析中的病例人群相似。在临床实践中，还需要考虑患者意愿、操作方便程度对选择的影响等循证决策证据之外的要素。

总结来说，临床经济学分析的研究结果可以给医疗卫生支付者和决策者提供重要的参考信息，能帮助优化医疗资源配置，同时也可以促使临床医生在临床诊疗过程中作出更合理的临床决策。

本 章 小 结

临床经济学研究的目的是在临床实践中对不断出现的新的诊疗措施进行科学的评价，从对社会是否有利的角度作出经济分析，提出经济学上的依据，达到以最合理有效的方式分配和利用有限的卫生资源的目的。临床医师应熟悉临床经济学评价中的基本概念，掌握临床经济学评价方法，并应用于临床实践。

（陈世耀）

第十九章

循证决策分析

学习目标

1. **熟悉** 临床决策分析概念与模型。
2. **了解** 如何阅读与评价循证决策分析研究文献。

第一节 临床决策分析概述

临床实践中，待决策的问题往往比较复杂，如某一诊断方法虽然准确性高、可靠性好，但同时费用昂贵或会产生新的创伤；手术治疗虽然可以控制疾病进展，延长患者的寿命，但同时会对健康造成新的、严重的损害，影响患者的生活质量。医生可能会依据临床经验权衡利弊作出治疗决策，但是，这是一种简单的、粗线条的、甚至"含糊"的决策方法。有时交给患者或者家属去决定，即使医生告知各种诊断以及治疗方式的好处和风险及相关数据，患者及家属会综合考虑治疗效果及自身的经济承受能力做决定，但这同样是非定量的、非科学的临床决策方法。这两种临床常用的决策方式难以全面考虑和准确衡量各方面因素对结局的影响，也就难以给出具有说服力的答案。这里要讨论的是建立在定量分析基础上的决策，它可以帮助医生更全面、更系统、更科学地分析和解决决策问题。那么，在临床经济学中，应该如何更准确地判断疾病诊断，合理选择诊断试验？如何更加综合地、客观地评价治疗的利弊？

决策（decision-making）是为解决目前所面临的问题，从若干可选行动方案中选择最佳行动方案的过程。临床医生需要随时为患者的诊断、治疗作出临床决定。这些临床决定亦即临床决策（clinical decision）。科学的决策强调根据有关研究结果，在充分收集所有诊治方案的科学证据的基础上，通过建立模型，使用合理的定量分析方法，充分评估不同方案的风险和效益，将各备选方案的不确定性及利弊有机地整合在一起进行综合比较，实现定量决策，以减少临床不确定性和利用有限资源取得最大效益的过程，这也是一直强调的用循证医学的思维方法进行临床决策，即循证决策分析过程。

第二节　决策分析的实施

一、决策分析的基本步骤

循证决策过程包括以下 5 个基本步骤：①提出需要解决的临床问题；②文献检索；③建立模型，分析比较预期结果；④选择方案与实施方案；⑤后效评价。决策可以针对一个具体的患者，通过决策分析为患者选择最佳处理措施，也可以针对属性相同的群体，通过决策分析确定一线或者首选处理措施、备选处理措施。

二、构建决策分析模型

决策树模型和 Markov 模型是临床最常用的两种决策分析模型。决策树模型最为常用，尤其在急性病或短期项目的决策分析中；在慢性病的决策分析中更多选择 Markov 模型。针对复杂临床问题，可联合决策树和 Markov 模型。

1. 决策树模型　决策树模型分析的步骤包括：①根据临床问题明确分析目的；②根据临床实践经验和文献阅读评价确定备选方案；③列出每一方案所有可能出现的重要的临床结局；④建立决策树模型；⑤依据文献资料确定分析时间框架和决策的评定标准；⑥确定每个方案的各种临床结局发生的概率；⑦明确结果指标及各种临床结局的损益值；⑧综合分析并评价方案；⑨对分析中所用参数可能存在的不确定性进行敏感性分析。

图 19-1 显示了决策树模型分析原理。

最右端的三角形表示最终结局，痊愈、健康生存的效用值为 1.0；死亡为 0；因为全胃切除对患者的生活质量有严重影响，效用值为 0.6；但对于非胃癌患者，手术后生活质量受影响的程度略轻，效用值为 0.8。按时间顺序从左到右画出树状结构，每个分枝代表在一段时间内的一个临床结果或决策。用不同的节点代表决策、临床转归或最终结局。通常用小方格表示决策点，代表决策者欲比较不同的方案，决策点发出的分枝代表所比较的不同方案，圆圈所示节点常称为概率节点，概率节点发出的分枝代表可能出现的事件或临床结局。

决策树分析需要根据具体疾病确定时间框架，分析期通常为一个疾病周期。接下来，确定各种临床结局的损益值，即对各种结果进行量化，建立决策树后，计算期望效用值，它的计算从决策树分枝的最右端开始，将概率和效用值相乘，再将一个节点上各分枝的数值相加，从右到左逐级进行，直到最后计算出每个方案的期望效用。

另外，需要对模型进行敏感性分析、阈值分析。缺少相关研究提供分析所需的参数是引起决策分析的不确定性的主要原因，也是影响临床决策结果可靠性的重要因素。敏感性分析可以每次仅对一个因素进行（单因素敏感性分析），也可以同时分析两个或者所有因素的共同作用（两因素敏感性分析、概率敏感性分析），分析的范围应根据临床数据的来源而定。

2. Markov 模型　慢性病的自然发展过程中存在疾病不同状态之间相互转换过程，但总的趋势是病情逐渐加重，发生并发症并最终导致死亡。决策树分析并不合适，Markov 模型适用于分析慢性病中反复发作的临床事件。Markov 模型分析需要进行大量的计算，可以采用相关的决策分析软件如 TreeAge Pro 等。

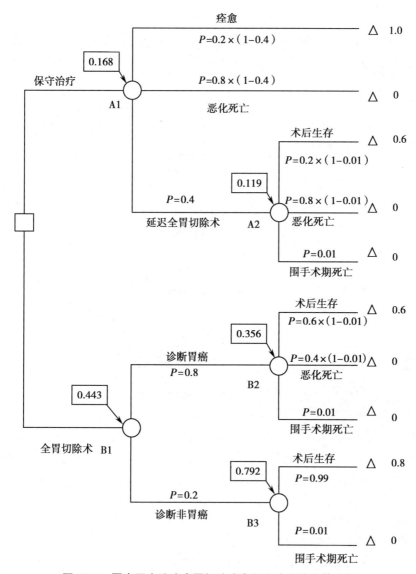

图 19-1 胃内巨大溃疡全胃切除或者保守治疗的决策分析

Markov 模型决策分析的原理是将所研究的疾病按其对健康的影响程度划分为几个不同的健康状态，并根据各自状态在一定时间内相互间的转换概率，结合每个状态上的资源消耗和健康结果，通过多次循环运算，估计出疾病发展的健康结局或费用。应用 Markov 模型进行决策分析的步骤包括以下几点。

（1）根据研究目的和疾病的自然转归设立 Markov 状态，确定各状态间可能存在的相互转换。通常根据研究目的和疾病的自然转归将整个疾病过程划分为几个不同的健康状态，即所谓的 Markov 状态。将所有可能发生的事件模拟成从一个状态向另一个状态转换的过程，并将所要分析的期间划分为相同的时间周期，称为 Markov 循环周期。在每个循环周期中，患者可能从一个状态转移到另一个状态。Markov 模型决策分析的原理如图 19-2 所示，在预防肝硬化食管静脉曲张破裂出血的决策分析中，图中六个 Markov 状态分别为：发生再出血之后的综合治疗状态（comprehensive state，再次内镜治疗或者再次 TIPSS 的综合治疗状态)、没有再出血以及肝性脑病的稳定状态(well)、单纯再出血状态(RB)、单纯肝性脑病状态(HE)、再出血以及肝性脑病同时存在的状态(RB+HE)以及死亡状态(death)。图中状态间的箭头表示患者在一个循环周期中可从一个状态转移到另一个状态。

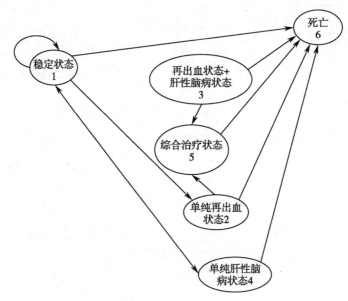

图 19-2　六状态 Markov 模型

（2）确定循环周期和每个周期中各状态间的转换概率。Markov 循环周期的时间长短通常根据临床意义设定。如肝硬化食管静脉曲张破裂出血，常用 1 年作为一个循环周期。确定了 Markov 状态及循环周期后，结合有关的临床研究或流行病学调查结果，估计出患者在各状态上停留的时间或转换到另一个状态的可能性。以后每个循环中状态间的转移概率可以是固定不变的，也可根据疾病的实际情况确定不同的转移概率。

（3）确定各健康状态的效用值。同样可根据具体疾病对患者的影响以及具体状态，以时间、疗效、安全性、生命质量和经济学指标分别制定。

（4）通过运算估计整个分析期的效用。首先计算出每个循环周期内各状态的分布概率。依据不同状态的概率和效用值计算每次循环的效用值和累积效用值。

（5）敏感性分析。与决策树分析一样，Markov 模型分析也应在基线分析的基础上进行敏感性分析，以判断分析结果的稳定性以及影响分析结果的主要不确定因素。

第三节　怎样阅读和评价决策分析研究的文献

对决策分析文献的评价与其他研究相似，应从以下几方面进行综合考虑。

一、研究设计是否合理，分析结果是否真实可靠

1. 所评价的方案是否包括了所有的重要策略和临床结局？　首先应明确决策树中有多少不同的选择措施，Markov 模型中有怎样的疾病状态转换，是否包括了所有的重要策略和临床结局。

2. 进行比较的临床方案是否为临床常用的方案？　在决策分析时，研究者不仅应指出对哪些临床策略进行比较，还应该对所比较的各种临床策略进行详细地描述。阐述方案各自的优点、缺点，说明比较的理由和存在临床选择困难的情况。

3. 是否考虑了所有有关的临床结果？　临床决策分析研究应建立在患者或者全社会的立场上，即应包括所有重要的临床收益和风险。应确信模型中所反映的权衡是当前患者以及社会所关注的，如治疗效果、不良反应、生活质量、成本 - 效果、依从性等。

4. 是否用明确的、合理的方法获得并确定分析所需的参数？　进行决策分析需要综合大量信息，研究者需检索文献、咨询专家和访问患者。首先需要全面检索文献，评价这些研究的真实性、有效性和一致性等，并进一步用定量分析方法（如 meta 分析等）估计临床事件发生的可能性或概率，并将这些概率分配到分析模型中各节点的分支上。决策分析应说明所用概率的文献检索情况、来源和推算方法，并将有关文献列出。

5. 效用值的设定是否合理，来源是否可靠？　效用值代表了决策分析中各种结局的定量测定值。作者应在文中说明赋值的方法。对可能的结局和效用值设定的情况了解得越清楚，效用值的赋值方法越可靠。

6. 在数据的选择上是否存在任何可能影响结果的不确定因素？是否进行了敏感性分析？敏感性分析是否合理？　决策分析所用的参数大多来自于已发表的研究结果，这些结果常存在估计不精确的问题，通常表现为置信区间很宽。应仔细了解作者对哪些因素和在哪些范围内作敏感性分析，并明确这些分析是否合理。

二、评价决策分析结果

在确定决策分析的方法合理、结果可靠的基础上，应进一步明确该研究所建议的方案可能给患者带来多大的收益，获得收益的可信度如何。

1. 在基线分析中得到的评价结果是什么？　基线分析（baseline analysis）指在分析中设定的概率或其他参数是分析者认为最佳的估计值，即最接近总体水平的估计值。决策分析是通过比较各方案可能获得的总的"期望效用"，选择效用最大的方案作为推荐的最佳方案。

2. 在分析中所用的证据强度如何？证据的不确定性是否会影响决策分析的结果？　选取研究设计较完善、方法可靠、质量较高的研究结果作为估计值。同时对模型重要参数进行敏感性分析。

三、研究结果的应用

如果研究各方面执行较好且临床患者情况与文献分析中的研究对象相符，那么，研究结论可以用于帮助临床医生进行临床决策。

第四节　循证临床决策分析案例

一、临床案例

患者男性，52 岁，肝炎肝硬化，食管胃静脉曲张破裂出血，肝功能 Child-Pugh B 级，经过积极补充血容量、降低门静脉压力、抑制胃酸、止血等药物治疗后出血停止。为了预防再出血，应该选择何种治疗？

通过查阅相关文献可以发现，肝硬化性门静脉高压患者发生食管胃静脉曲张破裂出血后，1 年再出血率在 50% 以上，出血死亡的风险也很高。药物治疗效果欠佳，手术治疗有诸多限制及弊端，内镜套扎联合药物治疗（EVL+β-B）和经颈静脉肝内门腔内支架分流（transjugular intrahepatic portosystemic stent-shunt, TIPSS）是临床医生为多数患者做出的选择，针对疗效、不良反应以及治疗费用，临床医师如何为患者推荐治疗措施？

二、临床问题

肝炎肝硬化门静脉脉高压食管胃静脉曲张出血患者，选择内镜联合药物治疗还是 TIPSS？

三、文献检索

通过检索相关数据库，可以检索到相应的文献：李莹，练晶晶，罗添成，等 . 预防肝硬化食管静脉曲张再出血的成本效果研究[J]. 中华消化杂志，2016，36（02）：113-118。

四、研究过程及研究结果

参考本章第三节进行文献评价（表 19-1）。得出结论：7 年的基线模拟研究结果显示（图 19-3），EVL+β-B 的期望花费为 7 444.25 美元 / 人，可以获得 1.98 个质量调整寿命年。覆膜支架 TIPSS 的期望花费为 13 151.69 美元 / 人，能够获得 2.34 个质量调整寿命年。在第 7 年，ICER=16 001.74 美元 /QALY，基于中国的意愿性支付阈值（WTP=3GDP，19 887 美元）可以得出，覆膜支架 TIPSS 较内镜套扎联合药物治疗有成本 - 效果优势。覆膜支架的价格在不大于 33 627.04 美元引入中国市场是具有成本 - 效果的。

表 19-1 1 年、3 年、5 年、7 年的基线分析结果

治疗方案	时间	成本 / 美元	LY	QALY	CER LY/ 美元 每 LY 每 QALY
EVL+β-B	1 年	4 492.47	0.95	0.64	
TIPSS		10 175.96	0.94	0.64	—
EVL+β-B	3 年	6 188.65	2.12	1.41	
TIPSS		11 560.49	2.25	1.51	42 655.63 55 963.19
EVL+β-B	5 年	7 026.18	2.71	1.79	
TIPSS		12 513.84	3.04	2.03	16 841.08 23 469.50
EVL+β-B	7 年	7 444.25	3.00	1.98	
TIPSS		13 151.69	3.51	2.34	11 274.48 16 001.74

单因素敏感性分析的结果（图 19-4）显示，内镜套扎联合药物治疗的再出血率是对 ICER 影响最大的因素，其次是 TIPSS 治疗的花费、肝性脑病效用值等。因此，选择内镜治疗，临床需要不断提高内镜治疗的效果；选择 TIPSS，支架费用是影响选择的重要因素，国家可以采用集中采购控制和降低支架等耗材费用。

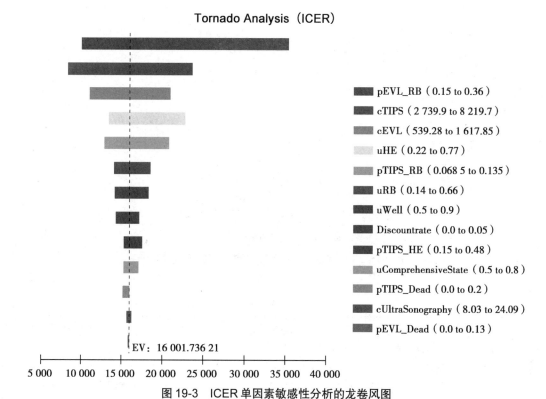

图 19-3　ICER 单因素敏感性分析的龙卷风图

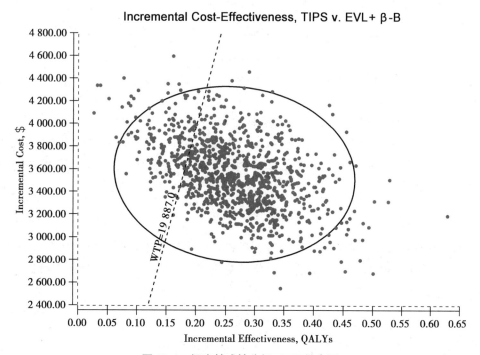

图 19-4　概率敏感性分析 ICER 散点图

　　研究进行了两因素敏感性分析（图 19-5）及阈值分析（表 19-2），结果显示，覆膜支架的价格不高于 5 401.52 美元时，TIPSS 具有成本 - 效果。

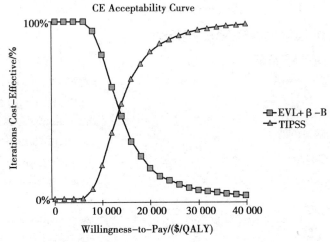

图 19-5　概率敏感性分析成本 - 效果可接受性曲线

表 19-2　阈值分析结果

变量	基线值	成本 - 效果分析阈值
内镜治疗组再出血风险	0.25	0.21
TIPSS 组再出血风险	0.10	0.13
覆膜支架价格	4 015.74 美元	5 401.52 美元
TIPSS 治疗花费	5 479.80 美元	6 865.58 美元
内镜套扎治疗花费	1 078.57 美元	658.63 美元
肝性脑病效用值	0.55	0.35

　　另外，研究进行了概率敏感性分析，通过 Monte Carlo 模拟运算，增量成本 - 效果图（图 19-4）显示，在中国意愿性支付阈值为 19 887 美元时，83% 的模拟显示 TIPSS 是具有成本 - 效果的。

　　由概率敏感性分析可接受性曲线（图 19-5）可以看出，若 WTP>13 920.9 美元 /QALY 时，大于 50% 的模拟显示 TIPSS 是具有成本 - 效果的。当 WTP 大于 39 774 美元 /QALY 时，大于 98% 的模拟显示 TIPSS 是具有成本 - 效果的，即几乎所有的患者进行 TIPSS 治疗都是具有成本 - 效果的。

本 章 小 结

　　决策分析在临床处理疾病的每一过程中，循证临床决策不仅让医疗工作者合理选择诊断措施，更让医疗工作者在处理患者时避免模糊和经验的处理方式，使临床决策更科学，患者利益和社会利益最大化。

（陈世耀）

第二十章

循证医学推动社会进步

学习目标

了解 现场调查、问卷调查、模拟试验、决策与推进观念及法规变化等循证实践过程。

中国机动车保有量正在逐年快速增长，伴随着交通事故频发，每年都有儿童乘客因故死亡，儿童道路交通伤害正成为一个重要的公共卫生问题。

循证医学实践并不局限于医疗决策的制定与施行，基于证据的更新和资料的收集生成的评估结果也能推进对于社会问题的理解、现行规定的反思，能充当法规制定的参考与佐证，从各个方面为患者健康及社会和谐服务。服务于人群的循证实践，需要明确现实存在的公共问题，通过调查研究分析问题、生成证据以推动观念变化并转化为法规，从而推动社会进步。

第一节 案 例 背 景

世界卫生组织（WHO）估计，到 2030 年道路交通伤害在全球疾病负担中将从 2004 年的第 9 位上升到第 3 位。2000 年我国 0～4 岁儿童因道路交通伤害死亡 10 642 人，5～14 岁儿童死亡 16 034 人。

资料显示，截至 2009 年底，全国机动车驾驶人为 1.997 7 亿人。随着我国汽车保有量的增加，如何防治儿童乘客伤害的问题将日益突显。开展儿童乘客安全研究是一项关于儿童乘客安全装置标准、规定、设计、伤害预防和法规制定上的重要课题。

第二节 提 出 问 题

这是中国儿童安全座椅约束装置和安全带使用与儿童道路交通意外伤害风险性的关系问题。

回答这个问题前，必须弄清楚以下几个问题。

1. 中国儿童乘客的实际乘坐方式如何？
2. 影响中国儿童安全座椅约束装置使用的因素有哪些？
3. 不同儿童座位或约束装置的使用和儿童道路交通意外伤害的发生有何相关性？

第三节 现场调查

一、中国儿童乘客的实际乘坐方式

我国缺乏对儿童乘客安全实践的直接观察研究,为了解国内儿童乘客的实际乘坐情况,研究者于 2009 年在上海进行了横断面观察性研究,通过对上海 G2 高速公路收费站路边车辆进行观察,了解儿童乘客的实际乘坐座位位置、约束装置的使用率和影响因素。研究者观察了 3 个上午 9—11 时的时间段,发现通过的车辆 93% 是小轿车,其余车辆占 7%,10% 的小轿车中有儿童乘客。二项回归法分别计算座位位置中正确的后排座位和其他座位位置的校正相对危险度(risk ratio, RR)值,比较有无约束装置使用的 RR 值(表 20-1)。

表 20-1 2009 年上海儿童乘客使用约束装置或正确后排座位的危险度

变量	危险度（95% 置信区间）			
	正确的后排座位		约束装置	
	未校正	校正	未校正	校正
年龄				
≤4 岁	**0.36（0.28～0.45）** $P<0.000\,1$	**0.35（0.28～0.44）** $P<0.000\,1$	0.73（0.39～1.36）	0.91（0.43～1.93）
>4 岁（参照）				
性别				
男	0.92（0.82～1.03）	0.96（0.87～1.06）	1.05（0.82～1.35）	1.07（0.65～1.75）
女（参照）				
使用安全带				
否	1.04（0.90～1.21）	0.99（0.87～1.12）	**0.09（0.01～0.64）** $P=0.016\,2$	**0.09（0.01～0.60）** $P=0.013\,7$
是（参照）				
车内儿童数				
一个	**0.74（0.64～0.85）** $P<0.000\,1$	**0.84（0.74～0.96）** $P=0.012\,4$	3.52（0.50～24.94）	3.33（0.55～20.01）
多个（参照）	0.94（0.72～1.22）	1.00（0.87～1.15）	0.94（0.49～1.81）	1.03（0.57～1.86）
后排座位				
否	n/a	n/a	1.11（0.67～1.84）	0.89（0.49～1.61）
是（参照）				
约束装置				
否	1.05（0.8～1.35）	1.07（0.82～1.39）	n/a	n/a
是（参照）				
成人乘客同行				
否	**0.77（0.57～1.04）** $P=0.083\,4$	**0.66（0.49～0.89）** $P=0.006\,6$	**5.09（2.94～8.82）** $P<0.000\,1$	**5.28（2.86～9.76）** $P<0.000\,1$
是（参照）				

注:儿童乘客由成人怀抱的后排乘坐不计入后排座位一栏中。

研究发现：在上海，高速公路上儿童前排乘坐较常见，约束装置使用率低。被成人怀抱的儿童乘客占 35.6%。不使用安全带的驾驶员驾驶的小轿车中儿童乘客使用安全装置的可能性低于同行使用安全带的司机（RR 为 0.09；95%CI 0.01～0.60）。除了驾驶员外，车内只有儿童时使用约束装置的可能性高于有同行成人的儿童乘客（RR 为 5.28；95%CI 2.86～9.76）。年幼的儿童（年龄≤4 岁）或车内若只有驾驶员时，儿童乘客较少被安排在后排乘坐（RR 为 0.35；95%CI 0.28～0.44。RR 为 0.66；95%CI 0.49～0.89）。单独出行的儿童后排乘坐的可能性低于有同行小伙伴的儿童乘客（RR 为 0.84；95%CI 0.74～0.96）。因此，正确乘坐座位位置、约束装置的使用可以显著降低儿童乘客的伤害风险。

二、中国儿童乘客安全装置使用的影响因素

为了解究竟哪些因素影响了儿童乘坐座位位置和约束装置的使用，研究者于 2008 年 10 月至 2009 年 10 月期间，随机选择了上海市松江区和浦东区的 5 家幼儿园进行家长问卷调查，通过家长问卷调查儿童家长对儿童乘客安全知识的掌握情况，进一步探究目前儿童乘客的主要乘坐方式以及影响儿童乘客安全的相关因素。

共有 1 010 位家长参加了问卷调查，参与率 100%。最终的统计数据含 970 位 3～7 岁儿童，由于乘坐座位、家长受教育水平和家庭收入等信息不全排除 40 位（5%）儿童，纳入和排除的儿童基本特征相似。研究发现 60.8% 的被调查者未使用安全装置，年龄≤4 岁的儿童和男童未使用安全装置的比例分别为 44.0% 和 56.0%。78.0% 的家长听说过儿童安全座椅等安全装置，但实际只有 57 份问卷表示拥有该类装备，约占 5.9%，曾使用者只有 12 例，约占 1.2%。29.4%（n=285）的儿童几乎每天乘坐小轿车，儿童乘客后排乘坐率为 83.1%（n=806），39.2%（n=380）的儿童曾使用某种形式的安全装置。

低龄儿童（≤4 岁）在前排乘坐的可能性更大（RR 为 0.82；95%CI 0.77～0.87）。相对于无驾照家长而言，有驾照的家长不愿意报告孩子在后排乘坐（RR 为 0.95；95%CI 0.91～0.99），但倾向于报告其孩子使用约束装置（RR 为 1.44；95%CI 1.18～1.75）。受过高等教育的家长更倾向于报告孩子在后排乘坐和使用约束装置（RR 为 1.08；95%CI 1.03～1.13）（表 20-2）。问卷调查发现家长对怀抱儿童乘坐以及安全气囊的影响等有认识误区；儿童乘客后排乘坐率较高，约束装置使用率低，提示家长缺乏儿童乘客安全方面的知识。

表 20-2　上海 2008—2009 年家长问卷调查儿童乘客车内使用约束装置或后排座位的危险度

变量	危险度（95% 置信区间）			
	后排座位		约束装置	
	未校正	校正	未校正	校正
年龄				
≤4 岁	**0.83（0.78～0.88）**	**0.82（0.77～0.87）**	1.05（0.90～1.23）	1.04（0.89～1.21）
>4 岁（参照）				
儿童性别				
男	1.03（0.97～1.09）	1.04（0.99～1.09）	1.06（0.91～1.25）	1.04（0.89～1.22）
女（参照）				

变量	危险度（95% 置信区间）			
	后排座位		约束装置	
	未校正	校正	未校正	校正
家长驾照				
有	0.96（0.90～1.01）	**0.95（0.91～0.99）**	**1.48（1.22～1.79）**	**1.44（1.18～1.75）**
无（参照）				
家庭收入				
高	1.05（0.99～1.11）	1.00（0.96～1.05）	1.17（0.99～1.37）	1.06（0.89～1.26）
不详	0.94（0.72～1.22）	1.00（0.87～1.15）	0.94（0.49～1.81）	1.03（0.57～1.86）
低（参照）				
父母高等教育				
是	1.03（0.97～1.09）	**1.08（1.03～1.13）**	1.16（0.99～1.36）	1.08（0.91～1.28）
否（参照）				

三、儿童乘坐方式与交通安全性的验证

不同儿童座位或约束装置的使用和儿童道路交通意外伤害的发生有何相关性呢？国外研究发现交通事故中坐在车内前排不使用任何约束装置的儿童受伤风险最高，坐在后排使用合适约束装置的儿童风险最小；不使用约束装置的儿童受伤风险要较使用约束装置的儿童高 3 倍以上。司机后面的位置比后排右侧的位置死亡风险下降 8.1%，后排中间的位置死亡风险最低，仅 0.27%，比司机的死亡风险低 65%～71%，相对危险度最低的是后排中间位置，为 0.29，最高的是后排右边的位置 0.35，尤其是在翻滚的时候。虽然后排乘坐可以降低儿童乘客伤害的风险，但使用约束装置的安全效果更好，儿童乘客使用约束装置坐在后排中间位置又比右侧降低 43% 的风险。国外一项对 11 506 次车祸中的 17 980 名儿童乘客的调查发现，单纯后排乘坐的安全性小于使用约束装置的安全性，前排乘坐对比后排乘坐增加了 40% 的伤害风险（OR 为 1.4；95% CI，1.2～1.7）。

采用 MADYMO 软件模拟车辆碰撞试验，研究者对问卷的部分内容和高速公路观察到的常见儿童乘坐方式进行了验证，评价儿童乘客不同乘坐方式的安全性。发现儿童乘客在后排正确使用合适的安全座椅的保护效果最佳，最不安全的乘坐方式是儿童在前排由成人怀抱。

第四节　推进社会观念和法规变化

一、国外儿童乘客乘坐位置和使用安全装置的有关证据

各国对儿童乘客采用约束手段的普及率存在一定的差异，目前在欧美国家都有相关法律规定儿童乘车必须使用儿童乘客约束系统。同时对儿童约束系统以及在车辆中的安装固定，美国、欧洲、日本等国家和地区也都建立了完整的法规体系，包括美国 FMVSS 213、欧

洲 ECE R44 号法规等。亚洲的日本、韩国、新加坡等国家和地区也都已有相关立法。国际上许多国家的经验显示,立法是预防儿童乘客伤害的一种有力手段,可将其视为对保证儿童乘客安全承诺的检验。

1997 年美国交通安全委员会推荐每个州修订儿童乘客安全法,强制儿童后排乘坐,到 2004 年有 7 个州通过了儿童后排乘坐的法案。美国北卡罗来纳州 1985 年通过《前排乘客安全带法》后,4～15 岁儿童乘客死亡和严重伤害发生率下降了 42%。密歇根州《儿童安全座椅法》颁布后,儿童乘客受伤住院率下降了 36%,头部外伤发生率下降了 25%,4 岁以下儿童乘客受伤的比例下降了 25%。新墨西哥州《安全座椅法》颁布后,5 岁以下儿童乘客的死亡率下降了 33%,非致命性伤害发生率下降了 12.5%。这些经验充分说明针对儿童和青少年采用恰当的干预措施可以显著降低他们在道路交通伤害中的死亡率和致残率,实践表明使用儿童乘客约束系统(儿童安全座椅)、加高座椅、改良安全带以及让儿童后排乘坐等措施可有效地减少儿童乘客致命性和非致命性的伤害风险。

二、循证医学促进我国对儿童乘客安全的关注

我国已是世界第一大新车消费国,因此对儿童乘客安全的关注应进一步提升。循证医学实践的结果能够协助阐明问题,促进观念的变化并引起重视。恰当的干预措施可以显著降低儿童和青少年在道路交通伤害中的死亡率和致残率,我国应该继续努力制定和改进儿童乘客安全法律,加强社区和家长教育促进儿童乘客的安全。

结合儿童乘客安全实践的直接观察数据、上海家长乘车安全问卷调查以及模拟车辆碰撞试验,研究结果能够促进社会问题的发现,从而推动观念改变,有助于法律法规的制定和修改。2012 年 7 月 1 日,我国第一部关于机动车儿童座椅约束装置的强制性国家标准——《机动车儿童乘员用约束系统》(GB 27887—2011)正式实施,其将有助于提高公众对于儿童乘车安全的重视;此外,也将对儿童安全座椅生产企业、汽车整车制造企业产生强有力的约束。2014 年 3 月 1 日起,新修订的《上海市未成年人保护条例》正式实施,条例规定,携带未满 4 周岁的未成年人乘坐家庭乘用车,应配备并正确使用儿童安全座椅;携带未满 12 周岁的未成年人乘坐家庭乘用车的,不得安排其乘坐在副驾驶座位。

本 章 小 结

循证医学推进社会发展。循证医学中,医疗决策包括医疗政策的制定等应在现有的最好的临床研究基础上作出,强调证据的与时俱进、不断更新,收集充分的、可信的资料,形成评估结果,再根据评估结果提出政策、法规的制定方法或建议,从而最终保证患者的利益,取得最佳的效果。与临床实践以患者个体为中心不同,公共卫生领域的实践对象是人群。在公共卫生领域中,为了找出某种事件的原因以及相关因素,构建恰当的需要回答的问题更为重要。医疗行为或某些决策的干预会引起关注,不论是医生还是患者都会提出对干预的进一步疑惑,应通过临床实践和研究判断医疗干预会对患者带来怎样的影响,这就需要通过循证医学的步骤来阐明。

本章节从循证的角度,提出儿童道路交通伤害这一重要的公共卫生问题,通过对中国儿童乘客的实际乘坐方式、家长问卷调查探讨儿童乘客安全的影响因素,模拟车辆碰撞试验实践评价儿童乘客不同乘坐方式的安全性,说明儿童安全座椅约束装置和安全带的使用与儿童道路交通意外伤害风险性的关系,并进一步结合国际上的立法等干预措施后对我

国儿童道路交通伤害现状进行改善，推进制定和改进儿童乘客安全法律，促进儿童乘客的安全。

循证医学对社会工作的开展乃至推动社会进步都有着重要的启示意义。循证医学重视研究证据的积累，缩短了研究与实践的距离。循证实践是推动社会发展并获得社会认同的一个可能策略，将日常主要以常识、经验为指导的实践，转化为主要以科学理论为指导的实践，最终实现社会进步。

（潘曙明）

1

Introduction

Learning objectives

1. **To master** definition and concepts of evidence-based medicine; steps in practicing evidence-based medicine; significance and influencing factors of individualized clinical decision making.
2. **To be familiar with** individualization: the combination of science and art.
3. **To know** approaches to individualized practice with this book and other relevant tools.

1.1 Definition and concept of evidence-based medicine

Evidence-based medicine refers to clinical medicine that follows evidence. It is the application of clinical epidemiology theory and methodology in clinical practice based on available evidence. The core concept entails a conscientious, explicit and judicious use of current best evidence from scientific researches in making decisions about patient care, with full consideration of patients' preference. The notion of evidence-based medicine was first proposed by Sackett and his colleagues as a novel medical concept, which integrates best research evidence, clinical expertise, and patient values into making clinical decisions for patient care. In 1991, one of the founding fathers of evidence-base medicine, Dr. Gordon Guyatt, coined the term "evidence-based medicine", which lead to the birth of Cochrane Collaboration and Cochrane systemic reviews, promoting the use of evidence-based medicine in making clinical decisions with the consensus of experts and the general recommendation of clinical practice guidelines. With the continuous development of modern medicine, accumulation of information and innovation of technology, clinical physicians encounter various challenges, such as how to choose an appropriate diagnostic method? How to provide patients with a safe, cost-effective treatment plan? How to accurately predict patient prognosis? In other words, it is also the core task of evidence-based medicine how to obtain clinical research results and practice evidence-based medicine after scientific evaluation to better serve patients.

Evidence-based medicine aims to integrate multiple evidences to form a comprehensive strategy to solve clinical problems. Evidence-based analysis of risk factors can provide insight to preventing the development and progression of disease; evidence-based analysis of early diagnosis can improve diagnostic accuracy; evidence-based analysis of different treatment methods can guide the selection of a more effective treatment plan; evidence-based analysis of disease prognosis can improve patient prognosis and quality of life; evidence-based analysis of medications can promote healthcare management and scientific decisions.

In 2006, Gordon Guyatt proposed five developmental directions in evidence-based medicine, which are still instructive nowadays.

1.1.1 Access to the latest evidence-based medicine resources

In today's information age, the biggest challenge clinicians face is how to formulate the most effective treatment plan for individual patients in a short period of time. Best evidence-based medicine resources are like an onion that needs to be peeled back layer by layer. In some cases, clinicians can make a clinical decision based on evidence-based recommendations in guidelines; at other times clinicians may need to dive deeper and consider different evidential strengths. If the evidential strength is weak, further exploration of systemic reviews may be warranted to view related evidence and conduct systematic review. Meanwhile, even though there are recommendations provided by guidelines and also integrated electronic resources such as UpToDate, Clinical Evidence, where deep information can be easily accessible, new evidence continues to renew itself. Therefore, clinical medicine should keep up with development frontiers. Artificial intelligence (AI) may be a solution but still needs to be adjusted with individuals.

1.1.2 Development of evidence-based guidelines

Evidence-based practice focuses on overturning the reliance on expert recommendations and providing clinicians with an unprecedented autonomy in interpreting and employing evidence in clinical practice. Evidence-based practice guidelines require experts to formulate in accordance with the norms. The process of guideline development includes: identifying an answerable question; defining clear eligibility criteria for literature searches; conducting systemic comprehensive searches; judging the methodology quality of relevant studies; appraising recommendations of evidences. It has become a consensus to formulate guidelines in accordance with GRADE standards. The formulation of guidelines should combine local policies and population characteristics. Guidelines evaluation usually applies AGREE II for quality evaluation.

1.1.3 Ensuring evidence-based practice

Although evidence-based medicine (EBM) advanced clinical practice into a new era, clinical guidelines alone cannot guarantee standardized clinical practice. How to enable clinicians to use high-quality evidence in clinical practice should be a problem that is worth attention of every country during social advancement of evidence-base medicine.

1.1.4 Ensuring clinical decisions are consistent with patients' values and preferences

The third element of evidence-based medicine is to fully consider patients' values and preferences. Given the same clinical problem, different patients may have different considerations based on their religion, environment or lifestyle.

1.1.5 Incorporating evidence-based principles into healthcare policies

Incorporation of evidence-based principles into healthcare policy research by combining healthcare technology assessment and cost-effective analyses will aid the development and establishment of healthcare policies.

1.2 Evidence and evidence evaluation

Evidence includes basic research evidence, clinical research evidence, and group research evidence. In clinical practice, evidence-based medicine pays more attention to clinical research evidence from the clinic targeting patients.

According to the type of clinical research, evidence can be divided into original research reports, such as case reports, case-control studies, cohort studies, randomized controlled clinical trials, and secondary research evidence, such as systematic reviews and meta-analysis, clinical guidelines, and database-based clinical studies. The practical experience of clinicians is also a kind of evidence. Evidence from simple clinical practice experience is very weak, but the combination of literature results and clinical practice experience is often more credible than the literature itself.

Evidence can be obtained through literature search, and there are a series of literature search strategies to help clinicians quickly obtain the evidence they need. But there is so much literature and evaluation which requires lots of time and efforts. A convenient method is to directly search for the latest clinical guidelines, systematic reviews published after the guidelines, and original studies published after the systematic reviews. This strategy not only omits the evaluation of the guidelines and systematic reviews including a large number of literatures, but also obtains results of the latest clinical researches.

Application of evidence obtained from the original study or the secondary study in evidence-based clinical practice needs to be evaluated. Evidence evaluation includes publication standards and application standards, and the latter is more emphasized in clinical practice. For example, evaluation of diagnostic test pays more attention to whether the gold standard and the diagnostic test are accepted at the same time and whether blinding is performed. As to intervention studies, it is focused on whether control is set, whether there is randomization and randomization concealment, whether the measurement is blinded, or whether measurement can be repeated. As to prognostic researches, it is concerned whether two cohorts for survival analysis have the same start point, whether the outcome setting is reasonable and measured by objective standard means, whether there are losses to follow-up, whether confounding factors affect the prognosis, etc.

The classification of evidence level and credibility is based on the type of clinical research, as well as various factors such as sample size and population representativeness. Clinical decision-making is usually not based on the evidence provided by the results of a single study, but on studies of multiple approaches (basic, clinical, and population studies), multiple research types (case-control, cohort studies, randomized controlled clinical trials, researches based on real-world data, meta-analysis, etc.).

1.3 Practicing evidence-based medicine

Evidence-based clinical practice emphasizes that it is necessary to follow the evidence and recommend the latest and best evidence evaluated and suitable for the patient no matter for diagnosis, treatment or prevention.

Practicing evidence-based medicine includes five steps.

1.3.1 Formulating a clinical question that needs to be answered and turning it into a scientific question is the most critical step in successfully answering clinical controversial questions. For example, a 40 -year-old male patient was diagnosed with early gastric cancer according to gastroscopy and pathology. Ultrasound gastroscopy showed the gastric cancer was located in the mucosal layer. How to treat it is a general problem, but the specific question is whether to perform endoscopic submucosal dissection or laparoscopic resection. In a scientific word, can endoscopic submucosal dissection replace laparoscopic resection?

1.3.2 Searching for effective evidence, that is, obtaining the best evidence by searching medical literature databases. The simple method is to consult relevant guidelines and further evaluate the evidence at the end of guideline recommendation items and the level of evidence. Update of guidelines is relatively slow so that the latest literature results published after the time point of including the evidence in the guideline could be searched and cited through evaluation.

1.3.3 Critically evaluating the validity and scientificity of evidence. Not only do original researches need to be evaluated, guidelines also need to be evaluated. Although different types of research design have different evaluation criteria, the evaluation of evidence involves scientificity, effect of results and the scope of the applicable population.

1.3.4 Comparing the characteristics of the population in the literature with those of target patients and making clinical decisions based on the combination of clinicians' personal experience with local medical conditions. When applying evidence, it is necessary to take into account evaluation to judge bias and the influence of bias on the result and to put forward reasonable decision-making expectations.

1.3.5 Evaluating the results of the treatment, including short-term or long-term outcomes. If it fails to obtain desired results, reconsider the clinical problem and perform the evidence-based practice process again.

Evidence-based practice needs to formulate clinical questions first. Reading reviews help understand the progress of solution to clinical problems. Evidence-based practice needs to convert clinical problems, or problems encountered in clinical settings, into specific answerable scientific questions. This is a process turning a general problem into a specific question, which can be defined by PICO.

P: Population, Patient and/or Problem. First, think about the patient and/or setting you are dealing with which is the target population of applied evidence.

I: Intervention, or exposure. Think of what measures to take. It may be a drug or intervention for treatment, or a test or screening program for diagnosis, or risk of exposure for identifying disease etiology. The more fully understood the intervention measures or the exposure, the more comprehensive the judgment.

C: Comparison. What may be an alternative to the intervention? If the control is different, the result will be different.

O: Outcome. The specific clinical outcome of interest. The outcome can be direct, such as hemostasis, or endpoint like survival and death, or intermediate results and alternative endpoints, such as serological indicators, changes of disease status shown by images. The focus is on survival and death for serious diseases while the focus is on complications for chronic diseases.

When formulating clinical questions, correctly clarifying the type of problems helps to find answers, including the explanation of symptoms and signs, etiology, diagnosis, treatment, prognosis, quality of life, cost-effectiveness and so on.

Before application, the evidence must be strictly evaluated. The best evidence should have the three characteristics of validity, importance and applicability. When applying evidence to treat patients, it is necessary to fully communicate with the patient about the obtained evidence, and implement it on the basis of the patient's understanding and consent. Clinical practice should take full consideration of the patients and their families, society, medical service providers, and financial situation of payers. For diseases that require long-term treatment or observation, not only the short-term cost-effectiveness and cost-utility situation, but also the medium and long-term disease treatment burden and prognosis should be considered. Physicians should provide sufficient evidence and information in all aspects, and communicate well with patients to make the best clinical decisions together.

Evidence-based medicine advocates combining the clinicians' personal clinical practice experience with the best clinical evidence to make the optimal decision for the diagnosis and treatment of patients. This is the basic requirement for a doctor. Doctors who ignore clinical practice experience may misuse the best evidence even if they get it, because application of the best evidence vary with different individuals, and clinicians should make choices adapted to different clinical characteristics and status of the individual patient. Without the best and up-to-date external evidence, clinicians may use outdated methods, failing to make optimal decisions or even doing harm. Today, evidence-based medicine advocates providing medical services to patients in a well-founded manner. The practice of applying the latest and best results of medical research to clinical practice has been accepted by the majority of medical staff and patients, and the evidence-based practice is passed on among medical students and young physicians.

1.4　Evidence-based medicine and precision medicine

Evidence-based practice is a decision-making process from general to individual. When applying universal theories to individuals, factors that need to be considered include biology, pathophysiology, sociopsychological factors, and economic factors. Evidence-based clinical practice follows evidence from clinical medical practice and various studies, representing population. Applying theory to practice is a process of popularization and application from the overall to the sample, from the universal to the individual. To correctly complete this process from evidence to individual implementation, evidence should be of validity and be correctly applied to the individual. Otherwise, not only will it not be possible to provide the patient with the most suitable diagnosis and treatment plan, but it will even do harm to the patient, which opposes the principles of evidence-based medicine. In the practice of evidence-based medicine, a misunderstanding is that it only pays attention to the evidence but not the scientificity and validity of the evidence. Another misunderstanding is that as long as there is scientific and authentic evidence, it is recommended or applied to all patients at all costs, ignoring the applicability of the evidence and the impact of related factors on practice, especially the specific conditions and values of the individuals. Therefore, in the practice of evidence-based medicine, how to combine the characteristics, requirements and values of each patient, and how to correctly interpret and individually apply evidence is of the utmost importance.

Individualization is the most suitable treatment that the clinician adopts for the patient's specific disease. It is decision made by the doctor on the basis of combination of his own clinical experience, recent research evidence and the pathophysiological condition of the patient's disease itself, as well as the patient's wishes. Evidence-based medicine attaches importance to clinical experience, but opposes relying only on experience and ignoring the latest reliable evidence. Evidence from randomized controlled clinical studies may be questionable because of its strict selection criteria and ideal treatment environment. How to combine evidence and clinical experience in individualized treatment is particularly important. Whether the research results can be used for their own patients to achieve the expected results is the most concerned issue for clinicians.

Biological characteristics and socio-economic status affect the efficacy of individual treatment, including biological characteristics, gender, concomitant diseases, race, age, and pathological characteristics of the disease. Clinicians should fully consider these factors when applying the results of randomized controlled clinical studies to individuals.

Individualization needs to consider the benefits, risks and compliance of intervention measures.

1.4.1 Can the treatment be applied to a certain patient?

When the treatment is not suitable for the patient due to his biological characteristic, the doctor should consider the effectiveness and safety of the treatment based on the changes in the social environment as well as the patient's compliance with the treatment plan. Generally, the compliance of patients included in clinical studies is much higher than that of common patients. For example, as to the management of hypertension, patients with different compliances have completely different treatment effectiveness. It is also necessary to consider whether the clinicians are competent in the treatment plan, especially in invasive operations and interventional measures including surgery and interventional therapy. The choice of treatment should also be based on the medical conditions of the hospital and capabilities of the doctor. If the hospital is not equipped with the optimal treatment conditions or the doctor does not have the qualifications to perform the operation, a second-line treatment should be chosen, with patient safety as the primary consideration factor.

1.4.2 Does the patient's benefit outweigh the risk?

Whether doctors can manage outpatients well is also a factor that should be considered when choosing a treatment. Patients receiving anticoagulation therapy should be followed up on the INR value in an outpatient clinic. However, some patients cannot be followed up on time due to economic reasons or long distances, which will increase the risk of bleeding. Therefore, whether to conduct anticoagulation therapy and the specific plan of anticoagulation therapy should be carefully considered.

1.4.3 Consider stratification and subgroup

Providing evidence for stratification or subgroup analysis is a prerequisite for individualization of treatment decisions. For example, a randomized controlled clinical study on whether people with elevated serum cholesterol require hypolipidemic treatment included patients with elevated serum cholesterol aged 30~70 years. The results showed that the use of statins can significantly reduce the risk of cardiovascular death. Then, a 32-year-old female patient came and her physical examination showed elevated serum cholesterol, blood pressure of 110/70mmHg and no family history of diabetes or heart diseases. Do you want to give her hypolipidemic medication? Later, another 69-year-old man came in with a 40-year history of smoking and his serum cholesterol was slightly elevated and his blood pressure was 140/85mmHg; his mother died of a heart attack 20 years ago. What should you do at this time? Obviously, these two patients belong to the low-risk group and the high-risk group of cardiovascular death events respectively. If they were treated with the same hypolipidemic treatment based on the conclusion of a randomized controlled trial (RCT) alone, the risk of cardiovascular death events might only reduce from original 2% to 1% for the young women while for the latter elderly man it might drop from 40% to 10%. The former is more recommended with healthy lifestyle guidance such as diet and exercise to achieve the effect of reducing blood lipids while the latter calls more urgently for medical intervention in addition to healthy lifestyle guidance.

1.4.4 Consider the values and wishes of patients

Full consideration of patients' values and respect to patients' choices are decisive factors for clinical decision-making. Two patients in exactly the same situation may make completely different decisions after fully understanding their disease and treatment status. For example, considering that taking aspirin can prevent cerebral embolism but increase the risk of gastrointestinal bleeding, most doctors choose not to use aspirin, while most patients choose to continue the medication because they cannot accept the impact of cerebral embolism on their quality of life.

The use of evidence-based medicine tools to assess specific diseases or conditions and then implement individualized evidence-based decision-making. UpToDate and many other medical sites and even mobile phones APPs offer state scoring tools for each disease that provide evidence for individualized treatment of a variety of disease risk prediction models. These scoring models are continuously updated and revised based on the latest evidence-based medical evidence. The risk score of this patient can be obtained by inputting individualized data, and thus guiding clinicians to make clinical decisions, formulating diagnosis and treatment plans, bringing great convenience to clinical practice.

Taking the model for end-stage liver disease (MELD) as an example, in 2000, Malinchoc et al. proposed this assessment in order to predict the survival time and prognosis of patients after transjugular intrahepatic portosystemic stent-shunt (TIPSS). The risk score is as follows: $R = 0.957 \times \ln(\text{creatinine mg/dl}) + 0.378 \times \ln(\text{bilirubin mg/dl}) + 1.120 \times \ln(\text{INR}) + 0.643 \times$ (cause of cirrhosis: alcoholic or cholestatic cirrhosis is 0 and the rest are 1). For example, for a patient with hepatitis C cirrhosis, serum creatinine 1.9mg/dl, serum bilirubin 4.2mg/dl, INR1.2, his risk score is calculated as follows: $R = 0.957 \times \ln 1.9 + 0.378 \times \ln 4.2 + 1.120 \times \ln 1.2 + 0.643 \times 1 = 2.003$. For the convenience of application, Kamath multiplies the score calculated by the above formula by 10, and the result is rounded to the nearest integer, that is, 20. Subsequently, he conducted a retrospective and prospective study, proving that the MELD model can be generally used to predict the prognosis of patients with advanced liver disease. The prognosis of patients with chronic liver disease can be predicted according to their various indicators, which helps doctors to evaluate the condition and decide treatment methods and time. The updated study found that serum sodium is an independent predictor of hepatorenal syndrome and also reflects the influence of complications of cirrhosis and portal hypertension. It improved the MELD scoring system by replacing it with the MELDNa model (MESO, MESO= MELD/SNa×10). With the accumulation of clinical research evidence, the existing scoring system is constantly modified and improved. This is the basis for the individualization of evidence-based decision-making, and advancing direction of evidence-based medicine.

Precision medicine was first proposed in tumor research to develop targeted drug treatments based on tumor molecular classification and characteristics. This proposal is an example of the specific application of the individualized concept of evidence-based medicine in the oncology field for decision-making on molecular classification. At present, in the development, evaluation and clinical application of tumor molecular diagnosis and targeted drugs, it is also necessary to follow the concept of evidence-based medicine. The first is that the treatment of tumor patients still needs to emphasize general biological characteristics and socioeconomic characteristics; the second is that clarifying molecular targets of tumor patients also needs evidence, especially randomized controlled clinical studies of large samples, multi-centers, and different tumors and different tumor patients. Each tumor molecular marker can be regarded as a clinical pathological state of the disease.

1.5 Elimination of the misunderstandings of evidence-based medicine

Evidence-based medicine is a concept that emphasizes decision-making based on the best clinical evidence, the experience of clinicians, and the wishes and values of patients. Evidence includes case reports, cohort studies, randomized controlled clinical trials, meta-analyses and guidelines. Whether carrying out primary researches, meta-analyses and other secondary studies, or formulating guidelines, publishing papers with databases, all these provide evidence-based medicine with evidence, but they themselves are not the essence of evidence-based medicine.

Although evidence-based medicine emphasizes evidence, more emphasis is put on the evaluation of evidence. The concept of evidence-based medicine runs through the whole process of clinical practice, from transforming raised clinical questions to scientific questions, to literature retrieval, evidence evaluation, applying evidence to solve clinical problems and evaluating aftereffects. These five steps reflect the whole process of evidence-based practice. Scientific evaluation of evidence and individualized treatment of patients are the quintessence of evidence-based medicine clinical practice, and patients' outcome is the ultimate criterion for assessing the process of evidence-based practice.

1.5.1 Misunderstanding 1

A large number of low-quality meta-analysis and network meta-analysis are incorrectly recommended as evidence. Meta-analysis is a secondary research method focusing on clinical controversial issues, such as reports of different positive or negative results, to evaluate the results of different studies. Meta-analysis can expand the sample size and increase the representativeness of the population. You can register on Cochrane and receive methodological guidance including establishment of a meta-analysis team, systematic retrieval and evaluation, writing and publication standards, and most importantly, the scientific interpretation and application of meta-analysis.

The quality of meta-analysis, especially that of original research sources, is currently a tricky problem, as well as excessive use and interpretation of results.

First of all, meta-analysis requires a team, including at least clinical experts, methodology experts, and 2 researchers responsible for literature search and evaluation. Clinical experts are responsible for topic selection, inclusion criteria in the literature, selection of results, and interpretation of results; methodology experts are responsible for literature retrieval strategies, evaluation standards, data synthesis, and results presentation. Secondly, systematic literature retrieval and quality evaluation of scientific literature are the key points. The correct application of methodology directly affects the results. High-quality literature is the basis of high-quality meta-analysis. Thirdly, publish the results of meta-analysis in a standardized format. If data is not suitable for integration, especially low-quality original research data, systematic reviews rather than meta-analysis should be selected. Avoid the misuse of low-quality meta-analysis results.

1.5.2 Misunderstanding 2

Guideline misuse, especially guidelines related to the use of products. First, the formulating guidelines may be affected by stakeholders and result in problems; second, the guidelines were taken advantage of by merchants or misinterpreted. Guidelines systematically formulated by experts help clinicians and patients make appropriate decisions based on specific clinical conditions. The significance of the guideline is to standardize clinicians' diagnosis and treatment, improve the quality of medical services, reduce expenses, and suggest the direction of future clinical research.

The process of guideline formulation includes: determining the importance and necessity of the problem and the scope of application of the guideline; setting up a group to establish the procedures for formulating the guideline; comprehensive data collection, systematic analysis, and grading of evidence; putting forward recommendations by objectively evaluating the results; organizing external experts to review and modify the guidelines; publishing the guidelines and updating them regularly.

Guidelines, with obvious regional and topical variations, also require quality evaluation. The guideline evaluation includes scientificity / rigorousness, effectiveness / safety, economy, usability / feasibility, conflicts of interest, etc. It can be evaluated by AGREE Ⅱ standard.

The formulation of evidence-based medicine guidelines also requires breakthroughs. The emerging new evidence provides a basis for updating the guidelines. The emerging new clinical problems are also the driving force for clinical researches.

1.6　Development and challenges of evidence-based medicine in China

China introduced clinical epidemiology in the 1980s, sent a group of clinicians to study in clinical epidemiology centers in the United States, Canada, and Australia under the funding of the Ministry of Health and the World Bank, and became a member unit of the International Clinical Epidemiology Network (INCLEN). After returning to China, experts from various regions have successively set clinical epidemiology courses for undergraduates and graduate students in various universities since 1986. The former Shanghai Medical University and West China Medical University were approved to become Regional Clinical Epidemiology Resource and Training Centers (R-CERTC) in China. With the support of INCLEN, a large number of clinical epidemiological clinicians have been trained bilingually, and have now become the backbone of evidence-based medicine across the country.

In 1996, Professor Wang Jiyao translated evidence-based medicine into Chinese for the first time. In 2002, she edited *Evidence-based Medicine and Clinical Practice*, which is the first monograph in China that systematically introduces evidence-based medicine and clinical practice. The Clinical Epidemiology and Evidence-based Medicine Branch of the Chinese Medical Association has further promoted the development of evidence-based medicine in

China. The development of evidence-based medicine discipline has evolved from participation of experts from a single discipline to a professional team with multidisciplinary cooperation and organic integration centered on solving clinical problems. Evidence-based medicine centers represented by West China Medical Center, Sichuan University and Lanzhou University are led by methodological experts, and more emphasis is placed on the construction and expansion of evidence-based medicine methodology; evidence-based medicine centers represented by Shanghai Medical College, Fudan University and Peking Union Medical University are led by clinical experts, and more attention is paid to the promotion, application and evaluation of the concept of evidence-based medicine in clinical practice and scientific research.

Evidence-based medicine is a basic subject of clinical medicine. Only by mastering the methods of evidence-based medicine can we better carry out clinical practice, serve patients, and continuously improve our own ability of diagnosis and treatment.

Summary

Evidence-based medicine provides a reliable basis for optimal clinical decision making by combining the best research evidence, physicians' clinical experience, and patients' personal values. Since progressing medical and public health development, evidence-based medicine has also been gradually refined and improved to create possibilities for individualized precisive medicine practice.

(Chen Shiyao, Liu Tianshu)

How to ask answerable clinical questions

Learning objectives

1. **To master** how to build clinical questions clearly.
2. **To be familiar with** sources and types of questions.

We often need health care knowledge to make our decisions and take actions. The first step to make evidence-based practice is to propose clinical questions that are answerable from clinical researches. We will use a case to show how questions are raised and formed.

The patient is a 58-year-old man with gastric cancer who undergone a radical D2 gastric resection. After surgery, pathological findings showed adenocarcinoma, infiltrated into serosa, four positive lymph nodes among 32 resected lymph nodes, margin (-) and the pathologic stage was pT3N1M0 (ⅢA). After surgery, the patient may have many questions to ask as follows:

How could I get gastric cancer? → Pathogenesis

Is there any need for me to receive adjuvant chemotherapy? → Treatment

How long can I survive? → Prognosis

Many questions could be raised around this case to help us better understand the disease. However, if we want to have solid and evidence-based answers, the first thing is to raise a good question. Asking answerable clinical questions is not only the first step of finding evidence, but also the first step of practicing evidence-based medicine.

2.1 Sources and types of clinical questions

2.1.1 Where and how clinical questions arise

Questions originate from clinical practice. To find new and useful answers to important unresolved problems, you need to know a lot about the problem and be clear about the boundary between current knowledge and the unknown parts. Without adequate knowledge in this respect, it is difficult to know whether one is headed in the right "next-step" direction. Thus, clinicians should keep curious and be good at observing, finding and resolving problems.

2.1.2   Type of Studies

Clinical questions cover targeted population, such as adults, children, emergency patients or long-term treated patients, important intervention measures and results, potential compared contents (comparison of standard therapy and new choice), and impact of medical economy. It is helpful to think about what kind of question you are asking when you have created a question. Different types of questions will be solved by the relative types of studies (Table 2-1).

Table 2-1   Recommended research type for different kinds of questions

Type of questions	Recommended type of studies
Etiology	RCT > cohort > case control
Diagnosis	Prospective, blind comparison with a gold standard
Prognosis	Cohort > case control
Treatment	RCT > cohort > case control > case series
Prevention	RCT > cohort > case control
Cost	Economic analysis
Quality of life	Assessment of quality of life

">", defers to "better than".

Etiology: how to identify possible causes and risk factors?

Diagnostic tests: how to select and interpret diagnostic tests based on factors such as precision, accuracy, acceptability, cost, and safety in order to confirm or exclude a diagnosis? Accurate index includes precision and accuracy.

Treatment: how to select treatments based on efficacy, cost and life value of your patient?

Prognosis: how to predict likely outcomes and complications?

Prevention: how to reduce the occurrence of disease by identifying and modifying risk factors and how to diagnose disease early by screening?

Cost-effectiveness: which intervention is more cost-effective?

Quality of life: how will be the life quality of the patient following this intervention?

2.2   How to ask questions

2.2.1   How to build the questions

Well-built clinical questions contain background and foreground questions.

New knowledge originates from asking answerable questions. To find new and useful questions, you need to know a lot about the general knowledge that would help us understand disease. Such "background" questions can be concerned about any disorder or health state, a treatment or intervention, other aspect of health care, psychologic or sociologic phenomena.

2.2.1.1　Background questions refer to general knowledge about disease, which have two essential components.

A question root (who, what, when, where, how, why), with a verb.

An aspect of the disease condition such as a disorder, test, treatment, or other part of health care.

For example: How did I get gastric cancer?

2.2.1.2　Foreground questions refer to specific knowledge to inform clinical decisions, which include four main elements:

Patient or Problem: What is the scenario about the patients you are dealing with? Try to identify all the clinical characteristics which influence the problem. Sometimes, basic features such as age, gender or race could be relative with the diagnosis or the treatment.

Intervention: What is the main candidate intervention? The main intervention should be defined broadly, including an exposure, a diagnostic test, a prognostic factor, a treatment, and so forth.

Comparison: What is the main alternative compared with the intervention? This might be nothing, or standard care. Comparison of two interventions can get more direct and clear evidence.

Outcome(s): What is my expected accomplishment? You should spend some time working out exactly what outcome is important to you and your patient.

2.2.1.3　Examples

Poor-formulated question (question 1):

Should **gastric cancer patients** receive **adjuvant chemotherapy**?

Patient　　　Intervention

Well-built question (question 2):

Comparison　　　Intervention　　　Outcome

Compared with **observation**, can **adjuvant chemotherapy prolong survival** in **gastric cancer patients with stage of IIIA (pT3N1M0)**?

Patient

In the above examples, there are two components lost in question 1 and the type of patients is unclear (without pathological stage), while the four elements are completed in question 2, which is an intact and effective question.

As clinicians, we all need both background and foreground knowledge in proportions that vary over time, depending primarily on our experience with the particular disorder at hand (Figure 2-1). When our experience with the condition is limited, at point A, the majority of our questions (designated in Figure 2-1 by the vertical dimension) might be about background knowledge. As we grow in clinical experience and responsibility, such as point B, we'll have increasing proportions of questions about the foreground of our patients. Further experience with the condition puts us at point C, where most of our questions will be foreground. Note that the diagonal line is placed to show that we're never too green to learn foreground knowledge, or too experienced to outlive the need for background knowledge.

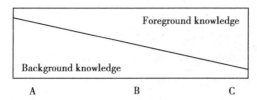

Figure 2-1   Our proportions of background and foreground knowledge vary over time

A. When the physician's experience is limited, the majority of questions is about background knowledge. B. As experience accumulates, questions about foreground increase. When the physician's experience increases to C, most of questions is about foreground knowledge.

2.2.2   Selecting questions to answer

We need to know how to start when there are more questions than the limited time may allow. We would find many questions at one time since our patients' illness burdens are large. So, the recommended strategy is to select questions. Selecting means deciding which of the many questions should be pursued. This decision requires judgment and we'd suggest you consider the nature of the patient's illness, and the nature of your knowledge needs. What kind of questions have priorities to be answered? The following questions can help us to filter the priorities.

Which question is the most related to the patient's well-being?

Which question could have a satisfactory answer?

Which question is most related to your clinical practice?

Which question is most appealing to you?

Which question could appear again in clinical practice?

Questions with priority to be answered are the most related to well-being, health, clinical practice. Meanwhile, we need to pay attention to the views of patients, so as to help us to collect evidence in favor of our patients and improve cure rate and the quality of medical service.

2.2.3   Determining the range of questions

The range of questions is very important to clinical researchers. If too wide or too narrow, the range of questions is not conducive to provide evidence for research or yield evidence to treat patients. The range of questions is usually associated with resources available, clinical implications and research quality. The following problems are not uncommon in clinical practice.

2.2.3.1   The range of questions is too wide

Questions of broad range are helpless to patients. For example, "Will cancer patients benefit from chemotherapy?" The range of this question is too wide as it is unknown what kind of cancer and what type of chemotherapy could be performed, which fails to provide useful information for specific patients. Questions of broad range will enlarge the sample size and increase research heterogeneity. However, on the other hand, research with wide range can provide more information and better utility but consume more resources.

2.2.3.2   The range of questions is too narrow

Questions of narrow range increase the opportunities of false positivity and false negativity for lack of information and eventually impair the validity of conclusions. Questions of narrow range have the same problem with subtype analysis since these narrow questions can be regarded as one subtype of those wide ones. Furthermore, such narrow questions have problems of generalized application though they may increase the research homogeneity.

Summary

Clinical questions originate from clinical practice, the purpose of raising questions is to serve for clinical decision-making. To ask answerable questions requires us to know a lot about the problem, understand the elements of building clinical questions, make sure the types of questions and precisely know the boundary between current and unknown knowledge. Proposing good questions are the basic skills of learning evidence-based medicine. Well-formulated questions can help us focus on the requirements in the daily clinical practice.

(Liu Tianshu, Chen Shiyao)

3

How to get useful evidence

Learning objective

To master literature analysis; use of evidence-based medicine databases.

An important feature of evidence-based medicine is to optimize medicine related decision-making based on quality evidence. Therefore, ways to obtain high quality evidence is of particular importance, and earn their predominant place in this chapter. The evidence here refers generally to well-designed and well-conducted research, from which we can extract useful information in several different ways. First, this can be done by literature analysis, mostly employed in latest research or ones less covered, which includes assessing the evidence qualities and integrating the results of original research, and analysis of qualitative and quantitative systematic reviews. Second, make full use of evidence-based medicine databases, where important medical information has already been organized, stored, and managed in the manner of data structures, which is a critical mean of accessing reliable medicine evidences.

3.1 Review of medical literature

Literature is publications that record and spread knowledge. Medical literature refers to those involving knowledge of medicine. According to its classification standard, literature goes into three types: primary, secondary and tertiary.

Primary literature is also called original literature, usually covers first-hand research results, findings, inventions, and insights. Primary literature presents in many different forms, such as journal paper, dissertation, conference paper, patent specification, and Sci-Tech report. Secondary literature is written by gathering, screening and further processing primary literature, and usually presented as follows: abstract, index and content. Tertiary literature is made by another round of screening and processing of primary literature based on specific aims and information from secondary literature, and falls into forms of review, yearbook, guidebook and textbook.

3.1.1 Original clinical study

According to whether random assignment is designed, the original clinical study is divided into two types: observational study and experimental study. The research subjects of the first type carry various objective characteristics and can't be randomly assigned according to the factors to be studied. Results are obtained by systematically and objectively describing the factors studied or comparing and analyzing the results which were made possible by well-designed study. This kind of study is not related to medical ethics and easy to operate. However, bias can be introduced easily, which makes it not so reliable.

Observational study is divided into descriptive and analytical studies according to whether the control group is set. The descriptive study is to describe the distribution, occurrence and development of diseases or traits in different population, territory or time. No control group is set in this kind of study, such as case report and cross-sectional study. Study of this kind can just propose the hypotheses of etiologies, but not identify the relationship between the exposure and response. Different from that of observational study, analytical research is based on descriptive research an important feature of analytical study is that different groups are set to compare with each other, such as case-control study and cohort study. The aim of analytical study is to explore the association between potential pathogenic factors and the status of diseases or health, through the analysis, screening the pathogenic factors, which helps in further identifying or validating the hypotheses of etiologies.

Different from that in observational studies, the study population is randomly divided into experimental and control groups in experimental studies. Under the same condition, the two groups receive different treatments, which is to be measured in the experimental group, while no treatment or placebo in the control group. The results of both groups are compared and conclusions about the treatment, if there are any, are drawn. Since objects are assigned randomly and the factors involved are under control, conclusions from this kind of study are much more reliable.

3.1.2 Review and commentary

Review and commentary both fall into the category of tertiary document. These two types not only have a close connection, but also have differences. Review is a kind of comprehensive and descriptive literature, which collects and analyzes the latest achievements of a specific research domain in a period of time. By summarizing and condensing the data and results in the primary studies and then generalizing valuable information, review can reflect the progress of a research topic comprehensively, guide readers to quickly acquire general information of the topic in this period and suggest the problems to solve and the difference between domestic and foreign research groups.

Commentary is a kind of literature that comment on a special research topic, after systematically collecting, organizing, analyzing related materials. The aim of commentary is to make a comprehensive observation about the current scientific achievements and the stages of research, based on which authors give their own opinions and suggestions about the obstacles lying ahead, possible methods to overcome them, and versions too, as a reference to other researchers, possibly an aid as well.

In summary, review focuses on the comprehensiveness and description of a specific research aspect. Besides comprehensiveness and description, commentary also focuses on comment. Review is more widely applied than commentary, while the latter gives more valuable academic opinions.

3.1.3 Systematic review and meta-analysis

Systematic review is a secondary study, also called systematic accessing, based on collecting, organizing and analyzing data from primary research. Systematic review can generate more reliable scientific information and has a profound influence on related researches.

Although referred to as review as well, systematic review is much different from common review. Systematic review is quite strict on its requirements, and generally focuses on a specific scientific problem to be solved. After the detailed introduction of retrieval strategy, including search methods and tools, the published and unpublished documents and data should be comprehensively collected. Meanwhile, document collation and strict review should be conducted, according to the established criteria. To reduce bias, blind review or review by many researchers are usually performed, mainly focusing on the reality of the documents, the application value and the factors with possible influence on results. Systematic review constantly collects new primary data to update and supplement new information.

According to different statistical processes followed, systematic review is divided into two types, qualitative and quantitative systematic review. Qualitative systematic review just collects and organizes the results of primary studies, but does not process or combine data using statistical methods, while quantitative systematic review combines data using statistical methods after the results are collected, and is also called meta-analysis.

Meta-analysis can comprehensively analyze results from multiple researches in the same research field, which has significant advantages over certain problems, such as insufficient statistical efficiency due to small sample size in a single study, inconsistency of the same research conducted by different groups, and missed scientific observations due to different questions raised in different studies, and can answer the original research questions which were not put forward in the original research. Meta-analysis has attracted much attention in the field of medical research and is ideal evidence of evidence-based medicine, it is mainly used to merge the results of randomized controlled studies which is mainly used to examine the etiological hypothesis of case-control or cohort studies in primary observational studies and medical interferences.

When preparing systematic review, the first thing you need to do is to clearly define the contents to be reviewed, the search methods employed, and exclusion and inclusion criteria followed. Meta-analysis is used to combine all the qualified samples in the selected studies. For the combined results, sensitivity analysis should be conducted because the quality of the selected studies is closely associated with the reliability of the meta-analysis. To obtain high-quality combined results, the quality of the selected documents must be ensured. Heterogeneity test is important in meta-analysis. Fix effect model is used when the consistency of the selected studies is good, while random effect model is used if the heterogeneity is found in the selected documents where clinical significance still exists. Meta-analysis should not be used when serious heterogeneity occurs.

3.2   Components of a clinical research

3.2.1   Overview

Clinical research reports include the whole process of clinical research, results, evaluation of results, summary, discussion, and vision. Clinical research report is a form of summary and presentation of research work, which highly summarizes the whole process of research work and fully reflects the research results and values. Usually, in terms of ethics and science, clinical reports are comprehensive, detailed, and reliable, which are very good reference and evidence for clinicians on aspects of clinical practice and decision-making.

Clinical research reports, including biomedical scientific research papers, are highly concise on the content of clinical research. In 1978, the *Vancouver Declaration* drafted in Vancouver, Canada, agreed on the unified format of biomedical journal papers. In 1987, China also issued a national standard (GB 7713—87) for the format of scientific and technical reports, dissertations, and academic papers.

Generally, medical scientific research papers have the following parts: title, signature (authors, affiliation, etc.), abstract (Chinese and English), keywords, preface, body, conclusions, references, appendices and English abbreviations etc. The body, including introduction, materials and methods, results and discussion, is written in IMRAD format.

This section will focus on the body of the research report.

3.2.2   Body

3.2.2.1   Introduction

For a research paper, introduction is a statement of the purpose of this study. At the beginning of the paper, researchers are supposed to explain the problems need to be solved and their importance. Then, review available studies on this issue, and finally explain the difference of this research, compared with the ones done before, and focus of the study.

3.2.2.2   Materials and methods

This section should provide experimental details, including experimental design, subjects, materials, treatment, and protocols, etc. Materials and methods should be described in details and precisely, which can enable other researchers to repeat experiments with no more information than that offered in this part. Reproducibility should be a prerequisite for all experiments. For example, randomized, controlled, and blinded design methods are commonly used in drug research reports to group research subjects. Besides the detailed description of grouping methods, researchers also need to give sufficient information on the treatment of different groups, list full standards for efficacy and safety evaluation. Finally, list the information about data collection and processing, as well as statistical software and methods used.

3.2.2.3　Results

In this part, only results should be presented, in the forms of text description, figures, charts or tables, but not any comments or explanations. Results include statistically processed data, formulas, graphs, images, and pattern diagrams, which are accompanied by reasonable descriptions. All the data should be well organized to focus on the key or new points. The textual narrative and graphs should be reasonably coordinated, not repetitive, and clearly presented. The data should be organically integrated and clearly layered to highlight the main content and innovative results. Data is the proof for your argument, so present it as it is, even if it is not what you expected. Sometimes, negative results can be the place where great discoveries emerge, even if not, they can help with next round of experimental design and conduct.

3.2.2.4　Discussion

The discussion of a clinical report is meant to analyze the results and refine the important information, to seek the inner association between the data and possible mechanism, to theoretically discuss and explain the results of treatments and observations. Through rational analysis and deduction in discussion, researchers can lay the foundation for the conclusion to come, and bring up new questions and further research topics. Discussion should be made based on the actual results, and kept to the key points and the questions to be answered. Reasonable analysis and interpretation of the results must be evidence-based, not otherwise. When results are under discussion, not only the positive ones but also the negative or contrary ones should be explained. Even if the study does not produce any results, it is necessary to explain as well as you can.

3.2.3　Other parts of the report

3.2.3.1　Conclusion

The conclusion is to summarize the results and the analysis in a concise way, indicate theoretical and practical significance, where the content of the article is highly summarized.

3.2.3.2　References

References are essential for a research paper and should be the most important published literature. They help to understand and support the motive, process, achievement, and even rationale of the study topic. References are literature limited to those that have been read by the author and need to be cited as proof. References include journals, books, conference documents, technical reports, dissertations, patents, etc. The following is an example of a reference for a journal article:

HALPERN S T D,UBEL P A,CAPLAN A L. Solid-organ transplantation in HIV-infected patients[J]. The New England Journal of Medicine,2002,347(4): 284-287.

3.2.4　Clinical research report analysis

Further understand clinical research report format through the analysis of an example, a clinical characteristic study on child-specific dermatitis.

Limei Zhang. Analysis of clinical features of 298 children with atopic dermatitis[D].

Chongqing Medical University, 2010.

3.2.4.1　Introduction

In the beginning, the paper explains the importance of regional difference studies in the clinical characteristics of children patients with atopic dermatitis (AD). Subsequently, it reviews the past and present studies on regional differences in the clinical features of children with AD. Finally, it illustrates the differences and focus of this study, compared to the past ones.

3.2.4.2　Materials and methods

Data collection: 298 children, complied with the 1980 Hanifint-Rajka AD diagnostic criteria, were included in this study.

Clinical feature definition: Here you need to define, as the authors did,　the main characteristics and secondary features according to the diagnostic criteria and score the disease severity (OSAAD, the objective severity assessment of atopic dermatitis) according to the objective SCORD scoring criteria.

Methods: With informed consents signed by the patients or their legal supervisors, specially trained epidemiological investigators started to record the patient's clinical features and laboratory examination data. The contents of the survey are as follows: name, gender, date of birth, age, home address, and contact phone number, age of onset, first symptom, clinical manifestations and causes of disease progression.

Quality control methods in the process of data collection and input: Check and revise the questionnaire repeatedly to make it more operative; in this paper, investigators were trained and passed all tests before getting the job, and all patients were diagnosed by dermatologists through a medical history-assisted examination; apply double data entry and check to cut down human errors; check the consistency of the data; interview selected samples on telephone.

Analyze the age of onset, the seasons of exacerbation and remission, and the influence of AD on quality of life. Group the patients according to their age, and analyze clinical features, such as skin lesion types, severity, predilection site, and secondary features, occurrence rate, etc. Finally, employ proper statistical analysis methods, like SPSS 26 statistical analysis software with χ^2 test, to determine any possible significant difference.

3.2.4.3　Results

In the results, the authors compared the age and gender distribution of the children, the time of onset, the location of predilection, the seasons of predilection, what happens, the severity of illness, and the incidence of minor and other symptoms. Finally, discussion was e made based on the results of the investigation. Reasonable analysis and interpretation of results are presented as difference discussion or cause analysis if there is no significant difference.

3.2.4.4　Discussion

Based on the results from this report, the authors came to the following conclusions:

The onset age of atopic dermatitis is young, with the incidence peaks in the first half year, and the onset rates decline along with aging.

Atopic dermatitis has a significant seasonality, which is more severe in winter and relieves in summer.

Children with atopic dermatitis are often accompanied by a family history of allergic diseases; the incidence of food allergy in children with AD is significantly higher than that of general population.

Different types of atopic dermatitis vary in types of skin lesions, areas of skin lesion involvement, severity of AD, and sites of predilection.

3.3 Database of evidence-based medicine

Evidence-based medicine (EBM) is clinical medicine following the scientific evidence, improving clinical practice and experience with objective evidence of scientific research, emphasizing that any medical decision-making should be based on the best scientific evidence, then make the best health care decisions for the patient. Therefore, aiming at the problems in the clinical work, we need to be constantly updated with latest literature, development, trend, and cutting-edge information of the specific problem.

From the initial manual retrieval, the evidence of EBM resources development has experienced a long process. With the rapid development of computer and network technology, it has gradually emerged from the time-consuming and laborious process into a fast and efficient one, greatly improved the ability of information obtaining. EBM database, a database containing clinical scientific evidence, is an important tool to get reliable scientific evidence, and organize, store, and manage medical information in the way of data structure.

EBM database is a retrieval system with its core based on clinical evidence. The aim is to establish a complete clinical data acquisition system and the ultimate goal is to collect and organize clinical evidence with scientific methods, making best platforms of clinical evidence for clinicians and researchers. Since the founding of the Cochrane Collaboration, the Cochrane Library, and the Clinical Evidence launched by BMJ in the 1990s, more and more evidence-based medicine resources have been available to clinicians. These resources rigorously evaluate the original clinical studies that are summarized and integrated using systematic reviews or meta-analysis, which greatly facilitates clinicians to conduct evidence-based clinical practice.

Commonly used evidence-based medicine database:

3.3.1 Cochrane Library is the main product of the international Cochrane Collaboration. It is published by the British Wiley InterScience company and information after 1996 is available. Built on the foundation of systematic evaluation of EBM and bringing together numerous databases, the Cochrane Library is the "gold standard" for evidence-based health care. It can help people involved in health care decision-making to keep abreast of all the latest evidence and provide them with the highest quality information about existing treatments and new treatments. It is intended for a broad audience interested in evidence-based healthcare, including clinicians, policy makers, researchers, educators, and students. The Cochrane Library is a database that provides high-quality evidence and is the main source of clinical research evidence, including Cochrane Database of Systematic Reviews (CDSR) and Database of Abstracts of Reviews of Effects (DARE), Cochrane Central Register of Controlled Trials (CENTRAL), Cochrane

Methodology Register (CMR), Health Technology Assessment Database (HTA), and United Kingdom NHS Economic Evaluation Database (NHS EED).

3.3.2 DynaMed database is one of the most comprehensive, widely used and famous evidence-based medicine databases which provide clinicians the most useful medical information, get the most needed information in the right way, and create the most useful clinical potential resources. The unique advantages of DynaMed database system include assessing all related research currently available, making every effort to present evidence with minimum bias; continuously updating and integrating new evidence to the database; accessible with either website or mobile devices for retrieving and reading. Based on the internal and external authenticity of researches, the quality of evidence can be ranked into 3 levels in DynaMed database, where evidence level 1 is the most reliable, based on patient-centered researches.

3.3.3 UpToDate database was founded in 1992, which belongs to the Wolters Kluwer publishing group, covering more than 10 000 medical topics in 20 field of medicine. The concept of UpToDate is to provide instant evidence-based clinical medical information to clinicians, rapidly answer clinical questions and provide treatment recommendations, decisions, and continuing education services. It also provides better medical information for patients. The editing process of UpToDate mainly includes the feedback, evaluation grading, evidence analysis, recommendation, expert review and updating. The content of UpToDate medical subject is divided into professional and non-professional version, and they directly provide the most personalized medical consulting services and continuing education without charge to keep consecutive attention.

3.3.4 MD Consult database was published by the world's largest medical group Elsevier in 1997. It is a clinical medicine online consulting platform, providing authoritative and constantly updated evidence-based clinical information resources for health care professionals. Its contents contain 15 disciplines, more than 1 000 clinical practice guidelines and more than 15 000 education handouts for patients. All over the world, more than 2 000 health institutions and 95% of American medical colleges have subscribed MD Consult database, which is an efficient plan for resource configuration in medical teaching, scientific research and clinical practices. The editing process of MD Consult database mainly includes retrieval, information classification, paper editing and reviewing, modifying, tracking and monitoring, integration update. It is the first to forge the database to a professional interaction platform, selecting different clinical subjects based on users' questions.

3.3.5 Clinical Evidence database was officially launched by the *British medical journal* (*BMJ*) publishing group in 1999. It was performed a comprehensive improvement and introduced its updated Database of Best Practice in 2009. The updated database not only fully integrated Clinical Evidence of diagnosis and treatment, but also added the content of basis, prevention, diagnosis, treatment, and follow-up in each of the key points written by clinical experts and authoritative scholars. It has covered about 660 clinical topics, more than 3 250 kinds of treatments, 3 000 diagnostic tests and 4 000 clinical practice guidelines. Clinical Evidence database is focusing on providing overviews to different disease conditions for clinicians and summary of interventions for disease prevention and treatment as well as bringing the best intervention on diagnosis and treatment to patients. The editing process of Clinical Evidence mainly includes the expert commission, peer review, quality assessment, publishing online and updating regularly. It is the first evidence-based medicine database with a Chinese version and the first one to edit the core content database into books for global distribution.

3.3.6　The ACP Journal Club is published by the American College of Physicians, mainly for internal medicine and its sub-subjects. The editorial staff will regularly screen more than 50 kinds of core clinical medical journals, involve high quality original research and system evaluation for clinical problems and outcomes, and then summarize in abstracts, propose valuable suggestions for clinical practice. It is mainly distributed in print or online version to help doctors to understand the new progress of medicine.

3.3.7　PIER (Physicians' Information and Education Resource) database mainly includes the diagnosis and treatment of diseases, screening and prevention, ethical and legal issues, and drug information. Its advantage is to use multi-level structure to guide clinicians to put into use of research evidence, and then acquire the effective practical advice through the database. The information of PIER database is showed on drill down format, that is, users can click on open instructions, step by step, to get more detailed information from summary data into the detail data. The new disease module is added and updated monthly to provide up-to-date information for physicians.

3.4　Evidence-based medicine search strategy

The search strategy is based on the correct analysis of the search information requirements, selecting an appropriate search system, determining the search path and search terms, clarifying the logical relationship between the search terms and the search procedure, and formulating a search query that meets the search requirements. The principle of search strategy development is comprehensive and repeatable. Being more and more occupied by clinical errands, clinicians find it more urgent to understand and master the way to make evidence-based medicine search strategies. Retrieving the latest and most valuable information directly from the vast biomedical databases can increase the search efficiency and save much time for clinical practice.

3.4.1　Steps of evidence-based medicine search strategy development

Determine the search range based on the search requirements.

Select appropriate search database.

Select appropriate search path, mainly using a combination of keywords and free words.

Choose 2-3 refined search terms that meet the search requirements. For example, classification number is the search term in classification paths, while in topic paths, search terms are usually title words, keywords, etc.

Make full use of Boolean operators, position operators, truncations, limiters, etc.

Pre-search, analyze and evaluate the quantity and quality of retrieved literature based on clinical questions.

Modify and refine search terms and search formulas based on pre-search results until search requirements are met.

3.4.2 How to develop a relatively good search strategy

For a specific disease, all disease names should be listed as search terms, and connected with "OR".

Multiple synonyms for intervention measures should be listed and connected with "OR".

For types of design included in the trial, multiple search terms should be used if available, connected by "OR".

Use the logical operator "AND" to connect three sets of search queries above.

If no appropriate results returned when three sets of search queries applied simultaneously, omit one set and try again.

3.4.3 The establishment of evidence-based medicine retrieval strategy

Search the MEDLINE database for the most up-to-date and comprehensive medical information resources related to treatment, diagnosis, etiology, prognosis, systematic reviews, and guidelines that meet the requirements of the EBM system review. Search steps are as follows.

Firstly, find out the content of the different topics you want by searching keywords, free words or a combination of both.

Adjust the retrieval methods to ensure recall rates (some literature may not be related when too much returned) or to ensure the search accuracy rates (when less literature returned, they should be more related to the topic, with higher missing rates).

Precision = (relevant items retrieved/ total amount of items retrieved) × 100%

Recall rate = (total amount of relevant items retrieved / total relevant items in retrieval system) × 100%

The use of more generalized search terms (such as a subject term) can increase the recall rate, but decrease the precision.

Improve precision as far as possible when using evidence; improve recall rate as far as possible when making evidence.

Examples of search strategy:

3.4.3.1 Retrieval model for treatment plan

Search strategy that ensures high recall rate: (diabetes) AND (randomized controlled trial [PTYP] OR drug therapy [MESH] OR therapeutic use [MESH:NOEXP] OR random* [WORD]).

Search strategy that ensures high precision: (diabetes) AND ((double [WORD] AND blind* [WORD]) OR placebo [WORD]).

Search strategy that balances recall rate and precision: (diabetes) AND (randomized controlled trial[PTYP]).

3.4.3.2 Retrieval model for diagnosis scheme

Search strategy that ensures high recall rate: (diabetes) AND (recall and precision [MESH]

OR recall [WORD] OR (diagnosis [MESH] OR diagnostic use [MESH] OR precision [WORD])).

Search strategy that ensures high precision: (diabetes) AND (recall and precision [MESH] OR (predictive [WORD] AND value* [WORD])).

Search strategy that balances recall rate and precision: (diabetes) AND (diagnosis).

3.4.3.3　Retrieval model for etiology

Search strategy that ensures high recall rate: (diabetes) AND (cohort studies [MESH] OR risk [MESH] OR (odds [WORD] AND ratio* [WORD]) OR (relative [WORD] AND risk [WORD]) OR (case control* [WORD] OR case-control studies [MESH])).

Search strategy that ensures high precision: (diabetes) AND (case-control studies [MH:NOEXP] OR cohort studies [MH:NOEXP]).

Search strategy that balances recall rate and precision: (diabetes) AND (risk[TW]).

3.4.3.4　Retrieval model for prognosis

Search strategy that ensures high recall rate: (diabetes) AND (incidence [MESH] OR mortality [MESH] OR follow-up studies [MESH] OR mortality [MESH] OR prognosis* [WORD] OR predict* [WORD] OR course [WORD]).

Search strategy that ensures high precision: (diabetes) AND (prognosis [MH:NOEXP] OR survival analysis [MH:NOEXP]).

Search strategy that balances recall rate and precision: (diabetes) AND (prognosis).

3.4.3.5　Retrieval models for system evaluation and guidance

Retrieval model for system evaluation: (diabetes) AND (meta-analysis[PTYP] OR meta-analysis[MH]).

Retrieval model for guidance: (diabetes) AND (Guidelines[MH] OR consensus development conferences[MH]) OR (Guideline[PTYP] OR consensus development conferences[PTYP]).

3.4.4　Adjusting search strategy

After the search strategy is formulated, it does not mean that the retrieval is done. In the actual retrieval process, more than one retrieval is usually required to achieve the desired results, which is why the retrieval strategy most likely needs to be adjusted. Adjustment usually means change databases or retrieval models, which depends on the databases available or search requirements, respectively. Under normal circumstances, if too many results are retrieved, the accuracy rate should be increased, which means to be more specific; if results retrieved are not enough, the recall rate should be increased by softening retrieval requirements.

3.4.4.1　Main methods to narrow down search

Use more specific search terms, such as subordinate words or subtopics that are more specific.

Increase the use of operator "AND" to improve retrieval accuracy.

Use logical operator "NOT" to exclude irrelevant search results.

Use keywords instead of free words.

Use fields to limit retrieval range, such as Title, Year, Publication Types, and Keywords etc.

3.4.4.2   Main methods to expand search

Use less operator "AND", and expand the retrieval range.

Include all synonyms, related words and near-synonyms, reduce the use of specific search terms and increase the use of "OR" operator.

Use category number for retrieval.

Use keywords and free words at the same time, or use all subtopics.

Reduce or remove limiter too restrictive.

Summary

In summary, the main resources of useful evidence for EBM are literature analysis and evidence-based medicine databases. Of which, literature analysis is mainly used in the search of cutting-edge information or on topics without much attention paid, where clinicians can retrieve original clinical studies based on specific clinical questions, and refer to the published systematic review analysis as well. In addition, plans like the Cochrane Collaboration have completed a large number of systematic reviews and established numerous databases based on that. Many excellent databases provide systematic high-quality evidence and are the main sources of clinical research evidence. Although searching for evidence is very important, the evaluation and grading of the quality of existing evidence is also an important part of the useful evidence collection process, especially when referring to original clinical studies. And yet, in the process of evidence-based medicine decision-making lays another two important elements, the doctor and the patient. Therefore, it is necessary to make the best decision based on the best evidence available, along with the clinical experience of the doctor and the patient's wishes.

(Sun Liangdan)

4

Appraising the evidence

Learning objective

To master the validity, importance, applicability of evidence.

Medicine demands critical thinking. A cornerstone of evidence-based practice is the capability to critically assess the quality of the evidence. In medical practice, critical appraisal involves the process of carefully and systematically assessing the outcome of scientific research (i.e., evidence) to judge its validity, importance and applicability. Without objective and comprehensive evidence appraisal, health care is evidence-free. In evaluating the evidence, one should have the knowledge of clinical study design and statistics, as well as the ability to analyze and tailor the study findings for the patients in front of us. Medical doctors should be trained to be truly well-informed critical thinkers.

After searching and retrieving the studies that are most able to answer the PICO question, one then will move on to the step of evidence appraisal. Contemporary healthcare relies not only on individual medical skills, but also on the best information of the effectiveness and safety of each intervention being accessible to healthcare providers. Thus, critically assessing the quality and usefulness of the evidence that is mainly from scientific researches turns to be a key step of evidence-based practice. The aims of critical appraisal are to determine the validity, evaluate the importance and assess the applicability of the evidence.

4.1   Levels of evidence and grades of recommendations

When viewing a volume of evidence relating to a question, it is important to understand that evidence is ranked in hierarchical systems, i.e., there are different levels of evidence which are not considered of equal value. However, it should also be emphasized that all levels of evidence are important and have their respective unique value.

Ranking the levels of evidence originally appeared in 1979 in a report by the Canadian Task Force on the Periodic Health Examination. Since then, many authors, organizations and journals have published several hierarchies mostly with 4 or 5 levels of evidence. These ranking systems have much in common: to rank studies according to the risk of bias (i.e., systematic error). Broad agreement exists on the relative strength of the principal types of epidemiological or clinical studies. Randomized controlled trial (RCT) and/or systematic reviews of RCT are ranked above observational study; on the other hand, expert opinion and anecdotal experience are ranked at the bottom of the evidence pyramid. The Oxford (UK) CEBM Levels of Evidence, among others, has been widely spread and accepted (Table 4-1). First released in 2000 and then revised in 2011, the Oxford CEBM Levels of Evidence, intended to facilitate clinical decision making with a simpler form (fewer footnotes), provides levels of evidence from studies about prevalence, prognosis, diagnosis, treatment benefits, treatment harms, and screening.

Table 4-1   Oxford Centre for Evidence-Based Medicine 2011 Levels of Evidence

Question	Step 1 (Level 1[*])	Step 2 (Level 2[*])	Step 3 (Level 3[*])	Step 4 (Level 4[*])	Step 5 (Level 5[*])
How common is the problem?	Local and current random sample surveys (or censuses)	Systematic review of surveys that allow matching to local circumstances[**]	Local non-random sample[**]	Case-series[**]	n/a
Is this diagnostic or monitoring test accurate? (Diagnosis)	Systematic review of cross-sectional studies with consistently applied reference standard and blinding	Individual cross-sectional studies with consistently applied reference standard and blinding	Non-consecutive studies, or studies without consistently applied reference standards[**]	Case-control studies, or poor or non-independent reference standard[**]	Mechanism-based reasoning
What will happen if we do not add a therapy? (Prognosis)	Systematic review of inception cohort studies[***]	Inception cohort studies[***]	Cohort study or control arm of randomized trial[*]	Case-series or case control studies, or poor quality prognostic cohort study[**]	n/a
Does this intervention help? (Treatment Benefits)	Systematic review of RCT or n-of-1 trials	RCT or observational study with dramatic effect	Non-randomized controlled cohort/follow-up study[**]	Case-series, case-control studies, or historically controlled studies[**]	Mechanism-based reasoning
What are the COMMON harms? (Treatment Harms)	Systematic review of RCT, systematic review of nested case-control studies, n-of-1 trial with the patient you are raising the question about, or observational study with dramatic effect	Individual RCT or (exceptionally) observational study with dramatic effect	Non-randomized controlled cohort/follow-up study (post-marketing surveillance) provided there are sufficient numbers to rule out a common harm. (For long-term harms the duration of follow-up must be sufficient.)[**]	Case-series, case-control, or historically controlled studies[**]	Mechanism-based reasoning

continue

Question	Step 1 (Level 1[*])	Step 2 (Level 2[*])	Step 3 (Level 3[*])	Step 4 (Level 4[*])	Step 5 (Level 5[*])
What are the RARE harms? (Treatment Harms)	Systematic review of RCT or n-of-1 trial	RCT or (exceptionally) observational study with dramatic effect			
Is this (early detection) test worthwhile? (Screening)	Systematic review of RCT	RCT	Non-randomized controlled cohort/ follow-up study[**]	Case-series, case-control, or historically controlled studies[**]	Mechanism-based reasoning

[*] Level may be graded down on the basis of study quality, imprecision, indirectness (study PICO does not match questions PICO), because of inconsistency between studies, or because the absolute effect size is very small; Level may be graded up if there is a large or very large effect size.

[**] As always, a systematic review is generally better than an individual study.

[***] An early structured cohort is a cohort in which all individuals enter the study at an early stage of a certain condition, such as the onset of symptoms, initial diagnosis, clinical manifestation of a pathological condition, etc. It is an important method to study the natural course and prognosis of disease by following up the early structured cohort.

Most of the evidence ranking schemes are simple and easy to use; however, they have also been facing criticisms and challenges for decades, mostly because of being simplistic: too much credit has been given to RCT in such hierarchies. In fact, observational studies can sometimes give us very sound evidence; while RCTs may not be the suitable design to answer some questions (e.g., prevalence, prognosis, or rare harms) or just cannot be conducted for ethical reasons. In some cases, even case-series and anecdotes will provide definitive evidence; on the other hand, RCTs or systematic reviews can also lead to an inconclusive result. In addition, not all RCTs are carefully designed and properly conducted; therefore, the results should be scrutinized cautiously.

Thus, more comprehensive evidence ranking system developed by the GRADE (grading of recommendations assessment, development and evaluation) working group is gaining more attention, and endorsed by many organizations. The GRADE working group defines both "quality of evidence" (Table 4-2 and Table 4-3) and "strength of recommendations" (Table 4-4) in multi-dimensional ways. By incorporating the risk of bias, effect size, consistency, indirectness, precision, etc. to rate the body of evidence, GRADE tends to be more accurate in evidence appraisal for systematic reviews, health technology assessment (HTA), and clinical practice guideline development, and has been widely used worldwide. However, the trade-off is the complexity of the GRADE system. It is time-consuming to master the GRADE approach, so is rating evidence by it.

Some points should be kept in mind when applying any schemes to rank evidence.

The levels will not tell us whether we are asking the right question. Even the best ever evidence cannot answer a mis-specified question.

The quality of evidence should not be judged solely by the study design.

The levels of evidence should not be directly translated into recommendations.

Table 4-2   Significance of the four levels of evidence in GRADE system

Quality level	Definition
High	We are very confident that the true effect lies close to that of the estimate of the effect
Moderate	We are moderately confident in the effect estimate: The true effect is likely to be close to the estimate of the effect, but there is a possibility that it is substantially different
Low	Our confidence in the effect estimate is limited: The true effect may be substantially different from the estimate of the effect
Very low	We have very little confidence in the effect estimate: The true effect is likely to be substantially different from the estimate of effect

Table 4-3   A summary of GRADE's approach to rating quality of evidence

Study design	Initial quality of a body of evidence	Lower if	Higher if	Quality of a body of evidence
Randomized trial	High	Risk of bias −1 Serious −2 Very serious	Large effect +1 large +2 very large	High (+ + + +) Moderate (+ + + −)
Observational study	Low	Inconsistency −1 Serious −2 Very serious Indirectness −1 Serious −2 Very serious Imprecision −1 Serious −2 Very serious Publication bias −1 Likely −2 Very likely	Dose-response +1 Evidence of a gradient All plausible residual confounding +1 would reduce a demonstrated effect +1 would suggest a spurious effect if no effect was observed	Low(+ + − −) Very low (+ − − −)

Table 4-4   The strength and direction of recommendation in GRADE system

Strength	Alternative term	Description	Factor	Direction
Strong		All or almost all informed people would make the recommended choice for or against an intervention. A strong recommendation implies that variability in clinical practice between individuals or regions would likely be inappropriate. Strong does not necessarily mean a priority recommendation	1. Balance between desirable and undesirable consequences of alternative management strategies. The closer the balance, the less likely a strong recommendation 2. Confidence in estimates of effect (quality of evidence). The lower the confidence, the less likely a strong recommendation	For Against

continue

Strength	Alternative term	Description	Factor	Direction
Weak	Conditional, discretionary, or qualified	Recommendations may be conditional upon patient values and preferences, the resources available or the setting in which the intervention will be implemented. Recommendations may be at the discretion of the patient and clinician, or qualified with an explanation about the issues that would lead decisions to vary	3. Uncertainty or variability in values and preferences. The less the confidence in estimates of typical values and preferences, and the greater the variability, the less likely a strong recommendation	For
			4. Resource use. The higher the resource use, the less likely a strong recommendation	Against

4.2   The principle and method of evidence appraisal

Evidence appraisal, also known as critical appraisal or critiquing the literature, refers to a deliberate and systematic examination of a published study, and making a reasonable judgment as to the validity of its methods, importance of the question and the findings, and application to clinical practice.

Despite plenty of criteria having been suggested, no universally accepted "gold-standard"instrument for critical appraisal exists. However, a structured approach with checklists in the process can potentially improve the quality of appraisal, and be useful to screen out researches of low quality or of little relevance. Some widely used checklists are listed below: CASP; Oxford CEBM; SIGN; SURE.

At the same time, guidelines exist for the transparent and accurate reporting of research. The CONSORT (Consolidated Standards of Reporting Trials) statement is an evidence-based, minimum set of recommendations for RCT. The statement comprises a 25-item checklist and a flow diagram. The checklist items focus on reporting how the trial was designed, analyzed, and interpreted; the flow diagram displays the progress of all participants through the trial. There are other reporting guidelines for observational studies (STROBE), systematic reviews (PRISMA), diagnostic studies (STARD), clinical practice guidelines (AGREE), etc. These statements and guidelines can not only guide the writing of a scientific report, but also help to critically appraise the respective reports. The EQUATOR database contains a comprehensive collection of these reporting guidelines with links to resources relevant to research reporting.

Generally, the following 4 major questions should be kept in mind whenever appraising a study.

Is this study necessary and relevant?

Does the study use valid methods to address this question? (Can I trust this study?)

Are the valid results of this study important? (Does this study matter?)

Are these valid, important results applicable to my patient or population? (Can I use the information provided by this study?)

A clearly focused question which is relevant to the field of interest is of first and foremost concern. Even with the most rigorous design and perfect conducting, a study is of little value if it does not address an important topic and add something new, or simply if it is not relevant to the current PICO question.

The assessment of necessity and relevancy is inevitably based on subjective opinion, as what might be crucial to some will be irrelevant to others. Nonetheless, the first question to ask of any study is whether its purpose and hypothesis are relevant to the specific field of work.

We need to determine whether the author has made it explicit why the study should be conducted. Look for, mostly in the introduction section of the paper, the problem statement and then the evidence for why the stated problem is really a problem. A good research question normally identifies three or four components (PICO): the group or population of patients, the studied parameter (e.g., an intervention), the outcomes of interest, and the comparison or control groups if applicable.

The following sections will show you how to assess the validity, importance and practice of a study providing it is necessary and relevant.

4.3   Internal authenticity evaluation of evidence

In scientific research, internal authenticity (internal validity) refers to the extent to which an estimation of effect based on a study is warranted. Schematically, truth in the study is a function of internal validity. The internal validity is assessed by the degree to which a study minimizes systematic error (or 'bias', systematic deviation of results or inferences from truth). Sometimes simply stated as validity, internal validity contrasts with external validity, the degree to which it is warranted to generalize results to other contexts.

The following questions aid to evaluate the internal validity of a research study.

4.3.1   Was the study design appropriate for the research question?

Different research questions can best be addressed by different study designs (Table 4-1, Figure 4-1). Generally, there are 2 types of research questions, either measuring frequency of events or assessing the association (e.g., the efficacy or effectiveness of an intervention). For the first type of question, an observational study rather than a RCT is the most appropriate design; while for the later, systematic review of well conducted RCTs or individual RCT might be the optimal choice. In case of a RCT being infeasible or unethical, non-randomized controlled trial followed by cohort study, case-control study and other observational designs can be the alternative.

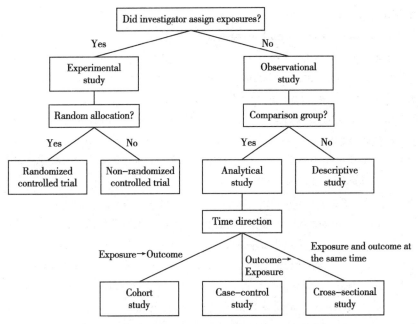

Figure 4-1　Algorithm for classification of types of clinical research

4.3.2　Did the study methods address the key potential source of bias?

Bias is systematic deviation of results or inferences from truth, which can be classified into 3 general categories: selection bias, information bias and confounding bias. Selection bias distorts result from procedures of selecting subjects, and from factors influencing study participation. For instance, differential selection of potential eligible participants or differential assigning groups biases the studies. Information bias is measurement errors in the needed information, which can either exaggerate or underestimate effects or frequencies. And finally, confounding bias refers to the distortion of a measure of the effect of an exposure on an outcome due to the association of the exposure with other factors that influence the occurrence of the outcome.

Glasziou et al proposed using the questions below to assess the internal validity of a primary study:

Recruitment: Were the subjects representative of the target population?

Allocation or adjustment: Was the treatment allocation concealed before randomization and were the groups comparable at the start of the trial (baseline)?

Maintenance: Was the comparable status of the study groups maintained through equal management and adequate follow-up?

Measurement: Were the outcomes measured with blinded subjects and assessors, and/or objective outcomes?

rammbo is a mnemonic for the elements from these questions.

Moreover, different study designs are prone to varying sources of bias, and call for different strategies and steps to minimize it. Thus, specific considerations and checklists for appraising studies with different study designs are needed.

4.3.2.1 Systematic reviews and meta-analyses

A systematic review is a secondary study with a meticulous, standardized protocol to identify, critically appraise and synthesize all the relevant studies on a particular topic. Meta-analysis can be used if applicable to combine the results from individual studies to produce a single pooled result. The risk of bias of a systematic review may arise from the selection, appraisal of studies and the quality of these primary sources. Publication bias results from the selective publication of investigations with positive findings, and it will distort overall perceptions of the findings on a specific topic.

The PRISMA (preferred reporting items for systematic reviews and meta-analyses) is an evidence-based minimum set of items providing a comprehensive framework for assessments of the quality of reporting in meta-analyses and systematic reviews that assess the benefits and harms of a health care intervention. PRISMA focuses on ways in which authors can ensure a transparent and complete reporting of this type of research. In addition, the CASP checklist for systematic reviews can be a practical tool for quick appraisal. Systematic reviews and meta-analyses are not confined to RCTs. The MOOSE (meta-analysis of observational studies in epidemiology) guidelines have been developed for meta-analyses of non-RCTs.

4.3.2.2 Randomized Controlled Trials

In RCTs, the integrity of randomization, treating equally across groups, assessing outcomes blindly or objectively, attrition rate, etc. are more of concern. The random allocation of participants into different arms in a trial eliminates selection bias and ensures that treatment groups are equivalent in terms of both known and unknown confounding factors; any differences in baseline characteristics (i.e. the potential risk factors), if any, between groups can only be due to chance. Therefore, the difference in outcomes should be ascribed to the effect of intervention plus chance. Statistically, the effect can be described and inferred based on certain models of probability distributions. If the outcomes are assessing blindly or objectively, information bias can be minimized.

However, study design alone will not guard against bias if crucial aspects of the study protocol are suboptimal and/or the study is poorly conducted. The potential for selective enrollment of patients into the study would be an important source of bias if the group to which individuals will be allocated is known or can be guessed. Allocation concealment is an important procedure to protect the integrity of randomization so that the treatment to be allocated is not known or easily guessed before each patient enters the study. There are many approaches of randomization that are known to effectively conceal the randomization sequence. The use of sequentially numbered, opaque sealed envelopes (SNOSE) is both cheap and effective. Centralized randomization by using a computer-generated allocation is efficient for concealed allocation especially in multicenter trials. Failure to conceal the allocation sequence will lead to a great distortion of the results. An intention-to-treat (ITT) analysis of the results of a trial based on the initial randomized treatment assignment and not on the treatment eventually received. ITT analysis is intended to avoid various misleading artifacts such as non-random attrition of participants from the study or crossover. Thus, ITT maintains the integrity of randomization at the stage of data analysis.

In RCT, study groups should be managed equally except for the investigated intervention. And all the outcomes should be measured objectively or blindly to avoid information bias.

The CONSORT (consolidated standards of reporting trials) statement provides a comprehensive tool with which to assess the standard of reporting in randomized trials. The CONSORT statement checklist and flowchart, as well as the aforementioned checklists of CASP, Oxford CEBM, SIGN, and SURE for RCTs, are very helpful for appraising RCTs.

4.3.2.3　Cohort Studies

Cohort studies involve following up two or more groups of participants longitudinally to observe the differences in the outcome of interest between groups. Cohort studies can be performed prospectively, retrospectively, or bi-directionally.

The major methodological concern with cohort studies is their high potential for selection bias and confounding. These problems are particularly significant when therapeutic interventions are studied. In this situation, the treatment that someone receives is determined by the patient's or doctor's preferences, current treatment paradigms or local policy. The participants in different groups would have been different in a number of ways, and these differences, rather than the treatment itself, might be responsible for the observed outcomes. Particularly, confounding by indication is a bias that occurs when the intervention of interest is selectively used or not used by those who developed the outcome of interest; a causal relationship between the intervention and its effect on disease outcome cannot be established. Although some potential confounding factors can be measured and accounted for in the analysis, the residual confounding is not possibly controlled in cohort studies. Residual confounding is the distortion that remains after controlling for potential confounders in the design and/or analysis of a study. There are three sources of residual confounding: additional confounding factors that were not considered; insufficient control of confounding; and misclassification of subjects with respect to confounding variables.

Objective or blind measure of outcomes independent of the exposure status is also crucial to avoid information bias in cohort studies.

The STROBE (strengthening the reporting of observational studies in epidemiology) statement is reporting guidelines for observational studies, including cohort, case-control and cross-sectional studies. In the appraisal of cohort studies, the SROBE statement and other checklists (e.g., the checklists of CASP, Oxford CEBM, SIGN, and SURE) can be helpful.

4.3.2.4　Case-control Studies

Case-control studies firstly select the cases with the outcome of interest (e.g., a disease) and the controls without the outcome. Then the data with respect to the potential exposures are retrospectively collected and compared between the case and the control groups. Case-control studies are the ideal design for the investigation of risk factors of a rare outcome (e.g., rare diseases).

Major methodological difficulties with case-control studies are the selection of both appropriate cases and controls, and the possibility of "recall bias"(a subjective interpretation of the causes of their outcome can alter their recall of the potential risk factors). To reduce the selection bias, the controls should be drawn from exactly the same source population as the cases, and the only difference between controls and cases should be that the controls have not developed the condition of interest (i.e., the only reason that a person would have been included in the case or control group is that he or she has or has not the specific outcome). And the same exclusion criteria, except for the outcome, are used for both groups; the cases and controls are defined clearly and differentiated from each other. To minimize the information bias, the exposure status should be measured in a standard, valid and reliable way; and the case ascertainment should not be influenced by the knowledge of exposure. Finally, the main potential confounders should be identified and taken into account in the study design and data analysis. The checklists aforementioned can be used to appraise a case-control study.

4.3.2.5   Cross-sectional studies

A cross-sectional study is a 'snapshot' of a particular population in which exposures and outcomes are assessed at the same time. Again, we can assess the validity of a cross-sectional study by the STROBE statement and other checklists.

4.3.2.6   Studies that assess the accuracy of diagnostic tests

These studies usually have a cross-sectional design, but possess many specific issues that should be considered, including participants enrollment, gold-standard, parameters measuring the accuracy of diagnostic tests, etc.

The STARD 2015 (standards for the reporting of diagnostic accuracy studies) provides a detailed flowchart and 30-item checklist for standardized reporting and appraisal of studies that assess the accuracy of diagnostic tests. Other checklists also provide similar and simpler tool for this type of study.

Hence, once identified the study design of a given paper, we should examine it for the risk of bias with one of the available design-specific critical-appraisal checklists, such as those developed by the critical appraisal skills programme (CASP), Oxford Center for Evidence-Based Medicine (Oxford CEBM) and Scottish Intercollegiate Guidelines Network (SIGN), etc. Separate checklists for the appraisal of systematic reviews, RCTs, cohort studies, case-control studies, diagnostic test studies, economic evaluations and qualitative research etc. are accessible on the websites as mentioned in the previous section, and most of the items of these checklists are derived from the Users' Guides to the Medical Literature series of articles that were originally published in the *Journal of the American Medical Association.*

4.3.3   Was the study performed in line with the original protocol?

Deviations from the planned protocol can affect the validity or relevance of a study. Common deviations include the changes of sample size, modifications in inclusion and exclusion criteria, variation in the provided treatments or interventions, changes to the employed techniques or technologies, and changes to the duration of follow-up. Any deviations from planned protocol should be scrutinized for the reasons and implications – will the internal and/or external validity be compromised?

4.3.4 Were the statistical analyses performed correctly, and do the data justify the conclusions?

Evaluating the appropriateness of statistical analyses for clinicians can sometimes be difficult. However, the methods and tools used in the statistical analysis should be described in appropriate ways in the methods section. In particular, the approach to dealing with missing data should be specified; patients lost to follow-up and missing data should be clearly identified in the results section, best be demonstrated in a flowchart.

The conclusions of the paper must be reasonable and logical based on the research data. In some cases, the authors may generalize their findings in a subgroup to a broader population. At times, a correlation can be misinterpreted as a causal relationship.

4.3.5 Are there any conflicts of interest?

Conflicts of interest occur when personal factors have the potential to influence professional roles or responsibilities, which should be openly disclosed. Identification of a potential conflict of interest is not synonymous with having an actual conflict of interest or poor research practice. During the process of critical appraisal, we should check, for a declaration, if any, about the source and role of funding for the study, and how this conflict was managed, is there a statement.

4.4 The importance of evidence

If a study can be trusted (internal valid), the next step is to ask whether the study matters, or how good/important a treatment, diagnostic test, etc. are. Normally, we would like to have one sentence with one figure to answer it; but in real life, one figure is far from enough to tell the whole story. Someone only cares about the hypothesis test. A P-value <0.05, so called statistical significance, will cheer them up and then say that it is an important finding. However, a P-value <0.05 is far from enough to tell the whole story again.

Four questions may aid to evaluate the importance of the findings of a study.

4.4.1 What is the primary outcome of the research? Does it make sense clinically?

An outcome is one of the possible results that may stem from exposure to a causal factor or from preventive or therapeutic interventions. The primary outcome is the outcome that a researcher considers to be the very most important and used to arrive at a decision on the overall result of the study among the many outcomes (i.e. the secondary outcomes) been examined in the study. The primary outcome is defined at the time of study design, providing a basis for the estimation of the sample size necessary for an adequate power to avoid false negative error. The primary outcome, together with the study hypothesis, is identified a priori and also reduces the risk of false-positive errors resulting from multiple statistical tests of many secondary outcomes. Especially, there is only one primary outcome in each RCT. And it is of utmost importance to differentiate a primary outcome from secondary outcomes. Statistical testing of secondary outcomes is associated with an increased risk of both false-positive and false-negative errors.

In clinical trials, "endpoints" are measurement and evaluation of what happens to people in the trial, and there are two types of endpoints: clinical and surrogate endpoints. According to the U.S. Food and Drug Administration (FDA), clinical outcomes are the most reliable clinical trial endpoints. They directly measure what matters most to people—whether they feel or function better, or live longer. Therapies can be recommended with confidence when clinical trials show that benefits, as measured by clinical outcomes, outweigh the adverse effects.

Surrogate endpoints are used instead of clinical outcomes in some clinical trials. Surrogate endpoints are used when the clinical outcomes might require quite a large sample size or take a very long time to study, or in cases where the clinical benefit of improving the surrogate endpoint, such as controlling blood pressure, is well understood. Occasionally, they can allow treatments to be assessed in situations where the use of clinical outcomes would be excessively invasive or unethical. In the evaluation of pharmaceutical products, commonly used surrogate endpoints include: pharmacokinetic measurements; in vitro (i.e. laboratory) measures; macroscopic appearance of tissues; change in levels of (alleged) "biological markers of disease"; radiological appearance, etc.

Clinical trials are needed to show that surrogate endpoints can be relied upon to predict, or correlate with, clinical benefit. Surrogate endpoints that have undergone this testing are called validated surrogate endpoints and these are accepted by the FDA as evidence of benefit. However, even a validated surrogate endpoint can sometimes be misleading. For example, in the Action to Control Cardiovascular Risk in Diabetes (ACCORD) trial, intensive therapy resulted in markedly lower glycated hemoglobin levels than standard therapy, but it did not significantly lower the rate of cardiovascular events, and the mortality was even higher. If the primary outcome in a study is of less clinical significance, or is not itself a direct measure of either harm or clinical benefit, special care should be taken. An ideal surrogate endpoint should have some features.

The surrogate endpoint should be reliable, reproducible, clinically available, easily quantifiable, affordable and exhibit a dose-response effect.

It should be a true predictor of disease (or risk of disease) and not merely express exposure to a covariable. The relationship between the surrogate endpoint and the disease should have a biologically plausible explanation.

It should be sensitive and have an acceptable positive predictive value—that is, a positive result in the surrogate endpoint should pick up all or most patients at increased risk of adverse outcome; and the positive result should always or usually mean that the patient thus identified is at increased risk of adverse outcome.

It should be specific and have an acceptable negative predictive value—that is, a negative result should exclude all or most of those without increased risk of adverse outcome; and the negative result should always or usually mean that the patient thus identified is not at increased risk of adverse outcome.

There should be a precise cut-off between normal and abnormal values, providing the surrogate endpoint is a continuous variable.

Changes in the surrogate endpoint should rapidly and accurately reflect the response to therapy.

It should be amenable to quality control monitoring.

A composite outcome is a combination of a number of individual outcomes (such as a number of different serious morbidities), which is frequently used as primary outcome in randomized trials. Although it can increase statistical efficiency and precision when used properly, such measures may prove challenging for the interpretation of results and bring greater uncertainty. Components can be unreasonably combined, inconsistently defined, and inadequately reported. In a systematic review posted on *BMJ*, in 11 of 16 trials with a statistically significant composite, the abstract conclusion falsely implied that the effect applied also to the most important component.

4.4.2   What is the magnitude of the effects in the study? Is it clinically relevant?

The term effect has two meanings: the endpoint of a causal mechanism (e.g. AIDS being an effect of HIV infection), or a change in a population characteristic (e.g. the disease frequency in a population) caused by a factor being at one level versus another. Often, disease frequency is measured in terms of risk (the probability of an event during a specified period of time), incidence rate (the number of new cases divided by the person-time at risk for a given time period) and odd (in a certain group of people, the number of people with the disease divided by the number of people without the disease), so the effect is the change in risk, incidence rate or odd, separately. And the effect size is the magnitude of the absolute arithmetic difference or the ratio of risks, incidence rates or odds between study groups, respectively (though actually the absolute difference measure of odds is rarely used) (Table 4-5). The effect size is the main finding of a quantitative study, and should be reported in a paper's abstract and results section. One should always ask whether the effect size is clinically relevant? Does a decrease of mortality of 0.2% or an increase of 12 days in median survival really make sense in practice? Does lowering the blood pressure of 1 mmHg really make difference for hypertension patients? We need a logic reasoning and judgment about the clinical significance of the effect size in the context of scientific and background knowledge.

Table 4-5   Common measures of effect size

Measure	Calculation	Remark
Relative risk or risk ratio (RR)	EER/CER	A relative risk of 1 means there is no difference in risk between the two groups. An RR of < 1 means the event is less likely to occur in the experimental group than in the control group. An RR of > 1 says the event is more likely to happen in the experimental group than in the control group

continue

Measure	Calculation	Remark
Odds ratio (OR)	(EE/EN)/(CE/CN)	OR approximates to RR when the prevalence of the disease is low (rare disease assumption)
Relative risk reduction (RRR)	|CER−EER|/CER or 1−RR	A RRR is the percent reduction in risk in the experimental group compared to the control group. If the event rate increases in the experimental group, the same formula can be used to calculate the relative risk increase. (RRI). This value is the absolute benefit increase (ABI) when the event represents a good outcome
Risk reduction (RD) or absolute risk reduction (ARR)	|CER−EER|	RD or ARR is the arithmetic difference between EER and CER. If the event rate increases in the experimental group, it turns to be the absolute risk increase (ARI).
Number needed to treat (NNT) or number needed to harm (NNH)	1/RD	NNT and NNH is the inverse of ARR and ARI, respectively. The NNT is the average number of patients who need to be treated to prevent one additional bad outcome. Similarly, NNH indicates how many patients on average need to be exposed to a risk-factor over a specific period to cause harm in an average of one patient who would not otherwise have been harmed

CE: control events; EE: experimental events. CN: control non-events; EN: experimental non-events. CER: control event risk (rate); EER: experimental event risk (rate).

Relative risk (RR) and relative risk reduction (RRR) are ratio-based measurements (Table 4-5). Special attention should be paid to the effect size expressed as RR or RRR. Because such measures (RR and RRR) cannot reflect the baseline risk (i.e. the event rate in the control group), thus it is not possible to discriminate huge effect size from small one. For example, a RRR of 50% can be found when the experimental event rate (EER) is 20%, and the control event rate (CER) is 40% (RRR=1−RR=1−0.2/0.4=50%). In this case, the treatment lowers a 20% risk of event (absolute risk reduction, ARR=40%−20%=20%), which is a considerable treatment effect and can be clinically significant. However, the RRR remains 50% when EER is 0.2%, and CER is 0.4% (RRR=1−RR=1−0.002/0.004=50%). At this time, the effect of the treatment is very tiny with merely 0.2% reduction of the risk of event (ARR=0.4%−0.2%=0.2%). Therefore, ARR is clinically more meaningful as it preserves the baseline risk, reflecting the absolute change of risk.

Number needed to treat (NNT), the reverse of ARR (1/ARR), is the average number of patients who need to be treated to prevent one additional bad outcome (i.e. the number of patients that need to be treated for one of them to benefit compared with a control in a clinical trial). NNT is an important and straightforward measure of the effect size of a health-care intervention, typically a treatment with medication. In the previous examples, an ARR of 20% corresponds to a NNT of 5, which means on average 5 patients need to be treated to prevent a bad outcome. On the contrary, when the ARR is 0.2%, the NNT turns to be 500 — on average 500 patients have to be treated to prevent only one case of the bad outcome.

Similar to NNT, number needed to harm (NNH) indicates how many patients on average need to be exposed to a detrimental effect of an intervention or a risk-factor over a specific period to cause harm in one patient who would not otherwise have been harmed. NNH is computed as 1/ARI. For instance, nutrient supplementation of beta-carotene in male smokers reportedly increased the risk of lung cancer. Suppose the absolute risk increase in five years is roughly 0.5%, then the NNH is 200 and it interprets as that if 200 male smokers take beta-carotene for 5 years, one case of lung cancer will be expected to develop on average.

Thus, the NNT and NNH provide us with a nice measure of the possible effort we and the patients have to expend to prevent or cause one more bad outcome, and help to balance the benefit of an intervention against the potential harm caused by it. To understand NNT and NNH correctly and comprehensively, we need to consider some additional points.

4.4.2.1 NNT, commonly expressed as a single number, is a point estimate. NNT usually makes sense only when the treatment has been shown to be statistically different to the control. We can also calculate the interval estimation according to the confidence interval (CI) of ARR. We will go into detail of interval estimates and confidence intervals in the following part of this section. For example, in a clinical trial taking itraconazole decreased the infection rate by 17% (ARR, 95% CI 4.7%~29.2%) in the first 6 months after transplantation, however increased 3% (ARI, 95%CI -13.2%~19.8%) of the mortality rate compared to fluconazole. In this case, on average 6 patients similar to the participants in the trial need to be treated to prevent one case of infection, the 95% CI is 3 to 21; The interval estimates provide the uncertainty of our estimates. On the other hand, for the statistically non-significant difference of the mortality, there are two 95% CIs of the NNH: $-\infty$ to -8, and 5 to $+\infty$.

4.4.2.2 NNTs always have a dimension of follow-up time associated with them. In the previous example, the NNT of 6 means compared to fluconazole, every 6 patients taking itraconazole will prevent one more infection in the first six months after transplantation. The NNT will definitely not be the same as to prevent one more case in the first year after transplantation. So, if we want to compare NNTs for different follow-up times, we need to make assumptions about them and a time adjustment to at least one of them.

4.4.2.3 NNTs is based on the comparison between the investigated and control interventions. Therefore, the baseline risk and the treatment in control group have a major impact on them. Our patients may have a different baseline risk of the outcome (e.g. poorly controlled diabetic patients are more vulnerable to infection), hence they may be of higher or lower risk of the event than the average patient in the clinical trial. The NNT should be adjusted for our patient's individual baseline risk of the outcome in daily practice.

4.4.3 How precise are the results?

The purpose of conducting a study is to estimate the true effect. However, the true effect can never be known realistically. The best we can do is to conduct a rigorously controlled study, and estimate the true effect by the observed effect in the study. This estimate is called a point estimate, a single value calculated from observations of the sample that is used to estimate a population value or parameter. The point estimate reminds us that, although the true value lies somewhere in its neighborhood, it is unlikely to be precisely correct. Less precision of the estimate means there are some random errors in the study. Random error is characteristically unpredictable in direction and amount, which may be due to the innate variability of the biological or sociological system being studied, or a lack of precision of the measuring instrument, or the innate variability in the way that different researchers or doctors interpret various data on certain patients, etc. As a principle, internal validity must take precedence over precision. However, a valid study with highly imprecise estimations can only lead to inconclusiveness.

A commonly used measure of precision is confidence interval (e.g. 95% confidence interval, 95%CI). The interval includes a range of parameter values within which all are compatible with the data under the standard interpretation of significance tests. The endpoints of a confidence interval, the lower and upper boundaries, are called confidence limit. The process of calculating the confidence interval is an example of the process of interval estimation. If the underlying statistical model is correct and there is no bias, a confidence interval derived from a valid test will, over unlimited repetitions of the study, contain the true parameter with a frequency no less than its confidence level. For instance, a 95% CI means that if there is no bias, the frequency with which the interval will contain the true parameter will be at least 95%. To put it simply, a confidence interval is a range of values within which one can be confident at least at a level of 95% that a population parameter is estimated to lie.

The construction of confidence interval involves statistical hypothesis tests. For example, if a 95% CI of RR includes the null value of 1, the null hypothesis that RR equals 1 cannot be rejected at the alpha level=0.05 ($P>0.05$). Another example is that if a 95% CI of ARD does not contain the null value of 0, the null hypothesis that RD=0 will be rejected at the alpha level=0.05 ($P<0.05$). However, an interval-estimation possesses more information than a P-value that measures the extent to which a hypothesis is compatible with the observed data. A confidence interval provides simultaneously an idea of the likely direction and magnitude of the underlying association and the random variability of the point estimate. On the other hand, however, the two-sided P-value indicates only the degree of consistency between the data and a single hypothesis, and thus reveals nothing about the magnitude or even the direction of the association, or the random variability of the point estimate.

The width of a confidence interval depends not only on the amount of random variability of the data, but also, to some extent, on the sample size of the study. The larger the sample size, the higher the statistical power to detect small effect, and the narrower the confidence interval. In other words, the precision of the estimates can be superior in larger studies.

The confidence limits (i.e. the lower and upper boundaries) also help us interpret the importance of the result of a study. For example, researchers in a study revealed one kind of eye drops lowered the intraocular pressure by 1mmHg more in glaucoma patients compared to traditional anti-glaucoma eye drops. The point estimate of 1mmHg can still be considered clinically relevant. If, however, the lower limit of the 95% CI is only 0.1mmHg which is far less important clinically, even the result is statistically significant because the 95% CI excludes the null value of 0mmHg, the study may not be considered definitive at the confidence level of 95%.

4.4.4 Are there any other explanations of the hypothesis test (e.g. false positive, false negative, or just a chance)?

We tend to believe the hypothesis tests in a study tell us the true stories, so do the confidence intervals. But that is not always real. Apart from the distortion caused by bias and confounding, one should bear in mind that there are two types of errors in statistical hypothesis test: type I and type II errors. A type I error is the rejection of a true null hypothesis (i.e. "false positive" finding), while a type II error is retaining a false null hypothesis (i.e. "false negative" finding). In other words, a type I error is to falsely infer the existence of something that is not there, while a type II error is to falsely infer the absence of something that is.

Pocock et al delineated the key questions that should be asked when the primary outcome is positive or negative (Table 4-6).

Table 4-6　Key questions to ask when the primary outcome is positive/negative

the primary outcome is positive	the primary outcome is negative
1. Does a P value of <0.05 provide strong enough evidence?	1. Is there some indication of potential benefit?
2. What is the magnitude of the treatment benefit?	2. Is the trial underpowered?
3. Is the primary outcome clinically important (if alternative outcome measures, combined outcome measures, are they reliable)?	3. Is the primary outcome appropriate (or accurately defined)?
4. Are secondary outcomes supportive?	4. Is the population appropriate?
5. Are the principal findings consistent across important subgroups?	5. Was the treatment regimen appropriate?
6. Is the trial large enough to be convincing?	6. Are there deficiencies in trial conduct?
7. Is the trial stopped early?	7. Is a claim of noninferiority of value?
8. Do concerns about safety counterbalance positive efficacy?	8. Do subgroup findings elicit positive signals?
9. Is the efficacy-safety balance patient-specific?	9. Do secondary outcomes reveal positive findings?
10. Are there flaws in trial design and conduct?	10. Can alternative analyses help?
11. Do the findings apply to my patients?	11. Does more positive external evidence exist?
	12. Is there a strong biologic rationale that favors the treatment?

After clarifying the magnitude and precision of the effect, clinicians can move on to the final question, that is, how to apply the findings to patients.

4.5　The application of evidence

If the evidence being assessed is shown to be both valid and important, the next step we need to do is to determine if we can apply it to the current patient. In this step, we need to integrate the evidence with our clinical experience and expertise, and with our patient's values and preferences. The following questions will help us to assess the applicability of the evidence.

4.5.1 Can this evidence be applied in the medical unit and current clinic setting?

Firstly, we need to consider whether the evidence can be applied in the current setting. Some new drugs may not be available on the local market or not be covered by medical insurance; some diagnostic tests may not be performed in the current setting due to lack of the specific instrument or detection kits.

4.5.2 Is the current patient more or less similar to the participants in the study?

In everyday practice, if the current patient before us meets all inclusion criteria and does not violate any of the exclusion criteria, and his or her demographic characteristics are similar to those in the study, we can then apply the valid and important results with considerable confidence. However, the patient before us may not be identical to those in the study. Often, they share some characteristics, while differ in others. Can the study results still be applied? Actually, most differences between our patients and those in the studies tend to be quantitative (e.g., different ages, different levels of risk for the outcome of interest) rather than qualitative (e.g., different immune status and response to infection, absolute contraindications). The best way we should do is to consider whether the current patient's sociodemographic features or pathobiology are so different from those in the study that the results are totally useless. If it is true, we should go on with the literature search for relevant evidence. Otherwise, the evidence can also be useful, though we need to estimate the individual expected effect if it is applied to the current patient.

4.5.3 What are the expected effects if the evidence is applied to the current patient?

Every patient has his or her unique risk factors for the outcome of interest, thus the expected effect in each patient may be different. If the effect of an intervention is shown to be clinically significant in the study, but the expected effect in the current patient is estimated to be minor, the intervention should not be used.

One approach is firstly to estimate the patient's expected event rate (PEER), the possible event rate if the current patient are not treated, then reverse the product of PEER and RRR or RRI of the intervention to yield an individualized NNT or NNH.

$NNT_{individualized} = 1/(PEER \times RRR)$ or

$NNH_{individualized} = 1/(PEER \times RRI)$

The individualized parameter, PEER, can be estimated based on:

the control event rate (CER) from the study;

CER from a subgroup with the characteristics similar to the current patient;

the calculation based on a valid clinical prediction guide (formula);

the data from other valid papers.

Once we estimate the expected effect of an intervention in the current patient, we may balance the likely benefit against the likely harm by the intervention via a measure, namely the likelihood ratio of being helped and harmed (LHH):

LHH=(1/NNT)/(1/NNH) =NNH/NNT or

LHH=ARR/ARI

For example, the age-related eye disease study (AREDS) formula of nutrient supplements containing beta-carotene decreased the progression of age-related macular degeneration by 28% in AREDS study. If the current patient is a smoker, the PEER can be 43% according to the study. On the other hand, beta-carotene had been shown to increase 0.5% of the risk of developing lung cancer in smokers in another study. The $NNT_{individualized}$=1/(PEER×RRR) =1/(0.43×0.28) =9; while $NNH_{individualized}$=1/ARI=1/0.5%=200. So LHH=200/9=22.2, which means even the patient might have a small increased risk of developing lung cancer, taking the supplements will still be over 20 times more likely to help him than to harm him.

4.5.4 What are the patient's values and expectations towards the intervention and the outcomes?

We should never forget that evidence-based medicine is the integration of best research evidence with clinical expertise and patient unique values and expectations. As the saying goes, one man's meat is another man's poison. The value judgement about the benefit of a good outcome and the harm of a bad event may be different from one another. Therefore, we need very good communication with the patient, to understand the patient's unique values and preferences, and to make sure he or she understands every detail of the intervention, the good and bad outcomes as well as the respective possibilities; then, we can finally make a decision. This collaborative process and shared decision making (SDM) allows us and the patients to make health care decisions together, taking into account the best scientific evidence available, the clinical expertise, as well as the patient's values and preferences.

Summary

Contemporary healthcare relies not only on individual medical skills, but also on the best information of the effectiveness and safety of each intervention being accessible to healthcare providers. Thus, critically assessing the quality and usefulness of the evidence that is mainly from scientific researches turns to be a key step of evidence-based practice. The aims of critical appraisal are to determine the validity, evaluate the importance and assess the applicability of the evidence.

(Yuan Yuanzhi)

Clinical research design

Learning objectives

1. **To master** the contents and principles of clinical research design.
2. **To be familiar with** different types of clinical research designs.
3. **To know** how to use different types of clinical research designs to solve clinical problems.

Case 5-1

Miss Ma, 21, was a junior student at a key university in Beijing. On April 19th, 2016, she attended the obstetrics and gynecology department due to abdominal pain. Blood routines showed that the total number of leukocytes was $14.51 \times 10^9/L$, neutrophil ratio was 74.5%, and C-reactive protein was 10mg/L (normally less than 0.5mg/L), indicating the presence of infection or inflammation. B-scan ultrasonography showed two pelvic space-occupying lesions, and the property of the one on the right side of the uterine fundus remained to be determined, possibly affected by the large amount of effusion in both the ovary and the pelvic cavity. Further transabdominal and transvaginal ultrasonography revealed that the bilateral ovaries increased in size, with solid cystic changes, and the cystic areas were arranged in a honeycomb pattern. A rich blood flow signal was seen in the solid areas of CDFI, and free fluids were seen in the abdominal cavity, with a maximum depth of 5.6cm. Taking into account the ultrasound results, clinicians considered the possibility of ovarian cancer. Further investigation of tumor markers CA125 showed an increased value to 151.5μl/ml (normally less than or equal to 35lμ/ml), but coagulation and liver and kidney function were normal. At the same time, thyroid ultrasound and breast ultrasound were performed on the patient. Multiple thyroid nodules with punctate calcification were found in bilateral thyroid glands. Bilateral hyperplasia of the breasts was found and the structure of the glands was disordered. Peritoneal MRI revealed bilateral cystic space-occupying lesions in adnexal areas. Cystic adenocarcinoma or cystadenoma was considered highly possible. PET-CT showed a small amount of peritoneal effusion and flaky low-density shadow was seen in the pelvic uterine area with slight increased metabolism and local bleeding density. The hepatobiliary pancreas, spleen and kidneys were not significantly abnormal.

Question: How should a clinician manage this patient?

Should the patient be diagnosed with ovarian cancer? What's the evidence for the diagnosis?

What causes this change? How should evidence for evidence-based medicine be obtained?

What interventions can be used to ease the patient's pain?

Clinical medicine belongs to the category of applied science, with the purpose of serving patients. The doctors' job is to identify the cause, confirm the diagnosis, and take appropriate treatment to maximize the patient's recovery or improve his prognosis. Clinical problems are problems that need to be solved in the medical practice. Clinical research questions arise from clinical practice. The solution to clinical research questions is helpful for raising the awareness of the disease and is expected to improve the diagnosis and treatment. The diagnosis of the disease is the first problem that clinicians must solve when facing the patient. The correct diagnosis is the basis of correct treatment, and the correct diagnosis depends on the understanding of the specific etiology, pathological mechanism and clinical manifestations. With the development of medicine, the progress of human society, and the changes of the natural environment, new and unknown diseases continue to emerge, which also keeps deepening our understanding of the etiology of the known diseases, and the changes in the living environment have also resulted in a big change of human disease spectrum. Therefore, cause diagnosis has been undergoing a constant transforming and deepening process. Etiology research in epidemiology explores the causes of disease as well as the interactions between related factors. In etiological study, what needs to be emphasized is that exposures related to the outcome (disease) must occur before the outcome. However, these factors are not necessarily the real cause of the outcome. The vast majority of chronic diseases, such as cancer, essential hypertension, diabetes, and atherosclerosis, are the result of a combination of genetic and environmental factors. The study of etiology provides the basis for the clinical diagnosis, treatment and prevention of the diseases, with the hope of maximizing the benefits of disease prevention and control. Table 5-1 outlines the types of etiology study commonly used in clinical research.

Table 5-1　Summary of common design types for etiology study

Types	Subtype 1	Subtypes 2	Features	Uses
Observational study	Descriptive study	Case report	Fast, with no control and no design	Providing cause cues
		Cross-sectional study	With design but no control	Descriptive distribution, searching cause cues
	Analytical study	Case-control study	From effect to cause, grouped according to whether the subject has the disease or not	Preliminary diagnosis of causality

continue

Types	Subtype 1	Subtypes 2	Features	Uses
		Cohort study	From cause to effect, grouped by exposure	Verification of causality
Experimental study		Randomized controlled trial	Randomized grouping, human intervention	Verification of causes, study of drug effects and side effects

The case of a young female patient above is used as an example to discuss and introduce the common etiological research methods.

5.1　Statement of clinical research problems: case report

Case report is detailed clinical reports on an individual case or a few cases, covering the patient's clinical manifestations, differential examination results, laboratory tests and examination results, treatment and prognosis of the disease, which usually include the author's analysis and discussion of the patient's etiology, diagnosis and treatment. In the reports some hypotheses of suspected diseases are raised from these abnormal cases. The exploration of possible causes from abnormal findings is often the first clue to find serious or rare adverse reactions of the clinical drug in actual clinical work.

Take the above-mentioned patient with suspected ovarian cancer as an example. This is an example of a young female patient atypically suspected of ovarian cancer. Both ovarian ultrasound and nuclear magnetic resonance made the clinicians highly suspect ovarian cancer. There were multiple endocrine organs involvement, but PET-CT did not find obvious hypermetabolic foci and dyscrasia commonly found in patients with advanced ovarian cancer. Through detailed examination and report of clinical characteristics and laboratory tests of this patient, it was found that the ovarian changes and ascites similar to the manifestations of ovarian cancer might be the result of other medical problems of the patient, whose clinical symptoms were significantly different from those of common ovarian cancer patients. After a further investigation of the patient's medical history, it was learned that the patient recently took drugs to delay the menstrual cycle. Considering that the use of drugs could not be excluded as a cause, the clinicians advised her to stop the drug. On April 21, 2016, gynecological ultrasound results suggested that bilateral ovarian enlargement seemed to result from ovulation. There was only a small amount of pelvic fluid this time, an obvious reduction compared with the previous results. Five days later re-examination of gynecological ultrasound showed an increase of bilateral ovarian volume, with no obvious abnormalities in uterine sonogram. Blood routine returned to normal and abdominal pain disappeared.

A review of relevant literature shows that no clinical drug side effects of this symptom have been reported. This case report indicates that the drug may have a serious adverse reaction. The research questions raised have attracted the attention of researchers. A subsequent cross-sectional study of the population living in the similar environment as the patient was conducted to determine whether adverse reactions were caused by individual differences in the patients or whether there was a certain prevalence in the population. Therefore, an in-depth etiology study ensued.

In actual clinical and scientific research, we often come across a large number of special cases. The analysis of the diagnosis and treatment of these cases form case reports that often provide us with certain ideas. For example, in this case, the patient was easily misdiagnosed with ovarian cancer in clinical practice, but there were multiple changes in the endocrine system, and the clinical general condition was good, with no dyscrasia present in patients with ovarian cancer. The discrepancy between this patient and ovarian cancer patients raised doubts about the diagnostic accuracy. Individual or a series of cases may provide initial clinical clues, but with only case reports, clinical research is limited by individual differences. Hence another common type of descriptive research is needed—a cross sectional survey.

5.2 Cross-sectional study

Cross-sectional survey is also known as status survey or prevalence study. According to the requirements of prior design, clusters or sampling methods are used to investigate relevant factors and health status at specific time points (time periods) and among specific groups of people, so as to provide clues and hypotheses for further etiology study. The main characteristics of cross-sectional study are as follows: during a cross-sectional study, the disease or health conditions and certain factors are obtained at the same time so that it is difficult to judge whether the etiological factors occur before or after the disease. Therefore, the causal relationship cannot be determined. Only a comparison of differences in prevalence can be provided. Besides, in cross-sectional study there is no pre-determined control group, so preliminary statistical analysis is based on grouping of subjects according to their disease status, that is, with or without disease. Furthermore, the difference in the length of the patient's course may lead to differences in the prevalence obtained during the survey. For example, if the observation lasts for a short duration, even if the effect resulting from the factors occurs, it may not be discovered during the period of time when the investigation is carried out, thus leading to an underestimation of the prevalence rate, which may result in greater bias.

Cross-sectional study, by helping researchers gather the distribution of research factors and disease status in the entire population and their characteristics, can make an overall description and provide clues for further research on disease etiology and risk factors. As in the previous case, the researchers further designed a survey questionnaire for girls of the same major in the patient's university who lived in similar environment. The questionnaire involved basic information, physical examination, and auxiliary diagnostic tests. Basic information included age, lifestyle, and whether or not having medication and methods of administration, whether or not having other concomitant medications. Auxiliary diagnostic tests included gynecological ultrasound examination of the survey subjects. If there was an increase in the proportion of ovarian changes among the subjects who had a history of medication, and there was a significant statistical difference from the non-medication exposure group, it would be possible, through analytical study, to preliminarily consider that the drugs for altering the menstrual cycle may be related to changes in the ovary (Table 5-2).

Table 5-2   Occurrence of ovarian changes among subjects with or without medication for changing menstrual cycle

Whether or not medication is taken	Number of people surveyed	Ovarian changes/%
Yes	128	6.25
No	128	0

We also conducted investigations on the frequency of medication to find the differences in the incidence of ovarian changes at different doses. It was found that the higher the frequency of application, the higher the incidence (Table 5-3).

Table 5-3   Occurrence of ovarian changes with medication for changing menstrual cycle

Frequency of medication	Number of people surveyed	Ovarian changes/%
Greater than 5 times	32	15.625 0
3-5 times	32	6.250 0
Less than 3 times	64	1.562 5

Based on the results of the above cross-sectional survey, we can see that the adverse reaction had a higher prevalence in patients with more than three applications of the drug, suggesting that the cause may be related to the frequency of application and the cumulative dosage.

As described above, a large-scale survey was conducted on the past health conditions and medication status in the patient's class, grade and school. Through investigation of the presence of similar conditions in the population around the patient and the history of medication before the onset of illness, it was found that ovarian changes also existed among the patient's classmates who had the medication history to postpone the menstrual cycle. On the one hand, the patient was given follow-up after removal of intervention factors. The patient's outcome highly suggested that her recent medication history was related to her ovarian performance. On the other hand, a cluster sampling survey of the specific group of female students who had similar lifestyle was conducted through a questionnaire. The description of ovarian changes in terms of population, area, and time dimensions enabled a more comprehensive understanding of the overall prevalence of ovarian cancer among this particular population. As to the further investigation on the causes of the disease, we are going to introduce two common analytical research methods of etiology study: case-control study and cohort study.

5.3   Case-control study

Case-control study is one of the most important methods in analytical epidemiological study. The basic principle is to take a group of patients who have been diagnosed with a specific disease as a case group, and a group of patients who are not suffering from the disease but are comparable to the case group in some aspects as controls. The patients' previous exposure to various risk factors and their clinical data are collected. The exposure ratios of the risk factors in the case and control groups are measured, compared and statistically tested. If the ratio of an exposure factor between the two groups shows a statistically significant difference, it can be initially considered that there is a statistical correlation between the factor and the disease. After assessing the effects of various biases on the results of the study, it is possible to propose an initial hypothesis by inferring whether one or some exposures are risk factors for the disease. Case-control study is a retrospective study, a research method that explores possible causes from the effect. The key to case-control study is the selection of controls. On the one hand, the control selection must ensure that the controls are representative, that is, they represent the general population that may produces the cases. On the other hand, it requires the comparability between the cases and the controls, which means that after the exclusion of research factors, the other factors in the case group and control group are as balanced as possible. The aim is to improve the effectiveness of the case-control study.

Take the aforementioned case of ovarian changes as an example. According to case-control study design, a cluster sampling survey of 161 female students of the same major was conducted. Altogether 32 similar ovarian metastases were found. Then the rest without ovarian changes were in the control group. The general information, medication history, medication season, eating habits, exercise habits, radiation exposure (application frequency of microwave oven, hair dryer), etc. of all the above-mentioned subjects were collected and analyzed. The exposure ratios of the factors in the case group and the control group were measured and compared, relevant indicators (such as OR) were calculated and statistically tested to determine which factors may be related to the occurrence of ovarian changes.

It is worth noting that the case-control study design grouped the patient's classmates based on whether they had ovarian changes, and then compared the previous exposure to this type of drugs, including the frequency of medication, dose, past habits, etc., with the objective to suggest clues of the causes. To verify the causes, a cohort study design is needed.

5.4   Cohort study

Cohort study is another important method in analytical epidemiological study. The basic principle is to group specific population according to whether they are exposed to a certain factor or according to different exposure levels. The outcome of the disease and the differences in disease outcomes between the different subgroups are compared to decide whether the exposure factors are related to the disease and to further determine the level of association. Cohort study is more effective than case-control study in verifying the etiological hypothesis. However, cohort study is an observational study. The exposure of factors is not random because these factors have been present before the study. Just as the above example shows, the patients were grouped according to whether they took medication, the dose and frequency of medication, and the patients were followed up. Cohort study, a study from cause to effect, has advantages in testing etiological hypotheses and can be used for in-depth research to verify the etiological hypothesis.

We set up a study cohort according to whether or not medication was taken and the frequency of medication, and followed up the changes of the ovary for 6 months after medication was administered. The results of the morbidity are shown in Table 5-4.

Table 5-4　Medications and follow-up outcomes

Whether or not medication is taken	similar Ovarian changes	Occurrence rate/%
Yes	120	5.0
No	240	0.2

5.5　Randomized controlled trial

Randomized controlled trial (RCT) falls into the category of experimental controlled study and is prospective study used in the population to evaluate the effectiveness of medical interventions. RCT assigns research subjects to different groups according to random principles and adopts different interventions. Through follow-up observation at appropriate time intervals, RCT compares the differences in the frequency of occurrence between the groups to evaluate the differences in the effects of different measures. RCT is prospective studies with human interventions involved. The subjects are randomly assigned to experimental or control groups that are comparable. Blindness settings adopted can effectively reduce the bias caused by observational bias and the patient's psychological factors. Observational outcomes are accurately recorded during follow-up, compliance and follow-up rate are improved, and the efficiency of causal validation is enhanced. RCT is currently the most rigorous and reliable test method for assessing the effect of medical interventions and determining causality.

Case report provides us with clues. We then carry out cross-sectional study, case-control study, and further cohort study to provide evidence and ideas for the research of epidemiological characteristics and causes of the disease. The patient took the drug that was already on the market, but given the results of the analytical study, it was highly suspected that the use of this drug is related to ovarian changes. It is therefore necessary to conduct post-marketing large-scale clinical trials according to RCT principles of randomization, control-group and blinding. The subjects with ovarian changes after medication should be randomly divided into continuing medication group and placebo group, followed by the observation of ovarian changes, so as to verify the relationship between drug effects and ovarian changes, which means to conduct clinical trials. If there is no significant change in the ovaries of the test subjects who continue to take the drug, and the ovaries of the placebo-treated subjects gradually return to normal, it can prove that the effect of the drug on the ovary does exist. The information should to be reported to the relevant department in time to take further measures.

To further prove the causal relationship between the drug that alters the menstrual cycle and changes in the ovary (since the drug is already on the market), the researchers collected the subjects who applied the drug clinically and had ovarian changes and grouped them randomly. The control group continued to use the drug, while in the experimental group, placebo drugs with similar medication traits and tablet traits were given to the subjects. Neither the subjects nor the researchers were aware of the medication status of the study subjects. Follow-up observation of their ovary changes lasted for one year. Clinical outcomes were recorded, improvement Rate was compared, and the results were assessed. The results are shown in Table 5-5.

Table 5-5   Occurrence of ovarian changes in the continuing medication and placebo groups

Grouping	Observation cases	Ovarian recovery cases	Improvement rate/%
Continuing medication group	60	2	3.33
Placebo group	60	10	16.67

Summary

In summary, the scope of clinical research involves various aspects including diagnosis, treatment, and prognosis. Common etiological research methods cover all design types of clinical epidemiology. In terms of causal verification strength, experimental studies are better than observational studies, and controlled studies are better than uncontrolled studies. However, the choice of research design is often determined by the different stages of clinical problems and the needs of the researchers. The case report is often the first step, which provides the researchers with certain clinical ideas and discovers certain clinical problems, but whether it has practical significance depends on further conclusions of the research protocol. Observational study does not involve human intervention measures. It only requires the signing of informed consent and privacy protection, without the need to consider other ethical medical issues. It is therefore easier to operate and closer to the real-life environment. However, the study itself is more susceptible to confounding factors and the reliability of the conclusion may be affected. Compared with observational study, experimental study is better at controlling bias and has more reliable conclusions. However, experimental study often involves ethical issues. Sometimes it is difficult to achieve real randomness, blindness and comparison. There may be a big difference between experimental study and the actual clinical practice and therefore its promotion in the actual clinical work may be limited.

For different clinical problems, researchers can choose appropriate design type for clinical research based on actual conditions and requirements. Each type of design has a close relationship with its verification strength (level of evidence). A more rigorous and scientific design can control as much as possible all kinds of biased interference. The conclusions obtained are not easily negated by later research findings and therefore are highly credible. If we can carry out clinical research going from the easy to the difficult and complicated, rationally select the type of clinical research methods, draw appropriate conclusions according to different verification strength, it will help us make a reasonable explanation of the disease cause, and then guide disease prevention and treatment.

(Sai Xiaoyong)

6

Data measurement: accuracy and precision

Learning objectives

1. **To master** outcome variables and methods of measurement and consistency test.
2. **To be familiar with** data types and description, concepts and control measures of random and systematic error.

Case 6-1

A task is set to study a drug's clinical efficacy and safety for acute cerebral infarction, and indicators required to be measured include baseline information such as gender, age, height, weight, temperature, pulse, respiration, blood pressure, blood routine, liver and kidney function, electrocardiogram, skull CT, stroke-related clinical score (e.g., NIHSS score, Barthel index, modified Rankin scale). The main outcome indicator is three-month modified Rankin scale score; secondary indicators are 8 days, 15 days NIHSS score, Barthel index, modified Rankin scale score,and, three-month NIHSS score, Barthel index.

Data measurement refers to quantification of related indicators for studied health disease states of individuals, groups. Take clinical research in stroke as an example: what can be measured by the instrument include height, weight, temperature, blood and other indicators; the severity of the disease can be quantified by the internationally recognized stroke scale. Qualitative index can be classified according to certain principles, such as gender divided into male and female, prognosis divided into good and bad and so on. Only with the quantification of measurements can appropriate statistical approach be applied to compare and analyze. Data measurement is throughout the research work and true and reliable measurement is important to guarantee high-quality research.

6.1 Data types and description

6.1.1 Types of clinical data

In clinical work, measurement results of clinical symptoms, signs, laboratory tests, clinical efficacy, prognosis and other data are divided into the following three categories.

6.1.1.1 Quantitative data

It is also known as measurement data, numeric data or scales data, it is obtained by measuring the numerical value of the observed object. Data values can be shown as consecutive numbers within a certain range of the number axis, generally with a unit. For example: height (cm), weight (kg), hemoglobin (g/L), white blood cell count ($\times 10^9$/L) and so on.

6.1.1.2 Qualitative data

It is also known as enumeration data, classified by certain attributes or characteristics of the observed object. The data does not have the meaning of the number and cannot be represented in the number line, including gender, blood type etc.

6.1.1.3 Level data

It is classified according to certain attributes or characteristics of the observed object, but there is distinction in classification, strength, weight, size, degree, neither quantitative data which is continuously distributed, nor qualitative data which is classified into independent categories according to properties and attributes. The distinction between grades neither is equidistant nor can be measured. For example, clinical efficacy is divided into cured, improved, invalid, death; education background is classified into illiteracy, elementary, middle, high school, college and university, graduate; urine protein is expressed as −, ±, +, ++, +++ and ++++ etc.

6.1.2 Data type conversion

In clinical studies, we sometimes make conversion of several types of data for clinical purposes. For example, three patients have three blood pressure measurements of 125/78mmHg, 143/98mmHg, 175/110mmHg respectively. Blood pressure is quantitative data, but based on the definition of hypertension, it can be divided into normal blood pressure and hypertension. Therefore, these quantitative data can be converted into qualitative data. During the multivariate analysis of outcome contributing factors, if the blood pressure measurements are considered as continuous variables, we can get the impact of every 1mmHg change in blood pressure on hypertension, which is of no practical significance in clinical work. Generally, we observe the clinical impact of 10 or 20mmHg change. For example, the systolic blood pressure can be divided into following groups: <120mmHg, ≥120mmHg and <140mmHg, ≥140mmHg and <160mmHg, ≥160mmHg. Thus, we convert the quantitative data into level data. All conversion must be in accordance with the nationally and internationally recognized standards or related documents.

6.1.3   Soft-sensing index quantization

Soft-sensing index refers to clinical indicator without objective and quantitative measurement, including pain, nausea, fatigue, insomnia etc. In most cases this type of variables can only be described qualitatively, such as have or not have, yes or no, light or heavy etc. It is closely related to the patient's subjective feelings, with the lack of objective and accurate standards, so it is prone to heavy measurement error. In clinical scientific research, such indicators should be quantitative as much as possible. Currently, on the one hand, we use new quantitative measurement to replace soft-sensing index, such as polysomnography (PSG) for an objective assessment of insomnia. We can make accurate and objective evaluation on insomnia with following indications: sleep latency, frequency and time of awakenings, two kinds of sleeping phase, the proportion of sleeping phase, the total time of sleeping. On the other hand, we use psychology, social medicine, personality measurement, life quality measurement for the quantification of soft-sensing index, which is expressed numerically and classified for statistical analysis. For instance, in the past, pain was often measured based on the patient's subjective expression; at present, the 5-point Rating Scales (RS-5) has been adopted domestically and internationally. Pain is classified into five grades, namely mild pain (1 point), pain causing discomfort (2 points), pain having a sense of distress (3 points), acute pain (4 points), severe pain (5 points).

6.2   Systematic error and random error

In practice, subject to subjective or objective factors, gap between the measured value and the true value, is known as measurement error. According to its causes and properties, it can be divided into random error and systematic error.

6.2.1   Random error

It is also known as accidental error, it refers to the error offsetting each other formed of minor factors by random fluctuations during the measurement. It is a type of inconstant, random variation of error. The causes are the effects of some unstable and random factors, such as room temperature, relative humidity and barometric pressure and other environmental conditions, analysis personnel operation, the unstable equipment, and other small differences. Random error is characterized that the size and direction are not fixed, but the error distribution is subject to statistical law, featured as single peak, symmetry and boundedness. Single peak means more small errors than serious errors; symmetry means equal probability of positive error and negative error; boundedness means a great error probability is almost zero. With the measurement number increasing, a margin of plus or minus of random errors can offset each other, the average error will gradually tend to zero. Due to multiple impact factors to random errors and complicated causes, it is hard to be avoided or measured. But due to the normal distribution, it can be analyzed with statistical methods.

6.2.2　Systematic error

Systematic error is caused by the measurement tool, theory defects, personnel's incorrect operation etc. It is repetitive, unidirectional, and testable. That is, under the same conditions, when measurement repeats, it will repeat. The measurement result of the system is high or low, and there are certain rules of the numerical size. For instance, the instrument's zero point is not accurate, or the instrument is not adjusted well, or due to an improper method by the operator, or reagent purity is not high enough and so on. As in the measurement of blood pressure, due to the use of different manufacturer's sphygmomanometer, or whether mercury contains air bubbles, or too wide or narrow beam arm band, it can cause measurement errors. And with a new nurse in the process of blood pressure measurement, it is possible that he/she is not familiar with the standard operation for blood pressure measurement and under inflate or deflate too quickly, leading to inaccurate measurement.

6.2.3　Control error

In clinical studies, because random error is hard to be avoided, we control systematic errors as far as possible. The measurer is required to carefully analyze measurement tools, environmental conditions, and measurement methods to identify the cause of systematic error, and then take measures to control it.

6.2.3.1　To minimize errors caused by the persons being measured, we need to explain measurement purpose for active cooperation and reliable conditions, unify measurement time and method, and strictly control measurement conditions.

6.2.3.2　To minimize errors caused by measurers, we train measurers prior to research, strictly unify measurement methods and techniques; during evaluation, we adopt objective evaluation indicators and methods as far as possible, such as life and death. For non-objective indicators, we should strictly define them. For instance, in the study on cerebral infarction prognosis, according to the modified Rankin scale score, we classify the level of prognosis into good (0~2 points), not good (3~5 points), and death; and adopt blinded measurements method as far as possible.

6.2.3.3　To minimize error during the measurement, we need to check instruments and reagents carefully before measuring, correct commissioning and installation, and if necessary, we use a central laboratory for testing.

6.3　Outcome index and selection of measurement tools

6.3.1　Outcome index

The clinical outcomes of a disease refer to important events occurring in the intervention, directly related to patients, and of clinical significance, including survival, death and disability etc. Outcome index refers to variable measured at a certain time reflecting the health or disease clinical outcomes. To determine whether an intervention is effective for a treatment, it is very important to select outcome index. Good outcome index should have the following characteristics: accurately reflecting the intervention's impact on the extent of improvement in symptoms, and reflecting changes before and after treatment; with strictly unified standards and clear definition, and unlikely to cause ambiguity; with excellent consistency for different studies to be compared.

According to the research project, outcome index can be classified, from the point of view of information sources, into doctor-based and patient-based index. From the perspective of interventions, it can be divided into primary and secondary outcome index. Primary outcome index refers to the main objective of evaluation and measurement in clinical studies, which is determined according to the main effect of interventions. Secondary outcome index is based on interventions' auxiliary or secondary effects. From the point of view of reflecting the health of the patient, outcome index can also be divided into endpoint index and substitution index. Endpoint index refers to clinical events with the greatest impact on patients, and with the most concern from researchers and patients for the development of the disease, such as death, fracture, recurrence, which has most reference value for clinical decision-making. Substitution index is used for the evaluation of intervention effect when endpoint index is not feasible (e.g., taking a long time). Based on epidemiology, therapeutics, pathophysiology and so on, it can replace important clinical outcome, laboratory or iconography measurement indicators, such as blood lipid level, tumor size. Substitution index must have sufficient evidence to support relationship with other clinical outcome indexes, and may predict disease outcome.

The selection of the outcome index should be based on the intervention characteristics, treatment goals and the disease features. For example, when we study the effectiveness of some medications for insomnia, the outcome index may adopt related scale, including the Pittsburgh Sleep Quality Rating (PSQI), Insomnia Severity Index (ISI), Sleep Dysfunction Rating Scale (SDRS), etc., with total or sub-score as the outcome index. Meanwhile, according to *Guiding Principles for Clinical Research of New Chinese Medicine* , the effect of sleep therapy is graded into four levels, namely clinical cure characterized by normal sleeping time with over 6 hours of night deep sleep, full of energy after wakeup; marked effectiveness with significant remission of insomnia, sleeping time increasing more than 3h, and improved sleeping depth; effectiveness in which insomnia is relieved but the increase in sleeping time is less than 3h ; finally ineffectiveness, which is characterized by unnoticeable remission or exacerbation of insomnia after the treatment.

6.3.2　Selection of measurement tools

Clinical outcome measurement tools include technical measurement, clinical measurement and patient-oriented measurement. Technical measurement methods include laboratory test, imagological and electrophysiological examination. Clinical measurement methods cover physical and cognitive damage inspection and the evaluation of activities such as walking. Patient-oriented measurement methods include self-reporting from patients and agents on health, life quality and subjective health feelings.

6.4 Consistency test

6.4.1 Consistency test

In actual clinical work, inconsistency in judgment on special examinations or disease diagnosis occurs among different medical staff. Firstly, the same medical worker may get inconsistent results when observing multiple objects twice; secondly, two medical workers make inconsistent observation judgments for multiple objects; thirdly, multiple medical workers make inconsistent observation judgments for multiple objects. Especially in a large multi-center study, it is necessary to understand the consistency of observations or judgments. If the consistency is poor, it illustrates that the reliability of the results is influenced by judgment inconsistency on repeated checks. We should take necessary measures to control the measurement error. If consistency is preferable, the results of repeated testing are reliable. It is hard to avoid observation inconsistency of repeated observations in practical work. On one hand, we should use appropriate statistical methods to evaluate the consistency of judgments; on the other hand, we should take measures to minimize the inconsistency, which involves consistency test.

Consistency test method is diverse based on the classification of information. For quantitative data, such as blood pressure measurement results, we adopt interclass correlation coefficient evaluation. For qualitative data, it is divided into two cases: binary variables, for example, with or without the symptom, positive or negative test result; polychrome variables, such as the effect (recovery, effective significantly, effective, and ineffective). The check for qualitative data consistency is more commonly used, and Kappa value is mainly used to judge the degree of consistency.

6.4.2 Kappa test

Kappa test is a method for consistency test after correcting opportunity possibility, suitable for two or more investigators on consistency evaluation such as investigator results, diagnosis, test results, etc. The higher consistency means the more reliable results.

Kappa $= (P_0 - P_c)/(1 - P_c)$, in which P_0 is called observation consistent rate, P_c is called opportunity consistent rate, which is consistent with the two test results caused by accidental opportunity.

For example, two radiologists read 100 patients' skulls CT to determine whether there is cerebral infarction. The results are shown in Table 6-1.

Table 6-1　The Analysis results of two radiologists on diagnosis of cerebral infarction with skulls CT

Doctor A	Doctor B		Total
	negative	positive	
negative	74 (a)	2 (c)	76 (a+c)
positive	4 (b)	20 (d)	24 (b+d)
Total	78 (a+b)	22 (c+d)	100 (n)

Observation consistent rate (P_0) =(a+d)/n= (74+20)/100 = 0.94.

Opportunity consistent rate (P_c) =[(a+b) (a+c)/n+(c+d)(b+d)/n]/n=(78×76/100+22×24/100)/100= 0.65.

Actual consistent rate =P_0−P_c=0.94−0.65=0.29.

Non-opportunity consistent rate =1−P_c=1−0.65=0.35.

Kappa= actual consistent rate/non-opportunity consistent rate =0.29/0.35=0.83.

Kappa value is generally between −1 to +1. If observation consistent rate is more than opportunity consistent rate, the Kappa value is between 0 and +1. On the contrary, its value is between −1 and 0. If Kappa = −1, it is completely inconsistent; if Kappa = 0, it illustrates that observation consistent rate is completely caused by opportunities. If Kappa = +1, that is real consistency, completely excluding opportunities consistent, but the possibility is extremely tiny in practice. The size of Kappa value is divided into six sections, representing the strength of the degree of consistency. When Kappa <0, consistency is poor; 0.00 to 0.20, feeble; 0.21 to 0.40, weak; 0.41 to 0.60, moderate; 0.61 to 0.80, high; 0.81 to 1.00, strong.

Summary

Clinical measurements continuously evolve in clinical and research work, and are important guarantees for high-quality research. Measurement data types include quantitative data, qualitative data and level data. We should convert measurement data types according to the actual situation of the corresponding clinical studies, and we should adopt quantitative measurements as a replacement of qualitative indicators as far as possible.

Measurement error is classified as random error and systematic error. For systematic errors, we should, to the best of our ability, find out the cause and then take measures to control it.

The selection of outcome index is an important factor for the treatment effectiveness of interventions to the target disease, which should be based on the characteristics of the intervention, goals of treatment, and the nature of the disease.

Consistency test is adopted by medical staff to determine inconsistent judgments for a variety of special check, diagnosis, etc. Kappa test is used for qualitative data; its value is generally between −1 to +1. The greater the value, the stronger the consistency.

(Liu Xuedong)

7

Identify bias: The estimate of internal validity

Learning objectives

1. **To master** the concepts of selection bias, information bias and confounding bias.
2. **To be familiar with** the control of these three biases.
3. **To know** the measurement of these three biases.

Validity is the extent to which a concept, measurement or conclusion is well-founded and corresponds accurately to the real world. The purpose of science including medical research is to reveal the nature and inherent law of things, so that the results of the study should be consistent with the real results. The collected data, the results of the analysis and the conclusions obtained must be consistent with the objective reality. Validity includes internal validity and external validity. Internal validity is an inductive estimate of the degree to which conclusions about causal relationships can be made (e.g., cause and effect), based on the measures used, the research setting, and the whole research design. Internal validity refers to the validity of the study itself. External validity refers to how a study's results can be generalized to a larger population. External validity concerns the extent to which the (internally valid) results of a study can be held to be true for other cases, for example to different people, places or times. Internal validity is the premise of external validity but external validity does not necessarily perform well when internal validity does due to poor sample representation.

Error is the difference between the results of the study and the true value. The common errors in epidemiological studies include random errors and systematic errors. Random error is the difference between the mean and the population parameters of the random sampling, so it is called random error. Random error is commonly found in the study of random sampling, which can be reduced by using the correct sampling method and increasing the sample size. Systematic error, also known as bias, refers to systematical deviation from the true value due to the influence of other factors in study design, implementation, analysis and inference process and making the error of the results or conclusions. System error can be avoided, and must be controlled.

Generally, bias is divided into selection bias, information bias and confounding bias.

7.1 Selection bias in the population

7.1.1 Conception

Selection bias is the systematic error caused by differences in the characteristics of the subjects selected for the study and those who were not selected, thereby making the sample obtained not representative of the population intended to be analyzed. This bias is easy to produce in the determination of research samples and selection of control group. It may also be produced if the loss or no response during the data collection occurs. Selection bias can occur in all kinds of epidemiological studies.

7.1.2 Types

The common types of selection bias are as follows.

7.1.2.1 Non-response bias

Selection bias occurs if the outcome or exposure situations of respondents differ from those who does not answer in a specified sample. It mainly occurs in cross-sectional study and experimental epidemiology study. In cohort study lost to follow-up is another form of non-response. For some reason, research subjects are not followed in accordance with the design plan. The accepted minimum response rate is 80%.

7.1.2.2 Susceptibility bias

In the study of the association between some factors and a outcome(including the onset of disease, disease recurrence, death, etc.), some factors may directly or indirectly affect the susceptibility of the subject to the studied outcome and exaggerate or reduce the strength of the association between exposure and outcome, which leads to the bias known as susceptibility bias.

7.1.2.3 Admission rate bias

It is also called Berkson bias. As to inpatients, it refers to the systematic error due to differences in admission rates for patients with different exposures and outcomes. In case control study, if cases/controls have different exposures than population-based cases/controls, OR will be biased (could be over or underestimated).

7.1.2.4 Prevalence-incidence bias

It is also called Neyman bias. In case control study, if the cases include both the prevalent and incident cases, but exclude the cases of severe illness, short course and quick death, or light, atypical cases, it may result in the formation of case samples different from that only includes incident cases, because these two vary in condition status, type, course and history of exposure; in addition, the prevalent cases may even change the exposure, which results in distorting the real relationship between factors and disease.

7.1.2.5 Detection signal bias

It refers to the situation in which a factor with no etiological relationship with the disease studied can lead to the occurring of disease-related symptoms or signs, enabling the patients to visit a doctor as soon as possible, which results in higher detection rate of the disease in these patients than that in the general population. Thus, the mistaken conclusion of the factor and the disease associated is derived. This bias may occur in a hospital-based case control study.

7.1.3   The control of selection bias

It is difficult to eliminate selection bias once it occurred. However, selection bias can be controlled and reduced in proper design and implement during the study. In the design phase, targets and sample populations need to be clear; if random sampling is required, real randomization should be ensured, so that the sample is representative. If the study subjects need to be randomly divided into groups (experimental epidemiology), the homogeneity among the groups should be ensured by randomization. Cases in case-control study should be selected from a number of hospitals as far as possible, or from both hospital and community or in-patient and out-patient medical records at the same time. Strictly, explicitly included and excluded criteria should be defined for the selection of the study subjects so that they can better represent the population. In the course of the study, cooperation of study subjects should be obtained by actively taking measures to reduce the non-response, loss of follow-up of follow-up study and non-compliance of the experimental study, etc.

7.2   The bias during measurement

7.2.1   Conception

Information bias refers to bias arising from obtaining the required information during the implementation of the study, also called observational bias or measurement bias. Information bias may occur in different types of epidemiological studies and can come from the investigators, study subjects, measurement methods, instrument, equipment, environment and others. Misclassification is measurement error. There are two types of misclassifications in epidemiological research: non-differential misclassification and differential misclassification. Non-differential misclassification means all classes, groups, or categories of a variable (whether exposure, outcome, or covariate) have the same error rate or probability of being misclassified for all study subjects. Differential misclassification occurs when the error rate or probability of being misclassified differs across groups of study subjects.

7.2.2   Types

The common types of information bias are as follows.

7.2.2.1   Measurement bias

It is the bias, or deviation from the truth that is caused when any measurement collected or from subjects is not completely accurate in the measurement of any kind of information including the instruments, methods, reagents and conditions used in the research are not standard and uniform, the index selection and setting are not reasonable, the operator's operating error, the data record is wrong and incomplete. Measurement bias may occur in any type of epidemiological study.

7.2.2.2   Recall bias

Recall bias is a systematic error caused by differences in the accuracy or completeness of the recollections recalled by study participants regarding events or experiences from the past between compared groups. Recall bias occurs when cases and controls recall exposures differently in case-control study.

7.2.2.3   Reporting bias.

It refers to selective revealing or suppression of information by subjects and the resulting systematic errors.

7.2.2.4   Exposure suspicion bias.

Exposure suspicion bias can occur when knowledge of subjects' outcome status influences exposure assessment (affects cohort studies). If the case group was carefully asked about the history of exposure to a factor, but the control group was not equally seriously asked the same questions, this may lead to the wrong conclusion in a case-control study.

7.2.2.5   Diagnostic suspicion bias

If the investigator knew the exposure of study subjects and is subjectively inclined to a certain outcome when making a diagnosis or analysis, thus leading to erroneous conclusions, the resulting systematic error is called diagnostic suspicion bias. It can occur when knowledge of subjects' exposure status influences diagnostic assessment (affects cohort studies).

7.2.3   The control of information bias

7.2.3.1   Strict information criteria

The research contents include outcome, exposure and confounding factors must be agreed and clearly defined and standardized, and even better, quantified and graded. It is necessary to develop strict and detailed data collection methods. The instrument and equipment used should be calibrated; the reagent should be in accordance with the test requirements. Unified questionnaire should be designed; investigators have to be trained to unify the survey standards and survey methods. Appropriate measures should be adopted to obtain the cooperation of research subjects, so that they can provide the necessary objective and accurate information for the study.

7.2.3.2   Blind data collection

Make sure interviewers and study subjects are unaware of exposure/disease status to avoid their psychological effect on information bias.

7.2.3.3   Objective markers of exposure

Objective indicators should be used as far as possible.

7.2.3.4   Investigative techniques

On sensitive issues, sensitive question survey techniques or methods should be adopted as far as possible, such as designing appropriate questionnaire and applying randomized response technique etc., to obtain reliable information and avoid reporting bias. Sometimes, questionnaires to inquire certain information can include seemingly unrelated variables to divert the attention of the investigators or respondents in order to reduce the influence of subjective factors on the objectivity of information.

7.2.3.5　Statistical processing

The information bias in the research data can be analyzed and evaluated with misclassification analysis.

7.3　Confounding bias

7.3.1　Conception

Confounding bias (also called confounding) refers to the systematic bias occurring in the study due to the influence of one or more of potential confounding factors, which covers or exaggerates the association between factors and diseases (events), so that the real connection between the two is incorrectly estimated.

Confounding factor is also called extraneous factor, a third factor, confounder or confounding variable that is related to both the exposure and outcome studied, and if the confounder distributes unevenly between groups compared, it may result in distorting (reducing or exaggerating) the real association between exposure and outcome.

7.3.2　Characteristics

A confounding factor has several characteristics. It must be related with outcome (in unexposed people); it must be correlated (positively or negatively) with exposure in the study population; and it must not be an intermediate step in the causal pathway between exposure and disease. If a factor with the above characteristics distributes unevenly between the compared groups, it will result in confounding bias.

7.3.3　Control confounding bias

7.3.3.1　Restriction

Restricting admission to the study to a certain category of a confounder is to avoid the effect of the confounder and estimate the association between exposure and disease correctly. However, restriction may reduce the sample obviously and limit the generalization of the study result.

7.3.3.2　Randomization

Use the principle and technique of randomization to assign the study subjects into groups with the same chance and ensure that potential confounding factors, known or unknown, be evenly distributed among the study groups to eliminate confounding bias.

7.3.3.3　Matching

Matching is a process that makes a study group and a comparison group in an epidemiological study comparable with respect to extraneous or confounding factors. Matching can control confounding and improve the efficiency of study but lose the chance to analyze the matching factor. Therefore, it is generally believed that the matching factors should not be too many and should be limited to the main confounding variables.

7.3.3.4   Statistics analysis

In the stage of data analysis, confounders can be identified and controlled with statistical methods including standardization, stratified analysis and multivariate analysis. Mantel-Haenszel stratification analysis methods may be used to control confounder and calculate the adjusted results. If there are more confounders to be controlled, multivariate analysis such as covariance analysis, logistic regression can be used.

7.4   Effect of bias

Bias is an important issue affecting the validity of epidemiological studies. Selection bias and information bias can occur in both observational studies and experimental studies, but the effect of information bias (recall bias) is more serious in retrospective study. Random assignment homogeneously allocates known and unknown confounding factors into each group to control the confounding bias in experimental epidemiological studies.

7.4.1   The effect of selection bias and measurement

Whether there is selection bias in a study, in theory, can be evaluated by comparing the distribution and effect value of the disease (event) and exposure in the two 2×2 tables for general population and study samples. The distribution of disease and factors of total population and sample and the probability of sample selection are shown in Figure 7-1.

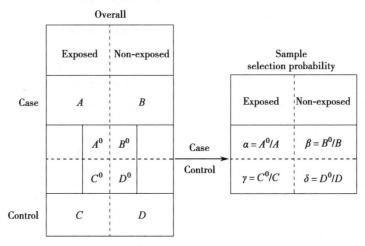

Figure 7-1   The demonstration of distribution of disease and factors of total population and sample
α, β, γ and δ represent probability of sample selection.

From Figure 7-1:

Odds ratio of total population $OR = \dfrac{A \cdot D}{B \cdot C}$.

Odds ratio of sample $OR^{0} = \dfrac{A^{0} \cdot D^{0}}{B^{0} \cdot C^{0}}$.

Based on probability of selection $OR^0 = OR \cdot \dfrac{\alpha \cdot \delta}{\beta \cdot \gamma}$.

The degree and direction of selection bias is:

Selection bias $= \dfrac{OR^0 - OR}{OR}$ 或 $\dfrac{\alpha \cdot \delta}{\beta \cdot \gamma} - 1$.

If it=0, that is $\dfrac{\alpha \cdot \delta}{\beta \cdot \gamma} = 1$, then there is no selection bias.

If it >0, that is $\dfrac{\alpha \cdot \delta}{\beta \cdot \gamma} > 1$, then there is selection bias, $OR^0 > OR$.

If it <0, that is $\dfrac{\alpha \cdot \delta}{\beta \cdot \gamma} < 1$, then there is selection bias, $OR^0 < OR$.

In cohort study, RR as indicator of association, then:

Relative risk of total population $RR = \dfrac{A \cdot (B + D)}{B \cdot (A + C)}$.

Relative risk of sample $RR^0 = \dfrac{A^0 \cdot (B^0 + D^0)}{B^0 \cdot (A^0 + C^0)}$.

Based on probability of selection in Figure 7-1 $RR^0 = \dfrac{\alpha \cdot A \cdot (\beta \cdot B + \delta \cdot D)}{\beta \cdot B \cdot (\alpha \cdot A + \gamma \cdot C)}$.

The degree and direction between RR^0 and RR is expressed in the following formula:

Selecting bias $= \dfrac{RR^0 - RR}{RR} = \dfrac{\alpha(A + C)(\beta \cdot B + \delta \cdot D)}{\beta(B + D)(\alpha \cdot A + \gamma \cdot C)} - 1$.

If $\alpha = \gamma$, $\beta = \delta$, then bias=0; That is there is no selection bias, otherwise there is selection bias.

7.4.2 The effect of information bias and measurement

7.4.2.1 Accordance

In general, repeat survey (measurement) is used to evaluate information bias. Use the repeated survey data to calculate kappa (κ) values (for the specific calculation method, please refer to the relevant books) so as to evaluate the consistency of duplicate detection as well as provide evidence for evaluating the internal validity of research results. It is generally considered that: $\kappa > 0.8$ is excellent; $0.6 < \kappa \leqslant 0.8$ is very good; $0.4 \leqslant \kappa \leqslant 0.6$ is moderate; $\kappa < 0.4$ is poor.

7.4.2.2 The degree and direction of information bias

The degree and direction of information bias of a study may be estimated according to the difference of real OR_T (objective tests, records) and the OR_O in the study.

Information bias $= \dfrac{OR_O - OR_T}{OR_T}$.

The magnitude of the value indicates the degree of bias.

If it = 0, then there is no information bias.

If it > 0, then there is information bias, $OR_O > OR_T$, it is positive bias.

If it < 0, then there is information bias, $OR_O < OR_T$, it is negative bias.

In general, non-differential misclassification will always bias towards the null, underestimating the link between research factors and the study of disease (events). However, the degree and direction of bias are difficult to estimate (over or under) when differential misclassification occurs.

7.4.3   The effect of confounding bias and measurement

The measurement of confounding effect for a potential confounding factor on an association between an exposure and an event can be conducted by comparison of the effect estimates (such as RR, OR, etc.) between the factor and the event (disease), and the adjusted effect estimates.

If there is a confounder (f), the estimated effect for a factor and disease studied are cRR (crude RR)   and cOR (crude OR) for cohort study and case-control study, respectively; the estimated effect after adjustment confounding, that is the estimated effect that have eliminated confounding are $aRR_{(f)}$ (adjusted RR) or $aOR_{(f)}$ (adjusted OR); $aRR_{(f)}$ or $aOR_{(f)}$ may be calculated with Mantel-Haenszel stratified analysis and other methods. The estimated effect RR of cohort study is as an example to illustrate the measurement of confounding.

If $cRR=aRR_{(f)}$; f has no effect of confounding, cRR is not confounded.

If $cRR \neq aRR_{(f)}$; f has effect of confounding, cRR is confounded.

If $cRR>aRR_{(f)}$; there is positive confounding, cRR over-estimated the association between exposure and disease studied due to effect of f confounder.

If $cRR<aRR_{(f)}$; there is negative confounding, cRR under-estimated the association between exposure and disease studied due to effect of f confounder.

The degree and direction of confounding:

$$\text{Confounding value} = \frac{cRR - aRR_{(f)}}{aRR_{(f)}}$$

If the value=0, there is no confounding. If the value $\neq$ 0, and if it >0, it is positive confounding; if it <0, it is negative confounding. The value indicates the degree of confounding.

Summary

Validity in research refers to the closeness of the observed results to the truth. The concept opposite to validity is error. The common errors in epidemiological studies include random errors and systematic errors, and the latter are also known as biases. The larger the error, the lower the validity.

In epidemiological studies, biases can in general be classified into three categories: selection bias, information bias and confounding bias. Selection bias is the selection of individuals, groups or data for analysis in such a way that proper randomization is not achieved, thereby ensuring that the sample obtained is not representative of the population intended to be analyzed. The common selection bias includes non-response bias, susceptibility bias, admission rate bias, prevalence-incidence bias and detection signal bias. Information bias refers to bias arising from measurement error. Information bias mainly includes measurement bias, recall bias, reporting bias, exposure suspicion bias and diagnostic suspicion bias. Confounding bias refers to the systematic bias occurring in the study due to the influence of one or more of potential confounding factors, which covers or exaggerates the association between factors and diseases (events), so that the real connection between the two is incorrectly estimated. When bias is suspected, its degree, direction, and the possible effect on the study outcome should be assessed. A number of methods can be used to control bias in the study design, implementation, and data analysis stage.

(Zhao Yashuang)

8

The causality and causal inferences

Learning objectives

1. **To master** the concepts of causality and risk factor, and the principles of causal inference.
2. **To be familiar with** the procedure of causal inference.
3. **To know** what causal models and DAGs are, and how to use them.

It is important to find out the cause of a disease, because the treatment and prevention will be more effective if the cause is clear. For instance, the discovery of small pox virus and its vaccine help eradicate the disease around the world; the clarification of low-density lipoprotein cholesterol (LDL-C)'s role in developing cardiovascular diseases and wide use of cholesterol-lowering drugs led to the marked decrease of the morbidity and mortality of coronary disease in western countries. How to discover the cause or risk factor of a disease? How to assess and evaluate a causal inference study? These are the critical questions we need to answer in this chapter.

8.1 Overview

The causality is the cause of the disease. The causality and causal inferences are one of the most critical issues in biomedical research, as human diseases can be diagnosed more accurately, or treated and prevented more effectively when the causes are clear. To clarify the cause of a disease needs collaborative efforts of multiple disciplines, and clinical epidemiology contributes to causal inferences from its perspective of human population and population-based investigation.

8.1.1 Sufficient cause and necessary cause

The causality can be defined as the relating of causes to the effects they produce, or the property of being causal. It can be further classified as sufficient cause and necessary cause. The sufficient cause is "a set of conditions, factors, or events sufficient to produce a given outcome". It is important to recognize that sufficient cause usually is not one factor but a composition of multiple factors. For instance, streptococci are the causal microorganism of streptococcal pneumonia, but mere contact of the bacteria is not sufficient to contract the disease, as which happens when the human immunity is also jeopardized. In this case, the combination of streptococci and low body resistance makes up the sufficient cause of *Streptococcal pneumonia*.

The necessary cause is "a causal factor whose presence is required for the occurrence of the effect". If there is no presence of the factor, the disease then will not occur. In the example mentioned above, if there is no contact of streptococci, the individual will not get *Streptococcal pneumonia*. Therefore, streptococci are necessary cause but not sufficient cause of the disease in this example.

Sufficient and necessary: if the factor is present, the disease always develops (the factor is sufficient), and the disease never develops without the factor (the factor is necessary), as illustrated in Figure 8-1. For example, trisomy 21 is the sufficient and necessary cause of Down's syndrome.

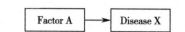

Figure 8-1　Factor A is sufficient and necessary cause of disease X

Sufficient, but not necessary: the factor can produce the disease alone (the factor is sufficient), but other factors can also do so by acting alone (the factor is not necessary), as illustrated in Figure 8-2. For example, high-dose radiation can produce leukemia, but not all leukemia are produced by radiation; there are other factors that can produce leukemia. Factor A is sufficient, but not necessary cause of disease X, either factor B or factor C is sufficient cause of disease X, but neither of them is necessary(in this case, disease X has no necessary cause).

Necessary, but not sufficient: as illustrated in Figure 8-3, each factor is necessary, but not sufficient to produce the disease by itself. For example, HPV is required to cause cervical carcinoma, but not every individual infected by HPV will develop the cancer in her life, as some other factors are also required. As illustrated in Figure 8-3, The combination of factors A, B and C is sufficient cause of disease X, and each of them is necessary, but not sufficient cause.

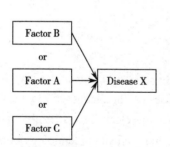

Figure 8-2　Factor A is sufficient, but not necessary cause of disease X

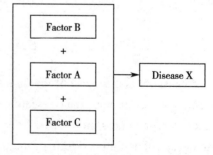

Figure 8-3　Factor A is necessary, but not sufficient cause of disease X

Neither sufficient nor necessary: if a factor is one of the causes of a disease, but the presence of the factor is not necessary before the disease occurs, and the presence of the factor does not necessarily lead to the occurrence of the disease, the factor is neither a necessary cause nor a sufficient cause. For example, hypertension is one of the factors that cause coronary atherosclerosis, but actually not every hypertensive individual will develop atherosclerosis, nor does every atherosclerosis have the history of hypertension. As illustrated in Figure 8-4, factor A and factor D together constitute a sufficient cause of disease X, but there are also factors B and E and factors C and F that constitute two other sufficient causes of disease X. Factor A is neither a sufficient cause nor a necessary cause of disease X.

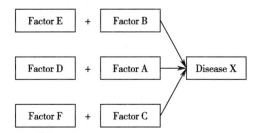

Figure 8-4   Factor A is neither sufficient nor necessary cause of disease X

In clinical medicine, a necessary cause has been identified for most infectious diseases and occupational diseases, etc. The causes of most non-communicable chronic diseases are multi-factorial, and they usually have multiple sufficient causes, each of which may have different combination of factors. In many chronic diseases, there may not be a necessary cause at all, or identified. Actually, their causes are usually not clear, with only one to several risk factors identified to be involved in their development.

8.1.2   Direct and indirect causes of disease

For some diseases, there are multiple factors that cause the disease. Some factors, causing the disease directly without any intermediate steps, are called direct causes or proximate cause; other factors, causing the disease only through an intermediate step or steps, are called indirect causes or remote cause. Direct causes are usually some biological, physical or chemical factors, e.g., *Mycobacterium tuberculosis*, toxicants in cigarettes and hypertension are direct causes of tuberculosis, lung cancer and atherosclerosis, respectively. Indirect causes are often some social, economy and culture factors etc., they are indirectly associated with the development of diseases, which contribute to the development of diseases indirectly through some intermediate factors (direct causes), e.g., low socioeconomic status (SES), poor healthcare system and low educational level, etc. may increase the susceptibility to diseases. As illustrated in Figure 8-5, factor A is a direct cause of disease X, while in Figure 8-6, factor A is an indirect cause to produce disease X through intermediate steps B and C.

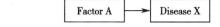

Figure 8-5   Factor A is a direct cause of disease X

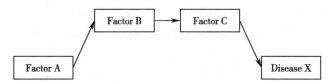

Figure 8-6   Factor A is an indirect cause of disease X

Direct and indirect causes are not categorical. They are just used to help us to understand the causal process between factors and disease development, some factors are straightforward, some factors have to go through some intermediate links to play a role. With the progress of scientific research, people have better understanding of the mechanism by which a disease develops, causing changes in the pattern of causative factors, more causal factors may be added in the process, and some factors deemed as direct causes may turn to be indirect ones.

8.1.3 Risk factors

The causal relationships are very complicate in many diseases, especially in non-communicable chronic diseases. Usually, the causation needs to be investigated by different disciplines. The establishment of the cause of the disease also requires corroboration of research findings from multiple disciplines. Epidemiology takes the population as the object of study and studies the cause of the diseases from a macroscopic perspective. Epidemiology is only one of the tools used to contribute to the clarification. More than often, the causation cannot be clarified by epidemiological studies alone. Many more evidences from other disciplines are needed to verify the causal inference. Risk factor is a term used in epidemiology to imply the causal relationship. A risk factor can be an aspect of personal behavior or lifestyle, an environmental exposure, or an inborn or inherited characteristic that, on the basis of scientific evidence, is known to be associated with meaningful health-related condition(s). It is an attribute or exposure associated with an increased probability of a specified outcome, such as the occurrence of a disease (may not be necessarily a causal factor, such as a risk marker). It is also referred to be a determinant that can be modified by intervention, thereby reducing the probability of occurrence of a disease or other outcomes (a modifiable risk factor and logically a cause of the disease).

8.1.4 Search for causes

When studying the cause of the disease, in order to facilitate the actual operation, people summarized a specific list of possible causes (Table 8-1).

Table 8-1　Possible causal factors

Category	Causal Factors
Host	
Congenital	Gene, chromosome, sex
Acquired	Age, growth, nutrition, physique, behavior, acquired immunity, previous medical history
Environment	
Biological	Pathogen, insects, ingestion or contact with plants and animals
Chemical	Nutrients, natural toxic plants and animals, drugs, minerals, heavy metals
Physical	Radiation, noise, vibration, atmosphere, geography
Social	Society, population, economy, family, life style, diet, hobby and interest, education, culture, healthcare, profession, politics, religion, custom

8.1.5 The causal models

The causal model is a commonly used tool in causal inference studies to build conceptual relationships between potential causal factors and occurrence of a disease based on current theories and experiences. It can provide a simplified framework for causal investigation. Due to different disease characteristics and research focus, there were many different causal models in history for different studies, for example, ecological models (including epidemiological triangle model and wheel model, etc.), web of causation model, and Rothman's sufficient-component cause model, etc.

Ecological models integrate individual and environment, providing a framework for pursuit of potential causal factors. Its holistic approach is strong, and its representative models include the epidemiologic triangle model and the wheel model.

8.1.5.1 The epidemiologic triangle model, as illustrated in Figure 8-7, emphasizes the interaction among pathogen, host and environment in the occurrence of a disease. If the three are balanced, the state of health is manifested; if the role of pathogenic factors is enhanced, disease occurs, such as the mutation of influenza A virus leading to the occurrence and prevalence of influenza; if the host resistance is reduced, disease can likewise occur, such as the emergence of infection in patients receiving immunosuppressive therapy; if the environment changes, the role of pathogenic factors can be

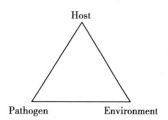

Figure 8-7 Epidemiologic triangle model

exacerbated or reduced, such as malnutrition in poor areas, tuberculosis prevalence. This model has been widely used in the cause of infectious diseases, and it clearly illustrates the synergistic role of the three elements: pathogen, organism, and environment in the development of infectious diseases. However, with the continuous socio-economic development, the disease spectrum of modern society has changed greatly, and chronic non-communicable diseases have become the most significant disease burden in today's society, with diverse and complex etiologies that are far beyond what can be covered by the epidemiologic triangle model.

8.1.5.2 The wheel model, as illustrated in Figure 8-8, is composed by the inner ring and the outer ring, the inner ring is the organism, including the natural characteristics of human (such as age and gender), nutritional status, immunity, endocrine level and heredity, etc., the core of which is genetic genes; the outer ring is the environment, including biological environment, physical and chemical environment and social environment, the biological environment includes various pathogenic microorganisms such as viruses and bacteria, as well as plants and animals as vectors of transmission, etc., the physical and chemical environment includes climate, water, atmosphere, soil, light, radiation and

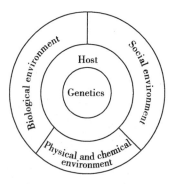

Figure 8-8 Wheel model

the physicochemical environment includes climate, water, atmosphere, soil, light, radiation and various chemical substances such as pesticides, insecticides and occupational pollutants, etc. The social environment includes socio-economic level, cultural level, political system, occupation, living conditions, spiritual factors, personal behavior, etc. The wheel model mainly emphasizes the interconnection and interaction between the organism (host) and the environment, which together lead to the occurrence of diseases, but the role or influence of each part of the wheel model on the occurrence of diseases varies for a specific disease.

8.1.5.3 The web model, as illustrated in Figure 8-9, build a web of causation by connecting different chains of causation, which is composed by multiple factors that have potential causal relationships or non-causal association among themselves, various factors in turn have different causal or correlational relationships with each other, reflecting the complexity of multi-causal diseases in the real world. The web model has the advantage of being intuitive and concrete, providing a practical theoretical framework for analyzing and calculating the relationships and effects among many factors, and has strong operability, but its analysis technique is more difficult.

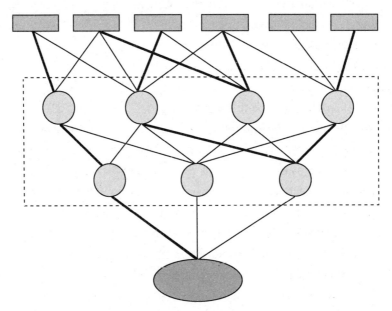

Figure 8-9　Web model

8.1.5.4 Rothman's sufficient-component cause model, as illustrated in Figure 8-10, shows that a disease has multiple sufficient causes including I, II and III, and each of them is composed by multiple component factors, e.g., sufficient cause I is composed by factors A, B, C, D and E, sufficient cause II by factors A, D, F and G, and sufficient cause III by factors A, B, E and H. Factor A is shared by all three sufficient causes and therefore is the only necessary cause of the disease. The sufficient-component model has some similarity compared to the web model, but it breaks down the full cause into several components and emphasizes more on the sufficiency and necessity of the causing factors.

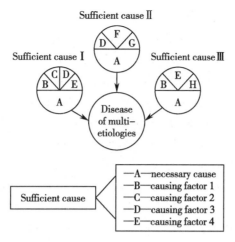

Figure 8-10　Rothman's sufficient-component cause model

8.1.6　Directed acyclic graph

Directed acyclic graph (DAG) is a useful tool to build a causal model. Its components include lines, arrows, factors and diseases. An arrow stands for causal relationship and timeline (directed), therefore arrows will not form a loop (acyclic), whereas a line without arrow head is a symbol of unclear association. DAG can delineate the relationships among factors and between factors and disease occurrence, which facilitates mathematical analysis based on the theoretical framework.

As illustrated in Figure 8-11, when the potential causal effect of factor L on disease Y is under investigation, other factors such as factor U and factor A must be considered at the same time. Factor L produces factor A, and factor A produces disease Y, which means factor L also has indirect causal effect on disease Y through intermediate factor A other than its direct causal effect on factor Y. Factor A is a mediator that does not need to be adjusted for when the

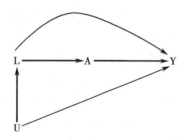

Figure 8-11　Directed acyclic graph

causal relationship of factor L on disease Y is calculated. However, Factor U is different. Factor U is the causal factor of both L and Y, which means factor U is a confounder of the relationship between factor L and disease Y, therefore factor U must be adjusted for when the causal relationship of factor L on disease Y is calculated, without adjusting for factor A.

8.2　The procedure and method of causal inferences

The study of causeal inferences follows certain scientific rules, and its basic process goes through the following three stages.

8.2.1　To propose a causal hypothesis

It is usually the first step and general method of scientific research in a study of causal relationship to identify a scientific question and propose a causal hypothesis to explain observations in the real world. To date, the etiology of many diseases, especially chronic non-communicable diseases, has not been clearly studied, while new diseases are emerging. The unknown etiology poses great difficulties for the correct diagnosis and effective prevention and treatment, forcing researchers to study the causes. Etiological research must be based on the epidemiology, clinical symptom, laboratory test results, and modern medical knowledge and methods. For example, when Severe Acute Respiratory Syndrome (SARS) ravaged the world in the spring of 2003, its etiology was unknown, but the clinical manifestations and transmission pattern were consistent with the characteristics of acute respiratory infectious diseases. Furthermore, based on the exclusion of bacterial, fungal, mycoplasma, chlamydia, common respiratory viruses, and influenza virus infections, scientists proposed that it is caused by a new virus with high virulence.

More than often, questions and hypothesis come from clinical practice. Logic methodology is often used to discover potential causal factors of disease, e.g., method of agreement, method of difference, joint method of agreement and difference, method of concomitant variation, and method of residues.

Method of agreement is to find common points from different phenomena or relationships. For example, although some patients with liver cancer have different dietary habits and living environment, they all have hepatitis B virus infection, suggesting that hepatitis B virus may be a cause of liver cancer. Although patients with food poisoning have different past medical history and behavior, most of them have a recent history of eating the same food, suggesting that the food may be the cause of poisoning.

Method of difference is to find differences from similar phenomena or relationships. For example, in a case-control study, patients with liver cancer in the same village were compared with others, and it was found that there was no or little hepatitis B virus infection among those who did not have liver cancer, suggesting that hepatitis B virus may be one of the causes of liver cancer.

Joint method of agreement and difference is the combination of homogeneity and dissimilarity methods, equivalent to creating a control group in the study to control for confounding factors.

Method of concomitant variation is a special case of method of agreement, where the frequency of disease occurrence changes accordingly when the exposure of a factor varies which may be the cause of the disease. Method of concomitant variation is subject to certain conditions, and can only be applied when the factor studied is a hierarchical or continuous variable and has a quantitative relationship with the probability of disease occurrence. For example, in the study of smoking and lung cancer, as the dose of smoking increased, OR or RR of lung cancer also increased, showing a covariate or dose-response relationship, suggesting that smoking may be the cause of lung cancer.

Method of residues is a special case of method of difference. When the exposure factors for a compound outcome event (A, B, C) are known to be limited to a specific category (a, b, c), and it is known by previous induction that b explains B and c explains C, the remaining a explains

A. For example, the incidence of liver cancer is not explained by hepatitis B virus infection and aflatoxin, but also by the unexplained part, which may be attributed to the "residual" factors within the exposure.

All of these methods are logically inductive and were mainly proposed by philosopher Mill in 1856 in his book *System Logic*. These methods can be applied in clinical epidemiological studies to facilitate the formation of hypotheses, the design of research protocols, and the drawing of etiological inferences. It is important to note that if the etiologic hypotheses do not include the true cause, these methods above will not only fail to provide effective guidance, but may also lead the etiologic analysis astray. It is certain that no one knows whether there is a true cause until the etiology of the disease is known, and this is just a reminder that the mere application of these methods does not prevent errors.

In addition to inductive methods, there are also the deductive methods which deduce the unknown through known laws. In clinical practice, when a hypothesis of etiology is proposed based on clues, the specific content or relationship that needs to be tested is deductively introduced according to the hypothesis, and then verified by empirical evidence. The more specific evidence or the more diverse the conditions of the evidence tested empirically, the more likely this hypothesis will be valid; conversely, the less likely the hypothesis will be valid (note: only the less likely, not excluded).

8.2.2　To test a causal hypothesis

A causal hypothesis must be testified by scientific investigations. Different disciplines have different profiles of methodology. The clinical epidemiology is based on the patient population as the main study population. In clinical epidemiology, the profile includes descriptive studies (e.g., case report, case series), analytic studies (e.g., cross-sectional study, case-control study, cohort study) and interventional studies (e.g. randomized, double-blind, controlled), etc., the scientific nature and strength of the argumentation are progressively stronger, as illustrated in Figure 8-12. Descriptive studies can provide threads for causal hypothesis, while analytic and interventional studies can testify whether the hypothesis is true or not. As interventional studies require more resources and are more challenging in ethics than others, case-control studies and cohort studies turn to be the mainstream methodology to testify causal hypothesis in clinical epidemiology.

For example, in the event of melamine-contaminated infant formula in 2008, pediatricians in Gansu first found a significant increase in the number of kidney stone cases among young children admitted within a short period. Finding that all of them had consumed a certain brand of formula, melamine was detected in several batches of infant formula produced by a certain group and it was proposed that melamine-contaminated infant formula might be the cause of this infant kidney stone. A subsequent cross-sectional study conducted in collaboration between clinicians and epidemiologists initially confirmed a

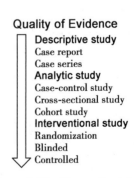

Figure 8-12　The methodology profile of clinical epidemiology

significant correlation between melamine-contaminated infant formula and infant kidney stones. In this instance, as prospective cohort studies and randomized controlled trials are contrary to medical ethics, no studies of higher level will be conducted for validation.

8.2.3 To identify causal relationship

In causal studies, the result may not be the true relationship between suspected causal factors and disease occurrence because of bias and/or confounding. The true relationship may be overestimated or underestimated, or there may be no relationship at all.

For example, in a case-control study to investigate whether coffee consumption causes pancreatic cancer, non-pancreatic cancer patients hospitalized in the department of gastroenterology were selected as normal controls, and coffee consumption was found to be a risk factor for pancreatic cancer. However, this conclusion was overturned by later studies because patients hospitalized in the department of gastroenterology tend to reduce coffee consumption because of other digestive diseases, making the proportion of coffee consumption in this control group lower than in the normal people, resulting in a spurious association between coffee consumption and pancreatic cancer development.

When a spurious association is excluded, the association between a suspected causative factor and a disease does not necessarily mean that there is a causal association between them. When the suspected causative factor and the disease occurrence are both associated with another factor, even if there is no relationship between them, there can be a statistically significant association, called indirect or secondary association. A secondary association is caused by confounding. For instance, a study observed an association between carrying a lighter and lung cancer, not because the lighter itself causes lung cancer (causal association), but because carrying a lighter is associated with smoking which is one of the main causes of lung cancer. The presence of smoking is a confounding factor affecting the relationship between carrying a lighter and lung cancer.

When sampling error, spurious association and secondary association are all excluded, the association between the suspected causative factor and the occurrence of the disease can only be a causal association and the etiological derivation can be performed.

When the results of different studies are not consistent, critical appraisal is needed to evaluate the quality of different evidence rigorously. The more high-quality studies supporting the causal relationship between potential factors and disease occurrence, the more confident we are of the causality. Actually, clinical epidemiological studies alone are not enough to ascertain a causal relationship. Studies from other disciplines, especially bench works at various levels (e.g., of animal, histological, cellular, and molecular, etc.), are needed to provide critical evidence to identify the causal relationship.

8.3 Causal criteria

8.3.1 Koch's standard

In 1882, Koch proposed the following 4-point principle to infer the causal relationship between etiology and disease onset.

The organism is always found in individuals with the disease (necessary cause).

The organism is not found in individuals with any other disease (specificity).

The organism, isolated from one who has the disease, and cultured through several generations, produces the disease in susceptible experimental animals (sufficient cause).

The same organism is isolated from the infected animals.

These postulates are very useful for infectious diseases, but not applicable for most non-communicable chronic diseases that are generally not of infectious origin.

8.3.2 Hill's standard

For diseases with multiple etiologies, Hill proposed the following 9-point principle to infer the causal relationship between cause and disease occurrence.

8.3.2.1 Temporality

The exposure of a potential causal factor must be present before the occurrence of a disease. This is the only criterion that is necessary for judgment of causality.

8.3.2.2 Strength of association

Relative risk, odds ratio and hazard ratio are often used to measure the strength of association. The stronger the association, the less likely is it caused by bias or confounding.

8.3.2.3 Consistency

Association is more likely to be causal if it is repeatedly observed by different investigators, in different populations and with different study designs.

8.3.2.4 Dose-response relationship

The greater exposure (dosage or time), the greater risk of the occurrence of a disease. Or, in some cases, the relationship pattern between the potential causal factor and the occurrence of a disease is consistent with the theoretical one (e.g., U shape).

8.3.2.5 Experimental evidence

If the intervention towards the potential causal factors prevents or ameliorates the risk of disease, it is strong evidence supporting the causal inference.

8.3.2.6 Biological plausibility

The relationship between the potential causal factors and the occurrence of diseases can be explained by known biological, physiological, pathological or other biomedical science disciplines.

8.3.2.7 Coherence

The coherence between epidemiological and laboratory findings increases the likelihood of a causal inference.

8.3.2.8 Specificity

A specific potential causal factor results in a specific disease, and a specific disease results from a specific factor.

8.3.2.9 Analogy

There exists similar relationship between similar factors and similar disease outcomes.

The first four points above are most important and often referred to in causal inference. However, most of the principles are not categorically needed, as Hill said, none of the nine points can support or nullify the causal inference without debates, none of them are indispensable either. Therefore, the causal inference needs to be judged by comprehensive considerations.

8.4   The critical appraisal of research articles on causal inference

The following principles need to be considered in critical appraisal of research articles to evaluate causal inference or effects of risk factors.

8.4.1   Are the results of the study valid?

8.4.1.1   Did the study use a research design that provides strong evidence?

Different study designs have various strength of evidence to support the scientificity and the causal inference or effects of risk factors. The evidence provided by descriptive studies is usually weak, while that by randomized controlled trials is strong as known and unknown factors other than the intervention between the groups being compared are distributed evenly by randomization therefore maximally minimizes the effect of confounding, and the strength provided by analytic studies (e.g., case-control study, cohort study, etc.) is between descriptive studies and RCTs.

8.4.1.2   Were there clearly identified comparison groups that were similar with respect to important determinants of outcome, other than the one of interest? Were there confounding effects on the causal inference?

Confounders may have significant effects on the causal inference. When they exist, appropriate measures should be taken to adjust for their effects. Some confounders are already known but some are not. Analytic studies (case-control or cohort studies) can only adjust for known factors, but RCTs can adjust for known and unknown potential confounders.

8.4.1.3   Were the outcomes and exposures measured in the same way in the groups being compared? Were they blinded?

Same methods should be taken to measure exposures and outcomes in the two groups being compared (intervention vs. control groups, exposure vs. non-exposure groups, or case vs. control groups) in causal inference studies. If blindness is taken in intervention and measurement, some bias will be prevented and validity preserved.

8.4.1.4   Was follow-up sufficiently long and complete?

There is a time effect relationship for any causative factor to cause disease onset. Some acute diseases develop rapidly after being exposed to causal factors, such as acute dysentery, but non-communicable chronic diseases usually need a long period to develop, e.g., atherosclerosis and tumors, therefore they need sufficient follow-up time to observe outcomes. If the follow-up time is too short, the results could be false negative.

On the other hand, if certain number of subjects are lost during follow-up, the validity of the study will be jeopardized, because the subjects who are lost during the follow-up may be different compared to those who chose to stay, and bias will be introduced. Usually, the proportion of subjects lost should be less than 20%. Otherwise, the validity of the studies will be seriously threatened.

8.4.1.5   Is the temporal relationship correct?

Causal factors must be present before the occurrence of a disease, so the temporality is a foundation of the causal inference. When evaluating cause studies, the veracity of the findings is high when it is clear that the presence of risk factors precedes the onset of the disease. The validity of trials and cohort studies is high because the temporality in these studies is clear, while the validity of cross-sectional studies is low as the temporality cannot be ascertained in them.

8.4.1.6   Is there a dose-response gradient?

The dose-response gradient means the levels of exposure (dosage, degree, time) are associated with various risks of disease occurrence. The pathogenic effects of harmful factors, such as chemical and physical, are correlated with the dose of exposure, and the greater the dose of exposure, the longer the time, and the greater the cumulative dose, the more pronounced the pathogenic effects.

8.4.1.7   Were the study results coherent with epidemiological distributions?

Epidemiology explores macroscopic aspects of pathogenic factors, organism and environment. If the distributions of exposures and diseases are coherent in time, space and population in the studies, then the exposures are likely to be the risk factors of the diseases.

8.4.1.8   Were the results of different studies consistent?

If studies in different areas, different populations, with different or similar methods have consistent results of causal association, and use relevant evaluation indicators to evaluate, then the causality is likely to be valid.

8.4.1.9   Were the causal inferences biologically plausible?

If there are biological evidences to support the causal inferences, the causality is likely to be valid.

8.4.2   Are the results of the study important?

Through the above analysis and evaluation of authenticity, if the results of an cause study have good authenticity, the results of the study should be further evaluated for clinical significance and value; otherwise, there is no need to evaluate its significance. The significance of cause study results is reflected in the following quantitative indicators.

8.4.2.1   Degree of association between exposure and outcome

The associations between exposures and outcomes can be expressed by relative risks (RR), attributable risks (AR) and attributable risk ratios (ARR) in RCTs and cohort studies, and odds ratios (OR) in case-control studies.

In judging the significance of RR and OR, it is often necessary to conduct sensitivity analysis, i.e., to observe whether the degree of association between suspected causative factors and disease occurrence will change significantly after adding different confounding factors for adjustment, so as to judge the reliability of the causal association. If the adjusted RR or OR is significantly smaller than the pre-adjustment RR or OR, the original result should be doubted; if the adjusted RR or OR remains the same or increases significantly compared with the pre-adjustment RR or OR, the authenticity of the causal association should be more convinced.

8.4.2.2   95% confidence interval for RR or OR

RR or OR is a point estimate of the association. The precision of the estimate, the 95% confidence intervals (CI) of the RR or OR, also needs to be clarified. If the 95%CI is narrow and does not include 1.0, then the association is precise and statistically significant.

Summary

The causality is the relating of causes to the effects they produce, or the property of being causal. It can be classified as sufficient cause and necessary cause, or direct cause and indirect cause. Risk factor is a term used in epidemiology to imply the causal relationship. When the risk factor is present, the probability of disease in the population increases; when the risk factor is eliminated, the probability of disease decreases The procedure of causal inferences usually includes identification of a scientific question, proposal of a causal hypothesis, testing by scientific investigations, and lastly, verification of the causal relationship. The causal criteria are used to judge whether an association is causal, among which the key elements are temporality, strength of association, consistency and dose-response relationship. When a research article on causal inference is critically appraised, a set of principles should be applied to assess its validity and importance.

(Liu Xiaoqing)

9

Diagnostic test evidence evaluation

Learning objectives

1. **To master** the concepts of a diagnostic test and diagnostic studies.
2. **To be familiar with** the commonly used indexes in evaluating accuracy of a diagnostic test: sensitivity, specificity, positive or negative result, the likelihood ratio and positive/negative predictive value; the evaluation principles of diagnostic test literature.
3. **To know** the calculation method and clinical significance of pre-test probability and post-test probability; the receiver operating characteristic (ROC) curve and its significance.

Clinicians diagnose patients every day. In addition to collecting history characteristics and doing physical examinations, choosing diagnostic test with high accuracy for patients and evaluating the clinical value of examination are also the keys to clinical diagnosis. In order to improve the level of clinical diagnosis and clinical research quality, it is necessary for clinicians to systematically learn and understand clinical diagnostic tests and research evaluation methods, and be familiar with the standard to judge the accuracy of a diagnostic test.

A diagnostic test refers to the test that is used to assess the patient's health, and make diagnosis and differential diagnosis of diseases according to laboratory test results of clinical trials, medical instruments and other examination means.

Diagnostic study is a test method of studying disease diagnosis, including the study of diagnostic methods, such as various laboratory tests, imaging examinations, radioactive nuclide, and endoscopy. Diagnostic study can be involved in all fields and links of clinical medicine. It is very important to make accurate and rapid diagnosis in clinical work. In order to improve the level and efficiency of clinical diagnosis, not only should the high-level diagnostic tests be applied clinically, but also the scientific evaluation and judgment of the diagnostic tests available should be made so as to help clinicians understand and apply them appropriately.

9.1 The common indexes and clinical application of a diagnostic test accuracy evaluation

9.1.1 The common indexes of a diagnostic test accuracy evaluation

9.1.1.1 Sensitivity (Sen) and missed diagnosis

Sensitivity(also known as sensitivity or true positive rate) refers to the proportion of people with the target disorder who have a positive test result. In other words, it refers to the proportion of positive cases diagnosed by the gold standard.

Missed diagnosis refers to the proportion of patients with the target disorder diagnosed as patients without the target disorder, which is also called the false negative rate.

The greater the sensitivity, the higher the proportion of positive result, it is easier to rule out the passivity of the target disorder if the result is negative, and lower rate of missed diagnosis.

9.1.1.2 Specificity (Spe) and misdiagnosis

Specificity refers to the proportion of patients without the target disorder who have a negative test result, or the percentage of cases with negative diagnostic test results using the gold standard diagnosis of no disease. Specificity is also called true negative rate.

Misdiagnosis rate refers to a diagnostic test that diagnosed a patient without the target disorder as a patient with the target disorder, which is also known as the false positive rate.

The truer negative cases, the higher the specificity, and the lower the misdiagnosis rate.

9.1.1.3 Accuracy (Acc)

Accuracy refers to the proportion of true positive and negative in total test cases of a diagnostic test.

Sensitivity and specificity are both basic characteristics of the accuracy of a diagnostic test.

In an ideal diagnostic test, its sensitivity and specificity should reach 100%. In other words, its false positive rate and false negatives rate should be zero.

Case 9-1

823 cases of patients with pulmonary lesions were checked by Chest X-ray, and a study of the diagnostic test accuracy by lung CT findings was made. Here we use this study (Table 9-1) to explain the common indexes.

Table 9-1   Evaluation of a diagnostic test with Lung Spiral CT

CT diagnosis	Real lung cancer patients	Unreal lung cancer patients	Total
Positive	a (385)	b (17)	a+b (402)
Negative	c (42)	d (379)	c+d (421)
Total	a+c (427)	b+d (396)	a+b+c+d (823)

Indexes calculation:

Sensitivity (Sen) = a/(a + c) × 100% = 90.16%

Missed diagnosis rate = 1 - sensitivity = 9.84%

Specificity (Spe) = d/(b + d) × 100% = 95.71%

Misdiagnosis rate = 1 - specificity = 4.29%

In this diagnostic study, the diagnostic accuracy of lung cancer by lung CT examination is:

Accuracy = (a + d)/(a + b + c + d) × 100% = 92.8%.

Accuracy reflects the sensitivity and specificity of a diagnostic test, the higher the accuracy of the test, the higher the sensitivity and specificity. However, accuracy can't reflect the features of either sensitivity or specificity alone. In clinical practice, what kind of diagnostic test should be chosen for specific diseases? What's the requirement of sensitivity and specificity?

In diagnosing peripheral lung cancer, due to the poor prognosis of malignant tumors, it is "bad news" to patients and patients' families once a clear diagnosis is made. Therefore, in order to reduce the misdiagnosis rate for all kinds of malignant tumor, inevitably, diagnostic tests with high specificity should be chosen.

While during the outbreak of SARS (severe acute respiratory syndrome), due to the serious infectious feature and rapid disease progression of SARS, in case of missed diagnosis, there will be catastrophic spread of the disease and life-threatening consequence to the patients. Therefore, in order to reduce the rate of missed diagnosis, the diagnosis of SARS patients should choose the diagnostic tests with high sensitivity.

9.1.2   Evaluation indexes and significance of the clinical application of diagnostic tests

9.1.2.1   Positive predictive value and negative predictive value

Predictive value is an index to evaluate the value of a diagnostic test, showing the clinical significance of the diagnostic test. It refers to the probability of a disease based on the known positive or negative diagnostic test result. Predictive value can be divided into positive predictive value (PPV) and negative predictive value (NPV).

Positive predictive value refers to the proportion of patients with the disease among all those who have a positive test. Negative predictive value refers to the proportion of patients without the disease among all those who have a negative test.

9.1.2.2   Positive likelihood ratio and negative likelihood ratio

Likelihood ratio is the ratio of the probability of a patient having a certain test result (e.g., positive or negative) in a diagnostic test to the probability of a non-patient having such a result, showing ratio of the probability of patients with the disease and without the disease. Likelihood ratio is divided into positive likelihood ratio (PLR) and negative likelihood ratio (NLR).

Positive likelihood ratio is the ratio of true positive rate and false positive rate in a diagnostic test, showing ratio of the probability of patients with the disease and without the disease when the result is positive. The greater the ratio, the greater the chance of disease. Generally speaking, when PLR⩾10, the diagnostic test has high clinical value.

Positive likelihood ratio (PLR) = sensitivity/ (1−specificity) = sensitivity/ misdiagnosis rate

Negative likelihood ratio is the ratio of false negative rate and true negative rate in a diagnostic test, indicating ratio of the probability of negative diagnosis and currently negative diagnosis when the result is negative. The smaller the ratio, the greater the value of test. It is generally believed that the diagnostic test has high diagnostic value when NLR⩽0.10.

Negative likelihood ratio (NLR) = (1−sensitivity)/specificity = missed diagnosis rate/ specificity

---

Case 9-2

Patient A, male, 45 years old, went to see a doctor because of "the pain in his right chest and back, which had lasted for six months". This patient felt dull pain in the right chest 6 months ago, accompanied by a dull pain in his back corresponding to the right chest. At night, the pain was felt obviously, accompanied by a cough, mostly dry cough, without hemoptysis or shortness of breath, etc. He has lost about 4kg weight since he was ill. He has been smoking for nearly 30 years, 15 cigarettes per day, and always coughs.

The lung CT examination was performed on the patient, which indicated crumb nodular shadows in the right lower lobe, and it's most likely peripheral lung cancer.

The result of patient A's CT examination is positive, then what's the probability that this patient is a real lung cancer patient? Here we interpret the results of patient A with the diagnostic results in Table 9-1.

Positive predictive value (PPV) = a/(a + b) ×100% = 95.77%

Negative predictive value (NPV) = d/(c + d) × 100% = 90.02%

Positive likelihood ratio (PLR) = sensitivity/ (1 − specificity) = 21.02

Negative likelihood ratio (NLR) = (1−sensitivity)/specificity = 0.10

It is concluded from the results of this study that:

According to the result of positive predictive value, the probability that patient A has lung cancer is 95.77%.

Lung CT examination has a high positive likelihood ratio, and patients with a risk of lung cancer is 20 times that without lung cancer.

9.1.2.3 Prevalence (Prev)

It refers to the proportion of people with the target disorder in the population where a diagnostic test is conducted.

Sensitivity and specificity demonstrate the probabilities of positive and negative result of a diagnostic test among sick patients and disease-free subjects respectively. However, clinicians need to know what the probability of illness and disease-free is when the diagnostic test results are positive or negative, which indicates the reliability of the diagnostic test. The positive result of a diagnostic test does not mean that the patient must be "sick". It suggests the probability of illness depending on the sensitivity, specificity of a diagnostic test and the prevalence of the target population (the probability of negative result that suggests "disease-free" is also affected by these factors). But the influence of prevalence is more important than that of sensitivity and specificity on predictive value. The lower the prevalence of the subjects, the higher the probability of disease-free will be suggested by the negative results, and the lower probability of illness will be suggested by the positive results.

When a diagnostic test is used in the target population with low prevalence, even the sensitivity is very high, the positive predictive value is low, which means more false positive cases may exist in positive results. Similarly, when a diagnostic test is used in the population with high prevalence, even the specificity of the diagnostic test is high, a lot of false negative results will still exist in negative results.

Therefore, clinicians must be aware that, when they interpret positive or negative result of diagnostic tests, the factors of different regions, population and prevalence should be considered. There will be differences in the meaning of the test results due to differences in subjects.

Case 9-3

A study was carried out to analyze the lung CT results of 126 subjects who were at high risk of lung cancer. In comparison with the research results in (Table 9-1), the factors that affect the evaluation index of the diagnostic test will be explained when interpreting the results of this study (Table 9-2).

Table 9-2　Lung CT diagnosis results of the lung cancer study

CT Diagnosis	Real lung cancer patient	Unreal lung cancer patient	Total
Positive	a (5)	b (8)	a+b (13)
Negative	c (2)	d (111)	c+d (113)
Total	a+c (7)	b+d (119)	a+b+c+d (126)

Table 9-3　Comparison of diagnostic test of lung CT between two groups with different prevalence

Study	Prevalence/ %	Sensitivity/ %	Specificity/ %	Accuracy/ %	Positive likelihood ratio	Negative likelihood ratio	Positive predictive value/%	Negative predictive value/%
1	97.2	90.2	95.7	92.8	21.0	0.10	95.8	90.0
2	5.5	71.4	93.2	92.0	10.5	0.31	38.5	98.2

According to the results shown in Table 9-3, among groups with different prevalence, when the accuracy of lung CT examination as a diagnostic test is almost the same, there is a big difference in the clinical diagnosis of patients with a positive or negative result of the diagnostic test. That is, the likelihood ratio of positive (negative) and the predictive value of positive (negative) are quite different.

Clinicians should note that the positive (negative) predictive value is the probability of being sick (not sick) when the test is positive (negative), which is influenced by the prevalence. The positive (negative) likelihood ratio is the ratio of the chance of being ill to the chance of not being ill if the diagnostic test is positive (negative). It is not influenced by the prevalence rate.

9.1.2.4   Pre-test probability

It is the clinician's estimate of the probability of the disease before applying a diagnostic test, i.e., the prevalence of the disease, and can usually be found in the literature.

9.1.2.5   Post-test probability

It is the predictive value of a diagnostic test under different prevalence scenarios, calculated from the pre-test probability of the disease to be diagnosed and the positive likelihood ratio of that diagnostic test after the test has been performed.

Sensitivity and specificity alone cannot reflect the full picture of the diagnostic test. The likelihood ratio reflects the characteristics of the diagnostic test by comparing the sick and healthy groups in the probability of the positive and negative results, and it is not affected by the prevalence, making it able to interpret diagnostic test more comprehensively and stably than mere sensitivity and specificity. Therefore, likelihood ratio is the ideal index for the comprehensive evaluation of a diagnostic test. And the post-test probability can also be calculated according to sensitivity, specificity, positive or negative result. It is helpful in making more definite diagnosis on the patients after the diagnostic test.

Case 9-4

Hypothesis 1: Patients A is one of the subjects in the study of Table 9-1. If his/her lung CT result is positive, the probability that he/she may be a real patient is calculated as follows:

Pre-test probability (prevalence) = 97.2%

Pre-test odds = 0.972 / (1 − 0.972) = 34.7

Post-test odds = pre-test odds × positive likelihood ratio = 729.7

Post-test probability = post-test odds/ (1 + post-test odds) ×100% = 99.9%

Conclusion: for patient A with a positive result of lung CT, his/her probability of lung cancer is increased from pre-test probability of 97.2% to post-test probability of 99.9%.

Hypothesis 2: Patient A is one of the subjects of Table 9-2. If his/her lung CT result is positive, the probability that the patient may be a real patient is calculated as follows:

Pre-test probability (prevalence) = 5.5%

Pre-test odds = 0.055/(1−0.055) = 0.058

Post-test odds = pre-test odds × positive likelihood ratio = 0.61

Post-test probability = post-test odds/ (1 + post-test odds) × 100% = 37.9%

Conclusion: for patient A with a positive result of lung CT, his/her probability of lung cancer is increased from pre-test probability of 5.5% to post-test probability of 37.9%.

9.1.2.6　ROC curve (receiver operator characteristic curve)

In a diagnostic test, ROC curve is drawn with the continuous data from multiple measurements by groups. When drawing, use the test sensitivity (true positive rate) as the ordinate, and 1−specificity (false positive rate) as the abscissa. Based on the data obtained from continuous grouping measurements, the calculated sensitivity and specificity are marked in the graph and combined into a curve, which is the ROC curve (Figure 9-1). Any point on the curve represents a sensitivity and specificity pair corresponding with the specific positive value of a diagnostic test.

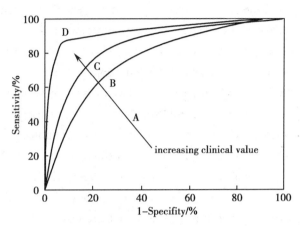

Figure 9-1　ROC curve

Take the ROC curve in Figure 9-1 as an example. The four curves of A, B, C, and D respectively represent the four diagnostic tests from A to D, and the clinical value of these diagnostic tests gradually increases. A good diagnostic test has the feature that its curve is away from the middle diagonal and very close to the top left corner (shown as curve D in Figure 9-1). A poor test is very close to the middle diagonal (shown as curve A in Figure 9-1). Usually, the accuracy of a diagnostic test can be evaluated by calculating the area under the curve (AUC). The larger the area, the better the test. Generally, the best cut point for the normal value is the point closest to the upper left in the curve. Meanwhile the area under this point is the largest. Using this point to distinguish between normal and abnormal, the sensitivity and specificity are the highest, that is, the cases of misdiagnosis and missed diagnosis are the least.

The ROC curve can be used to determine normal values and also to compare the advantages and disadvantages of different diagnostic tests by the area under the curve.

9.2　Standards for reviewing literature on diagnostic tests

To increase the scientific validity of diagnostic test studies and to improve the credibility of their findings, standards for reviewing literature on diagnostic tests have been established to facilitate the evaluation of diagnostic studies and help improve the efficiency and accuracy of diagnostic tests. The standards are made of the following eight parts.

Blind comparison and evaluation of a diagnostic test and the gold standard.

Analysis and evaluation that are included in the study cases.

The source of cases and the arrangement of study work.

Diagnostic test's repeatability and its clinical significance.

The normal value determined by the diagnostic test.

Application of the series test.

Narration of a diagnostic test method and analysis of its repeatability.

The practicability of a diagnostic test.

9.2.1 Whether the blind comparison is made between the diagnostic test and the gold standard

The gold standard of a diagnostic test in diagnostic study refers to the most reliable method currently recognized by the clinicians to diagnose a disease. It is also known as diagnostic criteria, which can distinguish between "illness" and "health". The gold standard in clinical diagnosis consists of the standards of etiological diagnosis, pathological diagnosis, surgical findings, special imaging diagnosis, clinical comprehensive diagnosis, and positive results obtained from the long-term clinical follow-up, etc. But it should be noticed that some gold standards are relative. With the progress in medicine as well as the deepening understanding of the disease, these relative gold standards are constantly being improved.

The choice of gold standard and its reliability directly affect the reliability of the diagnostic study conclusion. For the same group of subjects, using different gold standards may lead to different conclusions on a diagnostic test. Therefore, the gold standard must be selected strictly.

The accuracy assessment of diagnostic tests, that is, whether the diagnostic test accurately reflects the diseased or non-diseased subjects of the examination, is the key to the research. Accuracy assessment of a diagnostic test is mainly compared with the gold standard. In order to eliminate artificial bias, it is more scientific to apply the blind method to compare. Therefore, the diagnostic test under study should be blindly compared with the gold standard before clinical application and its sensitivity, specificity, positive and negative predictive value, accuracy and likelihood ratio should be calculated according to fourfold tables.

Case 9-5

In a diagnostic study, given the gold standard as sputum culture of *Mycobacterium tuberculosis* for tuberculosis, the diagnostic test to be evaluated is results of tuberculosis PCR test of blood sample, which is assessed as follows (Table 9-4).

Table 9-4　Results of Tuberculosis PCR Test of Blood Sample

TB-PCR	With tuberculosis bacterium/case	without tuberculosis bacterium/case	Total/case
Positive	45	5	50
Negative	8	62	70
Total	53	67	120

This study uses etiological diagnosis as the gold standard to scientifically evaluate diagnostic tests of tuberculosis PCR test of blood sample.

9.2.2 Whether the cases included in the study is representative

The study subjects of the diagnostic test should include the participants that use the gold standard to determine "diseased", namely case group, and the study subjects that use the gold standard to confirm the "no disease". Among them, the so-called "disease-free" subject of study refers to a participant who does not have the target disorder diagnosed by the gold standard, rather than a normal person who is completely disease-free.

Diagnostic studies with different application purposes should choose different study participants. For example, for the evaluation of screening diagnostic tests, general population can be chosen as the study subjects; while for clinical diagnostic tests, cases should be chosen as the study subjects. At the same time, cases should also cover different period, different degree of illness (mild, moderate, severe), with or without complications, typical and atypical cases etc., in order to make the results of the study representative. Control group can choose additional "disease-free" cases that don't have the target disorder, which is confirmed by the gold standard, but are easy to be confused with the disease in other cases, because such contrast is more valuable in clinical diagnosis, especially in the differential diagnosis. Normal persons usually should not be included in the "disease-free" control group, if they are included in the control group on the primary stage, the results should be responded with caution.

In case 9-5, the blood TB-PCR diagnostic test evaluation study, participants who accepted the blood test included mild, moderate and severe tuberculosis patients, as well as primary tuberculosis and secondary tuberculosis patients, so it is concluded that the evaluation results of the diagnostic test are scientific and credible in this way.

9.2.3 Whether the source of the participants is correctly described

Prevalence has a great influence on the final result, such as the predictive value of a diagnostic test. Participants come from different sources, that is, patients in different levels of hospitals have different demographic features, including different prevalence of a disease, which will largely influence the results of the study. For a certain diagnostic test, its sensitivity and specificity are relatively fixed. But in clinical work, we pay more attention to the positive predictive value of a diagnostic test. At the same time, we hope to reduce the false positive cases, and improve the prediction ability of disease diagnosis through the diagnostic test, and give full play to the efficiency of the diagnostic test. Given that the prevalence has more influence on the predicted values, one of the keys to improving the efficiency of a diagnostic test for clinicians is to choose groups with different prevalence to apply the appropriate diagnostic test.

Case 9-6

There are several different predictive values for groups with different prevalence in lung spiral CT diagnostic test.

For the crowd who had lung nodules, the pre-test probability is 97.2%, and the post-test probability is 99.8%; after lung spiral CT test, the predictive value only increases by 2.6%.

For the high-risk population who are smoking, the pre-test probability is 5.5%, and the post-test probability is 37.1%; after the application of this test, the predictive value increases by 32.1%.

Therefore, the sources of participants should be correctly described in the study in order to improve the scientificity and strength of research results.

9.2.4   Whether diagnostic test has a good repeatability

Repeatability is also called precision or reliability, that is, a diagnostic test should be operated repeatedly, and it is the precondition of the diagnostic test for clinical application. Repeated measurements of a diagnostic test should be relatively stable. In other words, when the same specimen is measured for many times, the results should be close, and the method should be reliable.

9.2.5   Whether the normal value of a diagnostic test is reasonable and reliable

Normal value should be accurately defined and clearly described, for normal value with different meanings can directly affect the data of normal value. When there is an overlap of the distributions of frequency test values for the sick and not-sick populations, scientific method should be adopted (such as normal distribution data using mean ± standard deviation, non-normal distribution with median or percentile, as well as the application of ROC curve, etc.). Then normal and abnormal point should be correctly differentiated, namely, to find the best point. The determination of the best point directly affects the sensitivity and specificity of a diagnostic test and other key indicators.

9.2.6   Whether the selection of joint test is rational and scientific

The joint tests of a diagnostic test include parallel test and serial test.

9.2.6.1   Parallel test

In order to improve the sensitivity of diagnosis, we can do several kinds of diagnostic tests for the same purpose at the same time. As long as one result of the tests is positive, the patient is afflicted with disease. The application of parallel test can improve the sensitivity and negative predictive value, but it reduces the specificity and positive predictive value; it also reduces the rate of missed diagnosis, and increases the rate of misdiagnosis. When applying this method clinically, we need to think carefully about the differential diagnosis to reduce misdiagnosis.

Evaluation method of parallel test (Table 9-5).

Table 9-5   Evaluation method of parallel test

Project	Results		Evaluation Results
	Test A	Test B	
Parallel test	+	−	+
	−	+	+
	+	+	+
	−	−	−

Test A: Sen = 80%, Spe = 60%.

Test B: Sen = 90%, Spe = 90%.

Parallel test calculation:

Sen = SenA + (1 − SenA) × SenB = 0.80 + (1−0.80) × 0.90 = 0.98.

Spe = SpeA × SpeB = 0.60 × 0.90 = 0.54.

Case 9-7

In order to diagnose tuberculous pleural effusion in patients with pleural effusion, hydrothorax indicators of LDH and ADA of a diagnostic study are tested (Table 9-6).

Table 9-6   Hydrothorax Diagnostic Test Results in Patients with Pleural Effusion

ADA test (A)	LDH test (B)	Pleural effusion patients with tuberculous	Pleural effusion patients without tuberculous
+	−	8	4
−	+	16	6
+	+	60	2
−	−	16	578
Total		100	590

ADA test (A):

Sen = (8 + 60) / 100 × 100% = 68.0%.

Spe = (6 + 578) / 590 × 100% = 99.0%.

LDH test (B):

Sen = (16 + 60) / 100 × 100% = 76.0%.

Spe = (4 + 578) / 590 × 100% = 98.6%.

Parallel test calculation:

Sen = SenA + SenB (1 − SenA) = 0.68 + (1 − 0.68) × 0.76 = 0.92.

Spe = SpeA × SpeB = 0.99 × 0.99 = 0.98.

The results show that the parallel test increases the sensitivity, but reduces the specificity.

9.2.6.2   Serial test

When a diagnostic test with high specificity is not available, in order to improve the specificity of clinical diagnosis, we can design a series of a diagnostic tests to be conducted in a certain order, and only when the results of the series of tests are all positive can we make a diagnosis that the patient is with the disease. Serial test can improve specificity and positive predictive value, but at the same time it reduces the sensitivity and negative predictive value, that is, it reduces the rate of misdiagnosis, but may increase the rate of underdiagnosis. Applying serial test is more appropriate when the specificity of multiple clinical diagnostic tests are not high.

Evaluation method of serial test.

The results of a series of diagnostic tests should be designed to be positive.

Calculation method: A, B, C, D... serial tests.

Sen (sequence) = SenA × SenB × SenC × SenD...

Calculate the sensitivity of the serial test.

Spe (sequence)1 = SpeA + [(1 − SpeA) × SpeB].

Spe (sequence)2 = Spe (sequence)1+ {[1 − Spe (sequence) 1] × SpeC}.

Spe (sequence)3 = Spe (sequence)2+ {[1 − Spe (sequence) 2] ×SpeD}...

According to this rule, the specificity of the serial test can be finally calculated.

Sensitivity, specificity and accuracy of the serial tests should be evaluated accurately, and at the same time, they should be compared with those of each individual test. The best joint test method can be chosen through the comparison among a series of similar tests.

Take the results of Table 9-6 as the calculation basis of joint diagnostic test and calculate sensitivity and specificity after series tests:

Sen (sequence) = 0.68 × 0.76 = 0.516 8.

Spe (sequence 1) = 0.99 + [(1−0.99) × 0.986] = 0.999 9.

The results show that serial test increases the specificity, but reduce the sensitivity of the test.

9.2.7   Whether the operation of the diagnostic test is carefully described

For the diagnostic test evaluated to be applied clinically, its specific operation should be carefully described, including operating steps, instruments and reagent specifications, any arrangement or restrictions before and after the test (such as diet, drugs, etc.), and evaluation method of the results, etc.

9.2.8   How is the clinical practicability of a diagnostic test

Comprehensive evaluation of clinical practicability of a diagnostic test should be made, including whether clinical application is convenient, whether the accuracy is high, whether the result is easy to determine, and whether cost benefit analysis is good.

Summary

The test with high sensitivity is mainly used to eliminate the disease-free participants, and the negative results are the most significant at this time. The test with high specificity is mainly used for the diagnosis of sick patients; the positive results are the most significant at this time.

The likelihood ratio of each diagnostic test can be applied to calculate the post-test prevalence so as to understand the prevalence when the diagnostic test results are positive or negative. It also can provide evidence for further diagnosis and treatment decisions, if necessary.

The selection of research participants directly affects the sensitivity and specificity of a diagnostic test. Cases group should include the cases with different severity, and control group should include participants that are confirmed to be without the target disorder by the gold standard, but with the disease that is easy to be confused with the target disorder, not healthy normal people.

The application of parallel test can improve the sensitivity and negative predictive value, but it reduces the specificity and positive predictive value; serial test improves the specificity and positive predictive value, but at the same time it reduces the sensitivity and negative predictive value.

(Wu Shangjie)

10

Therapeutic research

Learning objectives

1. **To master** the basic concepts and types of therapeutic research.
2. **To be familiar with** the evaluation principle of therapeutic research.
3. **To know** the characteristics, procedures and design of therapeutic research; the main factors affecting the results of therapeutic research.

The basic purpose of clinical medicine is to learn the occurrence, development and prognosis of diseases, take effective intervention gradually, avoid adverse outcomes and improve the prognosis of patients, increase cure rate and reduce morbidity and mortality. And this is also the main purpose of therapeutic research. Since the purpose of therapeutic research is to treat disease and improve prognosis, it is important that the results of the study be valid, as well as highly reproducible. Validity means the measurement actually represents what it aims to measure, unaffected by any bias factors. Reliability or reproducibility refers to the degree to which the research results can be repeated by other researchers. These two features are the key to therapeutic research.

10.1　The steps to design a therapeutic research

10.1.1　Select topics for therapeutic research

The core of a therapeutic research is selecting a topic. The selected topic should be a new idea with originality and novelty from clinicians in practical work. It always originates from keen observation and bold hypothesis. At the same time, the researchers should have deep understanding of the pathogenesis and epidemiology of the disease.

Topic selection is usually based on the following knowledge according to different research objectives.

Based on the understanding of the genetic, molecular, or cellular pathogenesis of diseases.

Based on the careful observation of a clinical phenomenon. Even when the pathogenesis of a disease remains unclear, the researchers could figure out some effective treatments.

Based on some inspirations from the results or conclusions of other researches, even some of which are incorrect.

10.1.2 The evaluation principles of therapeutic research

Therapeutic research is usually prospective. In order to ensure that the results are not affected by the known or unknown bias factors, and make the results of the study true and reliable to guide clinical practice, the three basic principles of being randomized, controlled and blind must be followed.

10.1.2.1 Randomization

Randomization is a method to allocate individual patients or persons who have been accepted for a study into one of the groups (called arms) of a study. Usually, there are two arms: one is called the experimental or treatment arm and the other is called the control arm. Another term for randomization is random allocation. This should not be confused with random selection, in which the investigator uses a process to recruit sample for the study. This is used to select a representative sample from the study population, usually in a survey. The correct assignment of clinical trial subjects to study groups is essential to ensure that the groups are identical at baseline and comparable across groups. The principle of randomization requires that each subject has an identical chance of being assigned to a test or control group. The purpose of this is to ensure that patients in the test and control groups have similar clinical characteristics and prognostic factors (both known and unknown), thus avoiding interference by the subjective will of the investigator or subject and increasing the correctness of the study results.

10.1.2.2 Control

To evaluate the authenticity of trial results, great emphasis is placed on the control and comparison of studies. Therefore, the establishment of controls is an important principle of clinical trials and a basic requirement of scientific research. The purpose of "setting up a control" is to set up a group of subjects with the same conditions and the same diagnosis to receive a test measure different from that of the test group, in order to compare the results with those of the test group, and to demonstrate the difference and the extent of the results between the two groups (or groups). The group of patients used for comparison (also called the control group) should have the same test conditions and observed indicators and effect criteria as the test group, except that they do not receive the intervention under study. Thus, the purpose of establishing controls is to make the baseline conditions of the study consistent and comparable, thereby eliminating the interference and influence of non-trial factors. The types of control group included: concurrent randomized control, non-randomized concurrent control, self-control, historical control, matching control etc.

10.1.2.3 Blind trial

In clinical trials, neither the investigator nor the subject of the trial knows the assignment of the test subjects, i.e., they do not know the group to which the subjects are assigned and whether they are receiving a test or control measure; this method of clinical trials is called blind trial. The purpose of a blind trial is to effectively avoid information bias and subjective bias of the investigator or subject. When evaluating subjective indicators, such as pain relief and shortness of breath relief, the use of blinded trials can overcome the subjective and suggestive biases of the investigator and the subject, and obtain accurate and reliable evaluation of the test results. Blinded tests can also be used for the analysis and reporting of study data.

10.1.3　Steps for therapeutic research

10.1.3.1　Selection of research subjects

In a therapeutic study, it is necessary to correctly determine the subjects and the diagnosis of the disease, which is crucial to ensure the repeatability of the research results. In specific studies, given the complexity of the research subjects and limited research conditions, it is impossible to enroll all kinds of patients for study at the same time. Therefore, inclusion criteria and exclusion criteria are usually determined according to certain research objectives, to limit the study to a defined range of subjects. Then through multi-level studies to accumulate comprehensive information, we can overcome the limitations of single research, recognize the overall rule.

10.1.3.2　Sample size estimation

If the sample size is too small, it is easy to get false negative results. However, if the sample size is too large, it will increase the unnecessary human, material, time and economic waste, increasing the difficulty of the research. Sample size estimation is mainly based on the sample size formula in statistics. The effects of the occurrence of errors (including false positive and false negative errors) caused by chance should be limited to an acceptable range, i.e., the occurrence of the type I error (α) and the occurrence of type II error (β) in the study should be limited to the acceptable range. Usually, when α is set as 0.05 and β as 0.1 to 0.2, then the test efficiency is 0.8 to 0.9, and the probability of error is appropriate and acceptable. Meanwhile, the effect of treatment is also important for sample size estimation. The greater the difference between the experimental group and the control group, the smaller the number of samples needed.

10.1.3.3　Measurement index and choice of endpoint

To determine the effect of therapeutic interventions, it is necessary to have a definite and objective measurement index. These indicators can be accurately determined, with good consistency, and can be quantified, easy to compare and analyze. As the measurement index of a therapeutic study, it is usually required to be sensitive to the reaction to the treatment, to accurately measure and determine the positive results of the treatment. The measurement index also should be related to the specific effects of treatment. At the same time, we should choose the economic and feasible test methods. Usually, the measurement indicators include soft and hard indexes. If the clinical reliability is poor, the repeatability is difficult to guarantee and it is not easy to quantify, the indicators are called soft indicators, such as the changes of patients' subjective symptoms and signs. Definite, objective, and easy-to-judge indexes known as the hard indicators, such as recover from illness, disability, mortality, and postoperative pathology, laboratory determination of quantitative indicators etc.

In order to observe the effect of the treatment, the choice of endpoints is also very important. Moreover, there should be a sufficient observation period to observe the short-term efficacy and long-term efficacy of the treatment. If the observation period is too short, it easily leads to false negative and false positive results. On the other hand, an extended observation period will have more impact on the final results and increase the difficulty of follow-up. Researchers must pay attention to this and find ways to solve it.

10.1.3.4 Methods for therapeutic research

Three principles should be followed in therapeutic studies: randomization, control and blinding. RCTs are the first choice for therapeutic studies. But other research methods are also the choice of therapeutic study according to different purposes, combining the objective reality of the researcher and the scientific nature and feasibility of the study, including cohort study, before-after study, quasi-randomized controlled study, and historically controlled trial e.

Randomized controlled trial

The design model of a randomized controlled trial is shown as Figure 10-1 and the analysis of results is shown as Table 10-1.

Design model:

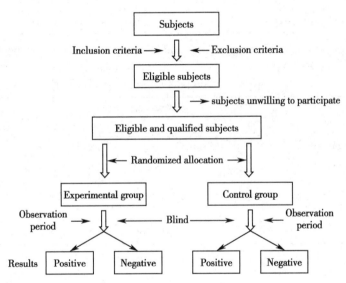

Figure 10-1　　Randomized controlled (blinding) research design model

Results analysis:

Table 10-1　　Quadruple tabular form of RCT

Group	Results		Total
	+	−	
Experimental group	a	b	a+b
Control group	c	d	c+d
Total	a+c	b+d	N

Example:

There are different opinions on the choice of treatment for patients with coronary heart disease. A study of 780 patients with coronary heart disease was conducted in a research center (Figure 10-2, Table 10-2 and Table 10-3):

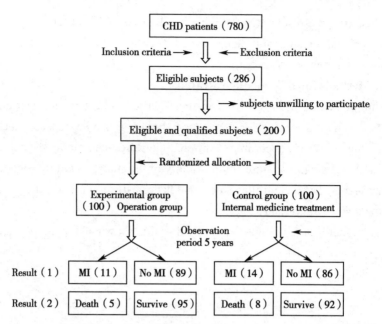

Figure 10-2　Randomized controlled (blinding) research design model

Table 10-2　Quadruple tabular form of RCT (1)

Group	Results (1)		Total
	+	−	
Experimental group	11	89	100
Control group	14	86	100
Total	25	175	200

Table 10-3　Quadruple tabular form of RCT (2)

Group	Results (2)		Total
	+	−	
Experimental group	5	95	100
Control group	8	92	100
Total	13	187	200

Conclusion:　Comparing the experimental group with the control group by χ^2 test, neither result (1) nor result (2) had statistical difference ($P>0.05$ in both). Clinically, the treatment of coronary artery bypass surgery cannot reduce the incidence of myocardial infarction or the mortality rate in patients with CHD for over 5 years.

Cohort study

Prospective cohort studies are generally used in therapeutic studies, where the observed population is naturally accepted and two cohorts are formed, and the interventions are not randomly assigned into the group by the investigator, but are naturally grouped and difficult for the investigator to control. The most important feature of prospective cohort studies is the ability to control for interferences that occur in the trial in a timely manner. As it is not randomized, it is difficult to ensure the balance between the number of two groups and the baseline situation. The design model of a cohort study is shown as Figure 10-3 and the analysis of results is shown as Table 10-4.

Design model:

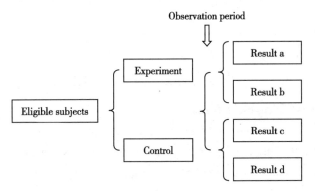

Figure 10-3   Cohort study design model

Results analysis:

Table 10-4   Quadruple tabular form of cohort study

Group	Results	
	good results	Bad results
Treatment group	a	b
Control group	c	d

Compare the experimental group and the control group by χ^2 test to clarify significance.

Self-controlled crossover study

Self-controlled crossover study is a prospective study method. Two different intervention measures are applied to the subjects at two stages. Then the effects of two interventions are analyzed. There is a wash-out period between two stages if necessary. The length of the wash-out period is decided according to the half-life of the drug, the treatments and objectives. Usually, this method is applied to chronic diseases or chronic recurrent diseases. The design model of a self-controlled crossover study is shown as Figure 10-4 and the analysis of results is shown as Table 10-5.

Design Model:

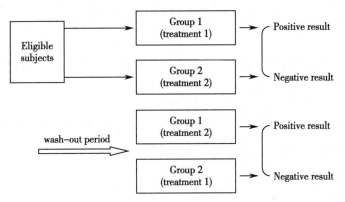

Figure 10-4   Self-controlled crossover study design model

Results analysis:

Table 10-5　Quadruple tabular form of self-controlled crossover study

Treatment	Positive	Negative	Total
Treatment 1	a	b	a+b
Treatment 2	c	d	c+d
Total	a+c	b+d	a+b+c+d

Quasi-randomized controlled study

Quasi-randomized controlled study and randomized controlled trial design are similar. The only difference is that the distribution of the subjects is in a quasi-random way. The patients are assigned to the experimental group or the control group according to the last number of their birthday or hospitalization number.

Due to the allocation, the baseline characteristics of the subjects are imbalanced due to the influence of the artificial selection bias. The reliability of the results is often not as good as that of randomized controlled studies.

Historical controlled study

Historically controlled study is to compare the results of the new interventions with those of previous studies. As the historically controlled study is not randomized in allocation or synchronously controlled, the comparability is not as good as RCT. But the cost and time of study are saved.

10.1.3.5　Analysis and interpretation of the results of therapeutic research

As to the analysis and interpretation of the research results, we must ensure the completion of data to carry out statistical analysis and results evaluation after the completion of the research. The results analysis includes: 1. The effect of bias and chance in the study, is it within the acceptable range? 2. What measures are taken to prevent bias effects, and how is the internal validity of the results of the study? 3. Is the statistical analysis method appropriate?

At the same time, it should be indicated the representative population the results can be applied to and the scientific and clinical implications of the research results as the results of the study are interpreted. Only through repeated practice and expansion of the research population, the validity of therapeutic study conclusions can be ultimately improved.

10.2　The main factors affecting therapeutic research

In addition to the choice of research methods, there are a variety of factors that may affect the validity of the study results. The researchers must be concerned about and control the influencing factors.

10.2.1　Comparability

Comparability means that the test and control groups should have complete similarity and consistency in characteristics other than the intervention being observed, i.e., to ensure relative balance in the baseline status of the study. It is necessary to adopt strict inclusion and exclusion criteria to select qualified subjects, and to strengthen the comparability of the experimental group and the control group with the method of matching and stratified randomization, which can directly affect the validity of the final results.

10.2.2 Sample size

Sample size directly reflects the impact of chance. A small sample size leads to the possibility of false positive and false negative results, and therefore decreases the credibility of the conclusion. Clinical therapeutic studies are often unable to enroll a large number of samples. So an appropriate sample size should be calculated to control the chance of false positive and false negative results to a minimum and acceptable range.

10.2.3 Control and placebo effect

Controls are essential and necessary for therapeutic research to determine effects, and strict controls are contemporaneous control cases that are exactly similar to the cases in the observation group. It is through the observation of a strict control group that the non-specific effects that occur in the test and control groups are eliminated and the true effect of the intervention to be observed is revealed.

In therapeutic studies, placebo is usually given to control cases to achieve a blinded effect. The effect of placebo in the control group, or even certain side effects, is called the placebo effect. It is a non-specific effect that can be caused by a variety of factors such as environmental and psychological, and its can also occur in the observation group. Therefore, it is possible to determine the specific and non-specific effects and the proportion of their occurrence in the test group by comparing the two groups, removing the non-specific effect and obtaining a true evaluation of the value of the observed treatment measures.

10.2.4 Bias and chance

The effects of bias and chance can seriously undermine the results of a study. Bias can occur throughout the course of a therapeutic study, including selection bias, information bias, and confounding bias, which can be avoided by the investigator through a sound, rigorous trial design. Chance, or sampling error, on the other hand, cannot be completely eliminated, but can only be controlled to a generally acceptable level by limiting the allowable level of type I and type II errors. In fact, all clinical therapeutic studies hoping to obtain true and reliable results have been centered around controlling bias and chance from the beginning.

10.2.5 Contamination and co-intervention

When the comparison is between two active treatments, contamination occurs when patients in one arm receive the treatment of the other arm. The difference between the treatment group and the control group was reduced, and therefore confuse the evaluation of the intervention effect.

Interventions other than the treatment under study that are applied differently to the treatment and control groups are called co-interventions. Co-intervention is a serious problem when double-blind trials are absent or when the use of very effective non-study treatments is permitted. The control of contamination and co-intervention is mainly dependent on the strict management of the researchers, especially the application of blinding in the treatment of the study. Double blind method can effectively avoid the occurrence of contamination and co-intervention.

10.2.6　Compliance

The degree of compliance in accepting and performing the prescribed medical measures (e.g., number of doses and duration of treatment) among the subjects included in the study is called compliance. Compliance might decrease if your patient is taking other medications or if the treatment requires multiple doses daily rather than single ones. Usually, in therapeutic research, the level of compliance of the observed subjects can be used to determine the level of study quality. A study attrition rate of > 20% is a rough guide to the number that may invalidate the final results. However, even a smaller percentage of patient drop-outs may affect the results of a study if not taken into consideration. Lack of compliance may influence outcomes since the reason for non-compliance may be directly related to the intervention.

10.3　Standards of therapeutic study assessment

10.3.1　Is it a real randomized controlled trial?

This is the most critical issue that determines whether the results of the treatment are real and effective. Only a true randomized controlled trial can really achieve a balanced distribution of known and unknown factors affecting prognosis, and ensure comparability, and ultimately reach a sound conclusion. Therefore, the following questions should be noted.

Is the assignment of patients to treatments randomized and is the randomization list concealed?

Does randomization produce comparable groups at the start of the trial?

Is there any contamination or co-intervention?

Are research participants "blinded"?

Of course, the results of other non-randomized studies are not excluded. Due to the limitation in implementing RCTs, the results of other non-randomized studies should also be considered. In this case, it is necessary to explain and define the validity of these results.

10.3.2　Are all the results of the study are reported and observed?

Therapeutic studies should have a clear purpose, relevant measurements, and ultimate criteria for judging effectiveness from the beginning of their design. Therefore, when evaluating and applying the study results, both positive and negative effects, i.e., effects and harms or side effects produced by the observed interventions, should be reported. All these elements should be available as comprehensive study results for the final analysis and evaluation of the study. At the same time, it should be evaluated whether blinding was performed, since blinding can effectively exclude information bias and thus can ensure the reproducibility and authenticity of the judgment of the study results.

10.3.3　Are the study subjects specific?

This is important for the research results to be applied correctly. The study report should describe the inclusion and exclusion criteria of the study subjects in detail. The clinical characteristics of the study subjects include age, sex, area, disease type, degree of disease and complications, etc. in order to make sure the intervention and prognosis can be applied to similar patients, while obtaining similar clinical results.

10.3.4　Is the clinical significance differentiated from the statistical significance of the research results?

When analyzing the study results, we must evaluate the difference between the intervention group and the control group statistically and clinically, which is vital to judge the value of the treatment.

Statistical tests estimate the probability that an observed association occurs due to chance or to the effect of interventions. When a statistical test shows the results are statistically significant ($P<0.05$), meaning that the results could have occurred by chance less than 5% of the time, and the true effect generated by the intervention itself was greater than 95%. Statistically significant differences are not related to the magnitude of efficacy, nor are they used to evaluate the efficacy of the intervention, its only significance is simply to evaluate the true extent to which such differences exist.

Evaluation of the clinical value of intervention includes drug prices, the frequency and severity of side effects in addition to the clinical efficacy of the intervention. This requires measuring the specific purpose of the study and specific metrics to be able to effectively evaluate the clinical significance.

10.3.5　Is the intervention in the research clear?

In order to ensure the validity and reproducibility of the study, the contents and methods of intervention in the research report should be as detailed as possible, such as drug dosage form, dosage, route of administration, duration of treatment and other auxiliary methods. The actual observation of the study, whether it is strictly performed and compliance is ensured, and whether it is strictly controlled to prevent contamination and interference, will affect the results of the test and should be detailed in the analysis report.

10.3.6　Are all the subjects included in analysis?

During the observation process of a therapeutic study, some of the patients under observation are often lost in the middle of the study for various reasons, called lost to follow-up. If lost to follow-up is beyond certain level, the validity of results may be severely compromised and conclusions may be misleading. The reason is that those lost to follow-up tend to have different outcomes than those who are retained. In the therapeutic studies, the rate of loss to follow-up should not exceed 10% of the total enrolled patients. If the rate is more than 20%, the results of the study may lose their validity. Therefore, only by careful and rigorous observation and tracking in research practice, the loss to follow-up rate should be minimized as far as possible to ensure the validity of the results of the study.

The order of these criteria represents their level of importance. They can help researchers and clinicians to evaluate the science and practicality of medical literature, improve their own research and guide the choice of clinical interventions.

Summary

The steps of EBM related to therapeutic measures include question raising → evidence query → evidence evaluation → evidence application → effect evaluation. The basic design principles of therapeutic research include randomization, control and blinding to ensure the validity of research results. The first choice of the methods for therapeutic research is randomized controlled study. Evaluation standards of therapeutic research include: Is it a real randomized controlled trial? Are all the results of the study reported and observed? Are the study subjects specific? Is the clinical significance differentiated from the statistical significance of the research results? Is the intervention in the research clear? Are all the subjects included in analysis?

(Wu Shangjie)

11

Prognostic study evidence evaluation

Learning objectives

1. **To master** the basic concepts of prognostic study.
2. **To be familiar with** the evaluation principle of prognostic study.
3. **To know** the types of prognostic study.

Clinicians are usually consulted about prognosis by patients, by colleagues or by themselves. For example, a 32-year-old female patient who was newly diagnosed with breast cancer and undergone a modified radical mastectomy. She and her family might ask: Will breast cancer relapse in the future? Can I get pregnant and have children in the future? Will pregnancy increase the relapse of breast cancer? As clinicians, we might consider how to interpret a postoperative pathological report. Should this patient be treated with adjuvant chemotherapy, radiotherapy, target therapy or endocrinotherapy? Actually, all these questions are about prognosis, that is, what is the relapse rate of breast cancer? Will pregnancy impact the prognosis of breast cancer?

In order to answer these questions, we need to understand the basic concepts and the types of prognostic studies, as well as to evaluate the validity, importance and applicability of the existing evidence about prognosis.

11.1 Basic concepts of prognostic study

Prognosis means the prediction/estimate of the outcome of disease (cure, relapse, deterioration, disability, complication or death) and the impact factors for the outcome. Prognosis is a part of natural history of illness referring to the development from the occurrence to the outcome, prognosis refers to the clinical course of the disease after the diagnosis is established and the many factors that influence this process. Prognostic studies investigate outcomes of patients and the contributing factors or rates of these outcomes among those diagnosed, include at least two aspects of rate estimation and exploration of factors affecting prognosis. Evaluations of rates include mortality, survival rate, cure rate, recurrence rate. Cure rate applies to diseases that would be cured while recurrence rate or remission rate applies to incurable illness. Mortality (or survival rate), or disability rate is suitable for severe diseases. Life quality is often added to chronic diseases. Health outcomes can be estimated by contributing factors such as subtypes of diseases and clinical index.

11.2　Types of prognostic study

Several types of studies can provide information on the prognosis of a group of individuals with a defined problem or risk factor, including cohort study (prospective or retrospective), case-control study, observational study, case series, expert opinion and case report. The quality of evidences for solving clinical problems varies with different types of prognostic studies. Therefore, it is important to master the different design methods of prognostic studies and to evaluate the advantages and disadvantages of different methods before obtaining evidence for prognostic studies and applying the evidence to judge the veracity of the results.

11.2.1　Cohort study

Cohort studies provide information on the prognosis. In cohort studies, investigators follow up one or more groups of individuals with the target disorder and monitor for occurrence of outcomes. Cohort studies derive outcomes (e.g., morbidity, cure rate, remission rate, recurrence rate and survival rate) from exposures. Cohort studies (prospective or retrospective) represent the best design for answering prognostic questions. The exposure existed before initiation of illness in prospective cohort studies and outcomes would be acquired during follow-up (Figure 11-1), while in a retrospective cohort study the exposure and disease both existed at the beginning (Figure 11-2), i.e., the study outcome has already occurred at the beginning of the study, thus exploring the causal relationship between past exposure factors and the current occurrence of a disease. The feasibility and reliability of retrospective cohort studies could be affected by the validity and completeness of history data.

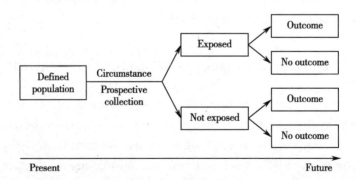

Figure 11-1　The design of a prospective cohort study

In the cohort study, the investigators define two or more groups of people according to the extent of their exposure to a potential cause of disease over time, patients are then followed up for a period of time to determine if they have a positive outcome. Therefore, the measures of an "exposure" and "outcome", as well as the follow-up time are the triple basic elements in cohort study.

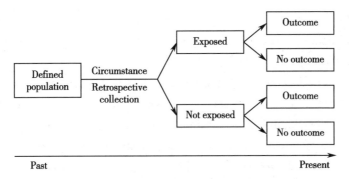

Figure 11-2   The design of a retrospective cohort study

Exposure is the most important element of prognostic study. Usually, participants are divided into two groups, the exposure cohort consisting of individuals with the putative causal event or condition and the unexposed cohort. They may be also divided into more groups characterized by different levels or types of exposure. The exposure should be a well-defined and quantifiable condition, making it easy to assign subjects to exposed and unexposed cohorts precisely. Prognosis of illness can be affected by lots of exposures carrying with different diseases; therefore, including all the potential exposures will be necessary to avoid deficiency. Clinical prognostic exposures are complex and interactive; hence, when the impact of multiple prognostic factors on the outcome cannot be clearly analyzed by applying single-factor analysis, multifactor analysis should be used. It is important to define and determine the outcome of events or endpoint, that is, the endpoint of follow-up (also known as a positive outcome) as precisely as possible, to avoid information bias. There is no difficulty in defining some results like death. For other outcomes, such as disability or remission of disease, they can be defined in a reasonably precise manner, but measurement of time is difficult. Censoring and positive endpoints are both outcomes.

Follow-up period is the length from beginning of study to the endpoint (positive outcome) or time of censoring. Observation of specific events requires that prognostic studies require a certain amount of follow-up time before a study endpoint (or positive outcome) can be observed. Follow-up period should be long enough to make positive endpoint occur. The length of follow-up period depends on natural medical history.

Survival analysis is the most common statistical method in prognostic studies. The beginnings of follow-up of prognostic studies are in sequencing, the same as the endings of the follow-up. Therefore, the length of follow-up periods is different in different cases. The outcomes include both endpoint and censoring when not achieving positive endpoint at the end of follow-up. Meanwhile, loss of follow-up can occur in many ways, especially when the follow-up period is very long. If the outcome is not inevitable, subjects may suffer from a competing risk and so be removed from follow-up. For example, if the endpoint of the study is death, some of the study participants may end the follow-up due to other causes. Most statistical methods for follow-up data treat losses to follow-up or competing risks as forms of censoring. At this point, average risk and occurrence time can be estimated using survival methods. Basic survival analysis involves stratification on follow-up time, including life-table analysis and Kaplan-Meier analysis. Among them, the life-table analysis is the basic method of prognostic analysis.

11.2.1.1　Advantages

A continuous period of time between study factors and outcome factors in cohort studies establishes a clear causal relationship between the two, providing strong information on clinical causality; the risk of developing disease from certain exposure factors can be measured directly; not knowing the outcome factors in the measurement fashion avoids bias in the measurement of exposure factors and also allows for the simultaneous measurement of known confounders to be controlled for in statistical analyses.

11.2.1.2　Disadvantages

It requires a lot of labor, material and time. Those with a low incidence of positive outcomes or those with a long cause-to-effect cycle require large samples and long follow-up to obtain a positive result. Some cohorts with special exposures have indeed been followed up for decades. Of course, lengthy studies of large population are expensive. However, should be noticed that if a cohort study has a very long follow-up period and exposure data were only collected at baseline, people may have changed their behaviors over the intervening years, often causes bias in outcome analysis. For example, smokers may quit smoking during the follow-up period, which jumps to an incorrect conclusion that smoking is not a risk factor for lung cancer.

11.2.2　Case-control study

Case-control studies are also used for prognostic study. Instead of identifying people on the basis of their exposure status and following up their development, we effectively start from the end. We select people with the target disease and a representative sample of people without the target disease from the same population and then ask them about their previous exposures (Figure 11-3), it is a research method that extrapolates from results to causes. For instance, if we want to know whether smoking was associated with lung cancer, we can compare people with lung cancer and controls without lung cancer to see if they differed in their smoking habits. Case-control studies are more time-efficient and economical, more suitable for assessing some rare diseases, and for assessing the relationship between multiple exposure factors and outcomes at once.

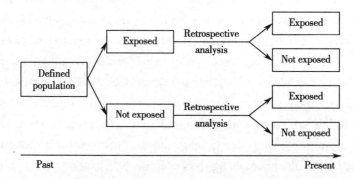

Figure 11-3　The design of a case-control study

Conventional wisdom about case-control studies is that their estimates and measures are not as valid as those of cohort studies. The vital problem in the design of a case-control study is selection of the control group. If the control group is not selected properly, it is easy to cause selection bias. Recalled bias is also an inevitable problem. Meanwhile, case-control studies cannot perform data of survival rates and are merely suitable for studies with minor impact in the analysis of disease prognostic factors. The following kinds of bias are common.

11.2.2.1 **Selection bias** is a type of bias generated from difference between those selected into the study and those not selected in some systematic way. For example, those who agree to participate in a study may be healthier (e.g., less overweight, lower levels of smoking and alcohol consumption, higher levels of physical activity) than those who refuse to participate. If this affects recruitment of controls (but not cases) for a case-control study, comparisons between cases and controls will cause selection biased.

11.2.2.2 **Recall bias** is a type of bias that systematic errors in the recall of previous exposures of study subjects due to distorted or incomplete memory of respondents resulting in clear exposure or not in case and control groups occur mostly in case-control studies.

11.2.2.3 **Interviewer (observer) bias** is a type of bias that arises in exposure (disease) measurement when an interviewer (or observer) is aware of the disease (exposure) status of an individual. For example, an interviewer may ask more detailed questions, and thus potentially get exposed factors, when they are talking to someone who they know to has disease. A clinician may be more likely to diagnose disease in someone they know has been exposed to a particular factor.

11.3   Evaluation rules of prognostic study

Evaluating validity, importance and suitability are very important in prognostic studies.

11.3.1   Is the study valid?

Population recruited should be defined clearly and representatively. The study population was accurately defined using accepted diagnostic criteria. The inclusion and exclusion criteria of recruitment in prognostic studies should be distinct to avoid selection bias.

Prognostic cohort studies need to be very clear about the starting point when including study subjects, because the stage and duration of the disease that the patient is in will directly affect the prognostic outcome. Prognostic outcomes are only realistic if the study subjects are at approximately the same stage at the time of inclusion. The study starting point should ideally be early in the disease course, or at least at the same stage of disease.

When a study subject withdraws from the original study plan for various reasons, it is called loss of follow-up. A substantial number of subjects lost to follow-up can raise serious doubts about the validity of the study because the outcome of the lost subjects is unknown. If the characteristics of subjects who lose in the follow-up period are more similar with the persons who do not, the bias will be minor. Loss of follow-up more than 20% of subjects is generally judged with skepticism, but loss of follow-up between 5% and 20% requires examination and reports on reasons of loss. If loss of follow-up is less than 5%, data of prognostic study can be credible.

The investigators should have clear criteria used to determine whether the outcomes have occurred, judgment criteria should be objective to avoid bias in clinicians' opinions when judging prognostic outcomes. To avoid measurement bias, the endpoints should have specific definition or criteria.

If the prognostic outcome is objective, such as death, a blind pattern may not be necessary. But often judgement of positive endpoints could be influenced by subjective factors, it is necessary to use the blind pattern. To eliminate potential bias in these situations, judgements should have been applied without knowing the patient's clinical characteristics and prognostic factors.

11.3.2　Are the results important?

The importance of prognostic study results is reflected by whether they report prognostic outcomes for the entire course of the disease, rather than for a particular time point. There are three ways in which outcomes might be presented: the percentage of survival at a particular point in time (such as 1-year or 5-year survival rates); median survival (the length of time by which 50% of study patients have died); survival curve that depicts at each point of time, along with the proportion of the original study sample who have not had a specified outcome.

Prognostic estimates should be accompanied by confidence intervals to represent the variation between sample and the true estimate. A 95% confidence interval is the range of values between which we can be 95% sure that the true value lies. You should take account of this range when extracting estimates for your patient. If it is narrow, you would believe that the study had enough patients to provide useful information.

11.3.3　Are your patients similar to those studies?

Is our patient so different from those in the study that its results cannot apply? Do the authors present the study subjects clearly? This guides us to compare our patients with those in the article, using descriptions of the study sample's demographic, clinical characteristics, diagnosis, inclusion and exclusion criteria. The more similar they are, the more confidently we can apply the results of the study.

Will this evidence make a clinically important impact on our conclusions about what to offer or tell our patient? Evidence regarding a person's prognosis is clearly useful in deciding whether or not to initiate a therapy. If, for example, the study suggests an excellent prognosis for patients with a particular target disorder who didn't receive treatment previously, our discussions with patients would reflect these facts and would focus on whether any treatment should be started. If, on the other hand, the evidence suggests that the prognosis is gloomy without treatment (and if there are treatments that can make a meaningful difference), our conversations with patients would reflect these facts and more likely lead us to treatment. Even when the prognostic evidence does not help make a treat decision, valid evidence can be useful in providing patients and families with information about what the future is likely to hold for them and their illness.

11.4　Clinical scenario

11.4.1　A clinical question

The patient was a 32-year-old woman who presented to the hospital because of breast lump. She was married but had not given birth to a child yet. The local physical examination showed a subcutaneous mass hard-fibrous texture of 1cm×1.5cm at the right breast. The patient was performed modified radical mastectomy of the right breast. The pathology came out to be invasive ductal carcinoma of the right breast with negative lymph nodes metastasis, estrogen receptor (ER) and progesterone receptor (PR) positive and human epidermal growth factor receptor 2 (HER 2)/ neu negative.

As a young and early breast cancer patient, she and her family might ask: Will breast cancer relapse in the future? Could pregnancy be possible? Will pregnancy increase the relapse of breast cancer? As clinicians, we first need to change the clinical questions into retrievable (containing key words) and easily answered ones. For example, we pose the following questions: Is there any difference between relapse rates of breast cancer patients with pregnancy or not? Is pregnancy a high-risk factor of breast cancer recurrence? Then, using the online retrieval device, we are able to identify an article comparing the difference of progression free survival between pregnant patients and non-pregnant ones after the diagnosis of breast cancer. At last, we need to evaluate evidence about prognosis for its validity, importance and relevance to our patients.

11.4.2　Examples of retrospective cohort studies

AMANT F, von MINCKWITZ G, Han S N, et al.Prognosis of women with primary breast cancer diagnosed during pregnancy: results from an international collaborative study[J].Journal of clinical oncology : official journal of the American Society of Clinical Oncology, 2013, 31(20).

11.4.2.1　Purpose

A previous meta-analysis showed a low recurrence rate in women patients with breast cancer diagnosed during pregnancy (BCP), but this finding is likely due to selection bias, as patients tend to choose pregnancy after they are recurrence-free. In addition, there are no studies exploring the effect of pregnancy in a specific patient population with estrogen receptor (ER) positivity. We aimed to determine the prognosis of patients with breast cancer diagnosed during pregnancy (BCP) of known ER status.

11.4.2.2　Patients and methods

In this cohort study, a multicentric registry of patients with BCP (from Cancer in Pregnancy, Leuven, Belgium, and GBG 29/BIG 02-03) compiled pro- and retrospectively between 2003 and 2011 was compared with patients who did not have associated pregnancies, using an age limit of 45 years. Patients with a diagnosis postpartum were excluded. The main analysis was performed using Cox proportional hazards regression of disease-free survival (DFS) and overall survival (OS) on exposure (pregnant or not), adjusting for age, stage, grade, hormone receptor status, human epidermal growth factor 2 status, histology, type of chemotherapy, use of trastuzumab, radiotherapy, and hormone therapy.

11.4.2.3 Results

The registry contained 447 women with BCP, mainly originating from Germany and Belgium, of whom 311 (69.6%) were eligible for analysis. The non-pregnant group consisted of 865 women. Median age was 33 years for the pregnant and 41 years for the non-pregnant patients. Median follow-up was 61 months. The hazard ratio of pregnancy was 1.34 (95% CI, 0.93 to 1.91; $P = 0.14$) for DFS and 1.19 (95% CI, 0.73 to 1.93; $P = 0.51$) for OS. Cox regression estimated that the 5-year DFS rate for pregnant patients would have increased from 65% to 71% if these patients had not been pregnant. Likewise, the 5-year OS rate would have increased from 78% to 81%.

11.4.2.4 Conclusion

The results show similar OS for patients diagnosed with BCP compared with nonpregnant patients. This information is important when patients are counseled and supports the option to start treatment with continuation of pregnancy.

This was a multicenter retrospective cohort study which enrolled primary breast cancer patients with known ER status. Primary outcome was disease-free survival, defined as time in months from the date of first diagnosis to any following events: local relapse, distant relapse, secondary cancer and death from any cause. To investigate the independent impact of pregnancy on outcome, we attempted to control for the following factors in a descending order: ER, nodal status, adjuvant chemotherapy, adjuvant hormonal therapy, age (<35 or ⩾35 years). A total of 311 pregnant patients were compared with 865 women with breast cancer who were not pregnant. For the total group (pregnant and non-pregnant patients together), median follow-up for DFS was 61 months. We did not find evidence of worse prognosis for women diagnosed with breast cancer pregnancy regarding disease recurrence (hazard ratio [HR], 1.34; 95% CI, 0.93 to 1.91; $P=0.14$). This study was to estimate the prognostic impact of pregnancy when breast cancer is diagnosed with known ER status in the largest series. The results of this study allow clinicians to support patients with BC on their pregnancy as there is no difference of disease-free survival between women with breast cancer pregnancy and patients who do not have associated pregnancies.

Summary

Prognostic studies are investigations of future events. The results of such studies improve our understanding of the clinical course of a disease and assist clinicians in making informed decisions about how to manage patients. Prognostic studies begin with the establishment of a disease diagnosis and examine the subsequent clinical course and the many factors that influence that course, including at least two aspects of rate estimation and exploration of the factors that influence prognosis.

Prognostic study designs include cohort studies, case-control studies, and cross-sectional studies. The level of quality of evidence for prognostic studies provided by different study designs is completely different. Therefore, before obtaining evidence for prognostic studies and applying the evidence, it is important to master the different design methods of prognostic studies and the advantages and disadvantages of different methods to subsequently judge the authenticity of the study results.

Evaluating validity, importance and suitability are evaluation principles in prognostic studies.

(Liu Tianshu)

Prevention and screening evidence evaluation

Learning objectives

1. **To master** the basic concepts of screening.
2. **To know** the principles for evaluating evidence of screening research.

In order to minimize the damage from diseases to population, modern preventive medicine not only emphasizes the prevention of diseases, but also aims to achieve early diagnoses and interventions. At present, the evaluation of effects of national screening tests mainly depends on indexes of authenticity and repeatability, such as sensitivity, specificity, Youden index and coincidence rate. However, insufficient attention is paid to issues such as the best interval period of screening methods as well as the health benefits and long-term effects of screening methods and strategies.

How to select the better screening methods and strategies of better social benefits under limited cost plan? How to find a screening method or strategy with less cost but still meeting the utility and effectiveness requirement? In what ways dose the screening test differ from the diagnostic test? To answer the above questions, this chapter will focus on the basic concepts and evaluation principles of screening.

12.1 Basic concepts

As a public health service, screening aims at the population at risk or already affected by a disease while unrecognizing the presence of the disease. For this purpose, questionnaire surveys and medical tests are conducted among the target population to determine further examination or treatment, thus decreasing the risk and harm of the disease. The concept of screening is similar but distinct from the concept of diagnosis. A diagnostic test is applied among people with clinical signs or symptoms who are seeking for diagnosis and conscious of their abnormalities. Whereas a screening test is carried out among patients at the early stage of a disease with subclinical symptoms or the population exposed to high risk factors, neither of them are aware of the danger.

The main purpose of screening is to identify asymptomatic or pre-symptomatic patients at early stage or individuals under high risk among the apparently healthy population. Therefore, the screening tests are performed on normal population or subjects within specified range, which are different from diagnostic tests directly aimed at a particular individual.

The value of screening is to provide effective secondary prevention before diagnosis and decrease the mortality and disability of the population by convenient and quick tests or examinations. It is one of the most important tools used for disease prevention and control by most developed countries. Also, screening could be performed to discern high-risk population for corresponding intervention and decrease the morbidity by the primary prevention.

Therefore, besides the effectiveness of the screening method (able to differentiate early-stage patients from healthy individuals), we should also judge the accuracy and value of a screening study by analyzing the level of improved quality of life for positive subjects after early diagnosis and interventions following screening.

12.2 Study design and evaluation principle

12.2.1 Principles of screening in practice

There are pros and cons in the application of screening. While identifying patients at an early stage and high-risk population, screening increases time at risk for target population and psychological burden for positive population. Therefore, at the beginning of a screening, the overall benefits should outweigh the harm, and the accuracy of screening method and the effectiveness of treatment should be evaluated. If there is currently no effective intervention for screening-detected early-stage patients, the implementation of the screening is meaningless.

A lead time is the latency between the detection of a disease and the time the patient sees a doctor for related signs or symptoms. The outcome of a disease with a longer lead time is better than a disease requiring a clinic visit after apparent signs or symptoms, because the patients have more time for diagnosis and treatment after being detected. For instance, hypertension and noise-induced hearing loss have a relatively long lead time, while pancreatic cancer with a short one. Since the diseases with a short lead time usually progress rapidly and leave limited time between detection and visiting a doctor, compared with starting the treatment on one's own initiative, there is no advantage for starting the treatment after being detected.

Currently, among all national and international principles of screening, *Principles and Practice of Screening for Disease* in 1968 by Wilson and Jungner for WHO screening work, is still the most frequently cited literature. Changes are made during practical application among different countries without replacement of the core content. The principles of screening practice in "Twelfth Five-Year Plan" national level official textbook of *Epidemiology* in general higher education undergraduate program are adapted from the 10 principles put forward by Wilson and Jungner. Compared with the original edition, our principles include clear limitations and explanations about the definition of target population, diseases for screening, public health issue for screening and concerned social benefits. In addition, ethical issues in screening plan are also discussed. Table 12-1 shows the comparison between the 10 principles by Wilson and Jungner and those cited in the national textbook. Only in accordance with the following premise principles can screening be of value and meaning in practice.

Table 12-1   principles of screening in practice

Comparison		Wilson and Jungner	Our textbook
Same	1.	The condition should be a local important health problem	
	2.	Facilities for diagnosis should be available for the disease or defect for screening	
	3.	There should be effective and acceptable intervention and treatment for patients or risk population with recognized disease	
	4.	There should be identifiable early signs or symptoms or indexes for a disease or defect or risk factor for screening	
	5.	The natural history of the disease, including development from latent to declared disease, should be adequately understood	
	6.	The total cost of screening, diagnosis and treatment needs to be balanced against the benefits	
Similar	1.	There should be a test or examination for the condition	Screening test should be quick, simple, economic, reliable, safe, effective and easy to be accepted by patients
	2.	The test should be acceptable to the population	There should be guaranteed manpower, material resources, funds and favorable social conditions to ensure the implementation and completion of screening
	3.	Case-finding should be a continuous process, not just a "once and for all" project	Case-finding should be a continuous process with successive and complete plan and should be carried on according to the plan
	4.	There should be an agreed policy on whom to treat as patients	Screening project should be acceptable and beneficial, respecting the privacy of target population with security measurements. The tested subjects should be treated justly, fairly and reasonably

Randomized controlled research plan could also be used to explore the value of screening in practice and early treatment. According to different target populations in screening and treatment as well as different time points for randomization, there are two kinds of randomized controlled research plans discussing the meaning of a screening project in practice with difference in the intervention time after screening (Figure 12-1).   For instance, one randomized controlled trial in New York had observed nearly 60 000 women around the age of 64 years old for 23 years. The prevalence of breast cancer was compared between women who underwent mammography screening and then received treatment and who did not. Compared with breast cancer patients in the unscreened group, the mortality rate decreased by 38.1% for breast cancer patients in the screened group at the 5th year of follow-up, 28.6% at the 10th year of follow-up and 22.7% at the 18th year of follow-up. Figure 12-1A shows the research procedure of this study. Another research plan in Figure 12-1B could be used as the major proposal of screening in pregnancy for subclinical hypothyroidism during prenatal care and assess the difference between early intervention after screening and symptomatic intervention.

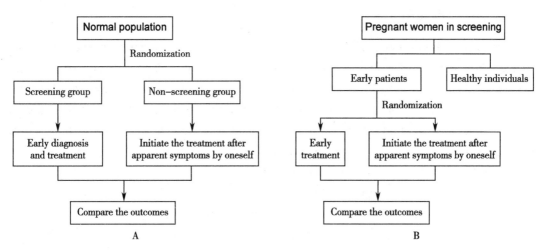

Figure 12-1　Randomized controlled research plans for screening

12.2.2　Types of screening

According to the range of target population and number of screening methods, screening can be classified into following types.

12.2.2.1　Population screening

Using the specific method to screen a whole population to find out possible cases among high-risk subjects and conduct diagnostic test or treatment. For example, pregnant women are initially screened using a glucose screening test, and those with abnormal results then undergo an oral glucose tolerance test to confirm the diagnosis.

12.2.2.2　Targeted screening

Conducting regular health examinations for people exposed to risk factors to achieve early detection and early intervention. For instance, regular pneumoconiosis screening among miners, asbestosis and lung cancer screening among asbestos workers and corresponding screening tests for workers exposed to lead and other poisonous or harmful substance.

12.2.2.3　Single screening

One screening test for one specific disease, which is the most popular screening type in use. For instance, conventional mammography screening for mammary disease.

12.2.2.4　Multiple screening

Application of multiple methods for screening or screening for various diseases at one time. For instance, in our country, free screening tests are provided to neonates for various kinds of hereditary or endocrine disease such as phenylketonuria, congenital hypothyroidism, glucose-6-phosphate dehydrogenase deficiency and congenital hearing disorders through assessment of heel blood and audiometry.

12.2.2.5　Case-finding or opportunistic screening

The screening subject visits or consults a doctor and the doctor supplements a screening test for another disease unrelated with present main symptoms.

12.2.3　The process of screening

Nowadays, the fundamental screening process has been uniformly approved by domestic and foreign scholars and has already been applied to the area of public health. Screening tests should be conducted among healthy or asymptomatic population to distinguish positive subjects from negative ones according to result of the test. Among positive subjects, diagnostic tests should be conducted to differentiate patients from non-patients. For patients and high-risk individuals, therapeutic or preventive interventions should be applied.

However, in real practice, the screening process is not that simple as it neglects the individuals with uncertainty results, such as a result not eligible for intervention but certainly not negative. Therefore, to design, evaluate and apply a screening plan, it is crucial to establish a definite and uniform standard for screening qualifications, such as age and sex of target population.

12.2.4　Screening models

Epidemiological screening model is a screening method based on materials from epidemiological surveys. Through establishing appropriate screening models, a large number of undiagnosed patients can be diagnosed and treated early. Meanwhile, the target population is greatly reduced to a smaller scale which simplifies the organization workload and saves a great amount of manpower, material resources and funds.

For example, the most common method of screening study on risk of diabetes is to analyze risk factors and evaluate the risk of developing diabetes for each individual. For each subject, the more risk factors with higher risk level mean a higher risk of diabetes. The screening model of impaired glucose tolerance among community population is such a convenient, economic and effective screening tool based on the risk factor scores.

Furthermore, mathematical models could also be used to establish screening models on the basis of epidemiological survey data. For instance, artificial neural networks could be used to set up a prediction model. Artificial neural networks could automatically derive quantitative rules from known data or conditions. When we input information from unknown samples, outcomes of a risk or an event could be predicted from calculations on the information to be assessed via artificial neural network. Shortcomings in traditional screening methods, such as low efficiency, time consuming, energy consuming and high cost, could be avoided by using artificial neural network as the preliminary screening method, hence more suitable for mass population screening. At present, artificial neural network has already been applied in the epidemiological screening for disease successfully. Gao Wei et al. are using this method to screen diabetic patients or high-risk individuals according to specific differences between patients or high-risk individuals and healthy subjects, such as obesity and family history of diabetes. Just by several simple and accessible indexes, artificial neural network can correctly identify 90% of subjects of abnormal blood sugar level, which reduces cost of blood sugar measurement for normal subjects. Its benefit cost ratio is 1.6 times that of regular screening plan (OGTT).

12.2.5   Evaluation principles of screening procedures

The core content of evaluation of modern screening procedures is the 7 evaluation principles proposed by Cochrane and Holland in 1971. These 7 criteria aim at 7 key elements of screening respectively, including simplicity, acceptability, accuracy, cost, repeatability, sensitivity and specificity.

Simplicity

The tests used by the screening program should be easy to administer and understand.

Acceptability

As screening is in most instances voluntary, it is essential that tests should be acceptable to the subjects.

Accuracy

The tests should give a true measurement of the attribute under investigation.

Cost

The expense of screening and benefits after tests should be comprehensively considered about.

Repeatability

The test should give consistent results in repeated trials on the same subject.

Sensitivity

The test should be able to identify subject with the disease or abnormality correctly.

Specificity

The test should be able to identify non-diseased subjects correctly.

12.2.6   Evaluation of screening results

To evaluate the value of any kind of screening test, we should first compare the result from the test with the result from gold standards, which means blind comparison between the result of the screening test in question and the result of an accepted and accurate diagnostic test. There would be 4 results after comparison: true positive (the results of the diagnostic test and the screening test are both positive), false positive (the result of the diagnostic test is negative while that of the screening test is positive), true negative (the results of the diagnostic test and the screening test are both negative), false negative (the result of the diagnostic test is positive while that of the screening test is negative).

According to results from the diagnostic test and the screening test, we can directly evaluate the screening test in the form of numbers through standardizing the evaluation by calculation formulas. Table 12-2 concludes the evaluation criteria according to authenticity, repeatability and benefits.

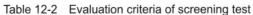

Table 12-2 Evaluation criteria of screening test

Categories	Criteria	Formulas
Authenticity	Sensitivity	Sensitivity (also called true positive rate): the ability of a screening test to identify individuals with disease
		Sensitivity = true positives/ all diagnosed positives×100%
		False negative rate (also called miss rate): the possibility of an individual with a disease to have a negative result from the test
		False negative rate = False negatives/ all diagnosed positives×100%
	Specificity	Specificity (also called true negative rate): the ability of a screening test to find non-diseased people
		Specificity = true negatives/all diagnosed negatives×100%
		False positive rate (also called fall-out): the possibility of an individual without disease to have a positive result from the test
		False positive rate = false positives/ all diagnosed negatives×100%
	Likelihood ratio	Positive likelihood ratio = true positive rate/false positive rate. The larger the ratio, the higher value of the screening test
		Negative likelihood ratio = false negative rate/true negative rate. The smaller the ratio, the higher value of the screening test
	Youden index	Youden index = (sensitivity + specificity) − 1. The ability of a screening test to differentiate patients and non-patients correctly
Repeatability	Coefficient of variation	When the test is based on quantitative assessment, coefficient of variation stands for reliability
		Coefficient of variation = standard deviation/mean×100%. The smaller the value, the better the reliability
	Coincidence rate	Coincidence rate (also called accuracy): when conducting the same test on the same study subjects twice, the proportion of subjects have the same results during two tests among total study population
	Coincidence test	Kappa test can be used to check the consistency of results of the same test performed at different locations or by different operators
Benefits	Predictive value	Positive predictive value: the proportion of diagnosed patients among all positive subjects from screening test
		Positive predictive value = true positives/all positives in screening test×100%
		Negative predictive value: the proportion of diagnosed non-patients among all negative subjects from screening test
		Negative predictive value = true negatives/ all negatives in screening test×100%
	Health economic evaluation	Cost-benefit analysis: to analyze the relationship between total cost of screening test and economic benefits acquired
		Benefit cost ratio (BCR) is the commonly used index
		BCR = total benefits/total cost. If BCR>1 then the screening is of practical values
		Cost-effectiveness analysis: to compare two intervention measures and evaluate cost and biological effect
		Incremental cost-effectiveness ratio (ICER) is the commonly used index
		ICER =increased cost/increased effect, indicating the increase in cost per unit effect increases. The smaller the ICER, the better
		Cost-utility analysis: to analyze the relationship between cost and life quality
		Quality-adjusted life year (QALY) and disability-adjusted life year (DALY) are commonly used indexes

One screening test should be able to detect a part of un-recognized patients among the population. The higher the detection rate, the more effective this screening. Apparently, when we evaluate the detection rate, factors such as the prevalence of the disease and time interval from the last screening of the same kind should be considered. Moreover, screening should be capable to improve the prognosis, decrease the morbidity, mortality and incident complications, and enhance the survival rate. The more improvement there is, the better effects of screening.

Theoretically, an ideal screening test should have high sensitivity and specificity at the same time. However, it is impossible to separate the two factors completely in actuality. When we try to increase the sensitivity of one screening test by regulation of critical point of the measurements, the specificity will correspondingly go down, vice versa. Therefore, it is very difficult to compare sensitivity and specificity of different screening tests. In addition, for multiple screenings, there would probably be no significant difference in screening effects by only comparing the sensitivity and specificity.

When it is unable to select an appropriate screening test based on sensitivity and specificity, evaluation of benefits becomes crucial. Benefit evaluation includes assessment of predictive value, identification of new cases and their prognosis status, and evaluation of health economics. Among them, economic benefits, namely social benefits are always neglected by clinical doctors. To evaluate the social benefits from screening methods and strategies, not only should we calculate the contribution to decreasing morbidity and mortality, but also changes in quality-adjusted life year (QALY) and disability-adjusted life year (DALY). DALY is defined by total healthy life years lost from onset of the disease to death. It is a quantitative assessment of lost healthy life years due to premature death, disability and dysfunction from the disease. The calculation of QALY should not only consider the subjective perception of changes in life quality, but also need to objectively reflect the harm effects of the disease on health and social resources. To evaluate social benefits of a screening test, we can calculate the loss of QALY and increase of DALY of different screening methods and combine the analysis with cost and best screening interval, to estimate the cost to increase each QALY and decrease each DALY. Health department could establish reasonable health policies based on the results of this analysis.

At present, most clinical doctors choose a screening test of good authenticity and high reliability when designing a screen procedure. As a result, most evaluations focus on sensitivity and specificity of the screening test, while effective model establishment and comprehensive effect assessment are neglected. Particularly, little attention has been paid to the health economic evaluation of a screening test. The essence of screening is to select representative samples in the smallest unit from big samples. If we blindly stick to the ideal sensitivity and specificity, we may ignore the basic definition of screening.

At present, the majority of screening strategies are single method for single disease or multiple methods for single disease. Taking advantage of multidiscipline, Lisong Liu et al. established a screening model based on combination of multiple disciplines, such as neurology, cardiology, endocrinology and etc., to screen population at moderate to high risk of stroke. Compared with screening models of single method or single discipline, the multi-method and multidisciplinary model ensures more comprehensive and objective evaluation of target population. However, to our knowledge, there is no available report about multidisciplinary screening model for multiple diseases. Further studies are needed to explore the application and estimate the effect of this screening model.

12.2.7 Bias of screening researches

Since screening test is a kind of trial, it could have selection bias, information bias and confounding bias (details in Chapter 7). Besides, there are some unique biases in screening test.

12.2.7.1 Lead time bias

The screening test has detected a group of asymptomatic patients who are unaware of the disease in advance. The result might deviate from the real situation because of lead time bias, if we have not considered this situation when comparing the survival period, mortality and cure rate etc. of patients detected from the screening with those of patients going to doctors on one's own initiative.

12.2.7.2 Bias from course of disease

The possibility of being detected by screening test is lower in diseases of shorter duration. This bias from course of disease should be considered when evaluating a screening study.

12.3 Application of evidence-based practice

Using Markov model, Guorong Li et al. conducted predictive analyses and provided strategic information for mass on-the-scene intervention or clinical trial of cervical cancer, to evaluate methods and strategies of cervical cancer screening from the view of cost-effectiveness and cost-utility. The following is their study methods and procedure.

12.3.1 Decide the screening test

Visual inspection with acetic acid (VIA) or visual inspection with Lugol's iodine (VILI) was the testing methods. With either one of them positive, electronic colposcopy should be conducted to collect the samples. The gold standard of screening for cervical abnormalities was the histopathological examination results (CIN2 as the positive result).

According to reports, the sensitivity and specificity of the above three screening tests were listed as follows: VIA (0.414, 0.945), VILI (0.4, 0.847) and colposcopy (0.814, 0.765).

12.3.2 Decide the screening strategy

There were 5 strategies on screening interval, including once in a life time, every one year, every 3 years, every 5 years and every 10 years.

12.3.3 Decide the screening model

Markov model was used to simulate 100 000 women, predict their situation in 20 years, compared with the non-intervention cohort and evaluate indexes such as cost and benefits as well as reduced number of patients and death among different screening strategies. From HPV infection to cervical cancer, 6 Markov statuses were set up as normal, HPV infection, CIN1, CIN2, CIN3 and cervical cancer. For the non-intervention cohort, only fees of treatment and follow-up were calculated, while expenditures of the intervention cohort included screening cost for whole population, fees of treatment and follow-up for CIN2, CIN3 and cancer, as well as screening cost for CIN 1 from different screening strategies (e.g., screening every 3 years) (Table 12-3).

Table 12-3   Effect and utility of screening cohort

Indication	Every year	Every 3 years	Every 5 years	Every 10 years	All life
Reduced incidence rate of cervical cancer /100 000^{-1}	616.66	569.99	501.73	319.13	54.6
Reduced mortality from cervical cancer /100 000^{-1}	2 826	2 368	1 934	1 129	379
Cost per QALY /Yuan	532	223	221	324	232
Cost per DALY averted /Yuan	490	208	208	309	213

12.3.3.1   Evaluation of screening benefits
Cost-effectiveness

As described in Table 12-3, using screening test of VIA and VILI followed by colposcopy, incidence rate and mortality of cervical cancer could be reduced by all the five screening strategies. During the 20-year period, the incidence rate of cervical cancer could be reduced by(54.5~616.66)/100 000, while the mortality could decrease by (379~2 826)/100 000. With decreasing screening interval, the number of reduced patients or deaths is increasing. However, increased QALY and reduced DALY are also going up. For the strategy of screening every 10 years, the cost of increasing one QALY is more than that in strategies of every 3 years or 5 years. This might result from the fact that the cost of cancer treatment is much higher than the cost of cancer screening. In addition, shown as lower reduced incidence and mortality rates as well as lower increased QALY by one screening in all life, screening interval should not be too long.

Cost-utility

As shown in Table 12-3, cost per QALY and cost per DALY averted are 532 yuan and 490 yuan respectively for screening every year, 223 yuan and 208 yuan for screening every 3 years, 221 yuan and 208 yuan for screening every 5 years, as well as 324 yuan and 309 yuan for screening every 10 years. Therefore, cervical cancer screening test of VIA /VILI combined with colposcopy has good cost-effect and cost-utility, and it is suggested to be conducted every 3 to 5 years in economically less developed regions.

12.3.3.2   Sensitive analysis

The sensitivity of VIA in the above study is 0.414, which is a bit lower than that in other references. This might be associated with clinical experiences of inspectors. According to this situation, sensitive analysis should be conducted when the sensitivity of VIA varies between 40%~75%. Compared with screening every 5 years, 10 years or once in all life, the cost of screening every 3 years does not vary much for different sensitivities. When the sensitivity of VIA is equal to 0.7, the cost per QALY for screening every 3 years is the same as screening every 5 years, though the reduced death number and patient number of cervical cancers are higher than those of the latter. Therefore, 3 years is the best interval for screening.

Summary

Screening is a preliminary detection method to differentiate healthy individuals and individuals with disease or high risk. For a screening study, we should first judge whether it is in accordance with the 10 primary principles of screening in practice to assess the practical value of the study. Then the screening procedure should be evaluated according to simplicity, acceptability, accuracy, cost, repeatability, sensitivity and specificity, while the screening result should be rated based on authenticity, repeatability and benefits.

(Xu Liangzhi)

13

Evaluation of adverse reaction research

Learning objectives

1. **To master** the evaluation methods of adverse reactions.
2. **To be familiar with** the concept and classification of adverse reactions; network meta-analysis.

During 1956—1961, thalidomide was used to treat vomiting during pregnancy in 17 nations and region. Thereafter teras events appeared in these nations, with short-limbed newborns looking like a seal, who were known as seal babies. There were more than 10 000 victims and over 5 000 babies died. The incident was a major event of serious adverse drug reaction in the history of public health.

13.1 The concept of adverse reaction

Drugs not only treat disease but also can lead to adverse reactions, so it is very important objectively and scientifically evaluating the safety and effectiveness of drugs. Adverse drug reaction is defined by the WHO Collaborating Centre for International Drug Monitoring as a harmful reaction which has nothing to do with the treatment purposes when the normal dose of drugs is used in the prevention, treatment and diagnosis of disease. According to the 63rd article of the *Provisions for Adverse Drug Reaction Reporting and Monitoring* issued by the Ministry of Health, adverse drug reaction is reaction unrelated to treatment purposes of qualified drugs under normal dosage and use. More comprehensively, adverse drug reaction should be defined as harmful reaction unrelated with the prevention, treatment and diagnosis of diseases when a variety of measures, means and methods are used.

13.1.1 Classification of adverse drug reactions

All drugs have adverse reaction, but individual differences lead to completely different results. The classification of adverse drug reactions is mainly based on mechanism, frequency and severity.

For mechanism, drug adverse reactions can be divided into dose-related adverse reactions and those unrelated with dose. The difference of them is whether there is a positive correlation between dose and adverse reactions in the isodose curve. The latter is usually caused by individual differences.

According to the frequency of adverse reactions, the Council for International Organizations of Medical Sciences (CIOMS) divides them into very common (frequency$\geqslant$10%), common (frequency 1%$\sim$10%), occasional (frequency$\geqslant$0.1%, <1%), rare and very rare.

According to the degree of harm, adverse reactions are divided into 6 levels: in Level 1 the harm is mild and patients get well after the drug is stopped, no treatment needed; in level 2, the harm is moderate and patients need treatment or intervention but not hospitalization, and recover easily; in level 3, the harm is severe, and patients require to be hospitalized for more than 7 days; in level 4, adverse reactions cause permanent damage (e.g. organ damage or disability); in level 5, they are life-threatening, and first aid is necessary (e.g. shock or suffocation); level 6 is death.

13.1.2　Drug safety research

A series of basic research must be carried out before clinical trials for any drugs, such as medicinal chemistry research for drugs' chemical structure, pharmacology and toxicology research for the mechanism of pharmacology and toxicology etc. Clinical trials of evaluating drugs' efficacy and safety are divided into the following 4 phases (Table 13-1).

Table 13-1　The main classification of clinical trials evaluating drug efficacy and safety

Phases	Purpose
Phase I	Preliminary human drug experiments, observation of the human body resistance and pharmacokinetic characteristics
Phase II	Randomized double-blind controlled experiment, preliminary evaluation of drug efficacy and safety
Phase III	Multicenter randomized controlled trials, further evaluation of drug efficacy and safety
Phase IV	The long-term clinical monitoring of post-marketing new drugs. The widely used drug research about curative effects and adverse reactions (including the common adverse reactions, rare adverse reactions, long-term adverse reactions)

So, the post-marketing safety monitoring of new drugs is important. If severe adverse reactions appear after post-marketing, the drug should be discontinued or recalled according to regulations.

13.2　Evaluation of adverse reaction

At present, various traditional evidence-based research and network meta -analysis about the efficacy and safety of therapies are emerging, and most of studies on safety involve adverse reactions. In this section, we will focus on the studies of adverse reactions, including their types, retrieval, and evaluation etc.

13.2.1 Evaluation indicators and study types of adverse reactions

Some original articles reported not only the efficacy and safety but also the adverse effects of the treatment. However, some treatments have long-term, rare and unrecognized adverse reactions. In order to evaluate the adverse reactions of drugs in a more standardized way, we should select the most common symptoms or signs that are considered very serious by both doctors and patients as the research indicators of adverse reactions, and consider both the long-term response and the short-term response. Most of the original research are randomized controlled trials (RCTs) about adverse reactions of medications. Therefore, in order to evaluate long-term, rare and unrecognized adverse reactions, we should take into account some original cohort studies, case-control studies, case reports, etc. to make a more comprehensive evaluation of adverse drug reactions.

13.2.2 The retrieval of adverse reactions

13.2.2.1 The data resources of adverse reactions

Reference books: *Meyler's Side Effects of Drugs*; *The Side Effects of Drugs* (SEDA).

Journal: *The Complete Drugs Reference*.

13.2.2.2 The retrieval strategy

We use subject headings, subheadings, and free terms for retrieval, and change retrieval strategy accordingly so as not to miss the related research. Here, we take MEDLILE for example.

Subject headings: drug toxicity; adverse drug reaction.

Subheadings: adverse effects; poisoning; toxicity; chemically induced; complication.

Free terms should be a few highly sensitive or specific adverse reactions of a disease. In addition to toxicity, side effects and harmful effects, we also choose clinical manifestations such as tiredness, fatigue, nausea and vomiting, etc.

13.2.3 The quality evaluation of adverse reactions

13.2.3.1 The diagnosis of adverse reactions

It is important and strenuous to evaluate the safety of a treatment by judging whether there is a causal link between adverse reactions and the treatment. To evaluate the causal relationship between medications and adverse reactions, the Karch and Lasagna method have been internationally used.

We can judge the causal link between drugs and adverse reactions from the following aspects:

Whether the time sequence of drug intake and adverse reaction is reasonable?

Whether the reaction belongs to the known adverse reactions of the drugs?

Whether adverse reactions abate or disappear after stopping or reducing drug using?

Whether symptoms appear after giving medicine again?

Give full consideration to other confounding factors such as pathological condition, drugs combination, and changes in treatment and so on.

The conclusion of causality between drugs and adverse reactions:

Sure

The time sequence of drug dependence is reasonable; the response is consistent with the known adverse drug reactions; after stopping drug using, reaction stops; symptoms appear after giving medicine again; other reasons cannot explain.

Very likely

Time sequence is reasonable; the response is consistent with the known adverse drug reactions; after stopping drug using, reaction stops; it cannot be reasonably explained merely based on patients' disease.

Possible

Time sequence is reasonable; the response is consistent with the known adverse drug reactions; patients' diseases or other treatments can also cause such adverse reactions.

Conditional

Time sequence is reasonable; the reaction is not consistent with the known adverse drug reactions; it cannot be reasonably explained merely based on patients' disease.

Suspicious

The above criteria are not met.

Besides the main method, the scoring calculation method is also a good way; APS(adverse drug reaction probability scale), also known as the Naranjo scoring method, is frequently used internationally. Of a total score of 12 points, $\geqslant 9$ is for sure, $5\sim8$ is likely to be relevant, $1\sim4$ is possible, $\leqslant 0$ is suspicious.

13.2.3.2　Evaluation of evidence for adverse reactions

Authenticity, importance and practicality are the three criteria used to test evidence. There are 4 ways to test authenticity: In addition to treatment and other related factors, whether the main clinical characteristics and baseline status of the patients included in the data are well defined and similar between groups; whether the evidence of adverse reactions is the result of blind observations; whether the observation follow-up time of adverse events is long enough and the data is complete; whether the evidence of adverse reactions meets the criteria for determining etiology or risk factors.

The purpose of evaluating the importance of adverse reactions is to confirm patients' extent of injury and degree of precision, which are reflected from the causal connection strength and the 95% CI.

If the authenticity and importance of adverse reactions are good, further consideration should be given to their practicality. Practicality means it is necessary to balance the advantages and disadvantages of the efficacy and safety of therapeutic measures; to prepare alternative treatment options; to communicate with the patient, combine the patient's opinion, and make a comprehensive consideration.

13.2.3.3　Quality evaluation of various types of studies on adverse reactions

The quality evaluation of adverse reaction mainly includes clinical trials of RCT experiments, case-control and cohort studies, case reports, etc.

There are mainly four factors affecting the quality evaluation of adverse reactions in clinical trials: monitoring method, time and frequency of adverse reactions; report results selectively; blind method; conflict of interest.

The quality criteria for evaluating evidence of adverse reactions in clinical trials mainly include evaluation in the implementation stage and reporting stage (Table 13-2).

Table 13-2　The quality criteria for evaluating evidence of adverse reactions in clinical trials

Stage	Contents
Implementation stage	Whether specific definitions of adverse reactions are given
	Whether methods for monitoring adverse reactions are reported (conventional methods or spontaneous reports, questionnaire or patient diary or tracking system)
Reporting stage	Whether control group data are reported
	What kind of adverse reactions are reported
	Whether any patients are excluded from adverse events in statistical analysis

The best study design for efficacy evaluation is the RCT trial. However, due to objective limitations, an RCT trial with a small sample size and short follow-up time is less reliable in providing information than a cohort study with a large sample size, good implementation and long follow-up. For the quality evaluation of adverse events designed as case control or cohort studies, please refer to the relevant chapters in this book.

There are 4 ways to test adverse reaction data authenticity.

Whether the case report has a good predictive value? If the case report does not have a control group, the adverse reaction might be a coincidence, which is not reliable.

Whether there is an explainable biological mechanism between the intervention and adverse reactions?

Whether the case report provides enough information for evaluation?

Whether the unreliable information could lead to error evaluation that has a negative impact on society?

13.2.4　Adverse reaction network meta-analysis

Network meta-analysis refers to the traditional direct (direct head-to-head comparison) and indirect comparison at the same time. Its main purpose is to comprehensively evaluate and sort evidence for all interventions simultaneously. Network meta-analysis can identify drugs and treatments with the highest relative safety and the least adverse reactions. The network meta-analysis software includes R and Stata. In addition to network diagrams, the output results of network meta-analysis generally include loop diagrams, ladder diagrams and rank ordering. It is worth noting that the interpretation of the final results should also be combined with actual situations.

Summary

Adverse drug reactions should be defined as harmful reactions unrelated with the prevention, treatment and diagnosis of diseases when a variety of measures, means and methods are used. Evaluation indicators of adverse reactions, types of included studies, and quality evaluation are the elements that need to be focused on. Network meta-analysis can identify drugs and treatments with the highest relative safety and the least adverse reactions.

(Rang Weiqing)

14

Applying evidence

Learning objective

To master the concept of evidence-based decision-making; the 5 steps of evidence-based decision-making.

Physicians are faced with different patients with all kinds of clinical symptoms in their daily work. They need to choose proper diagnostic methods, provide appropriate treatments, take appropriate nursing plans, analyze possible risk factors for disease development and give assessments on the prognosis. All the processes above are clinical decisions. Clinical decisions run through all aspects of medical activities. The accuracy of clinical decisions has a great influence on the quality and safety of the medical activities.

Traditional clinical decisions are always based on the physicians' knowledge and experience, or come from the experts' advice and opinions in authoritative books. While, with the progress of evidence-based medicine (EBM), the traditional clinical decisions and classic medical decisions are questioned. Firstly, clinical decisions based on experience and the experts' advice do not come from clinical high-quality researches which avoid some bias. Secondly, opinions from authoritative books have delayed effects and some new treatments could not be promoted while some ineffective or even harmful treatments are widely used. Thirdly, physicians from different medical institutions and regions cannot reach an agreement and sometimes even come up with contradictory clinical decisions, does not stand the test of time or space. Besides, many clinicians make arbitrary or variable clinical decisions. Even for one patient, the physician's clinical decisions may vary at different time. Fourthly, as the patients gain more access to the latest medical information and demand more high-quality medical care, they raise more doubts on the traditional clinical decisions.

In the era of "5P" medical model, which are "predictive, preventive, personalized, participatory and precision medicine", evidence-based decision-making could make clinical decisions more scientifically and effectively, and realize precision medicine which is "patient-centered" and minimally invasive.

14.1 The concept of evidence-based decision-making

Evidence-based decision-making is the clinical practice of following evidence, i.e., applying the principles of evidence-based medicine in clinical practice and making clinical decisions based on the best research evidence, clinical experience, and patient choice. Evidence-based decision-making contains three components: patients, physicians, and the best evidence. When patients seek for the help at diagnoses or treatments, physicians should make appropriate clinical decisions. In addition to using their own clinical experience and expertise, physicians should also update their knowledge, grasp new skills, search for the current best evidence. Then they should objectively evaluate the patients' conditions and take the expectations of patients into considerations. Finally, physicians should make appropriate clinical decisions in conjunction of the three components of evidence-based decision-making and thus effectively solve the troubles of patients.

Evidence-based decision-making is not merely a matter of science, but an economic and ethical issue in the case of limited resources. Applying evidence-based decision-making often encounters many difficulties. Firstly, physicians are faced with specific and complicated questions which cover the aspects of culture, society, politics and economy. Secondly, scientific and technological knowledge accumulated in the 21st century may be more than that in the past several thousands of years. Needless to say, it is very difficult to find the definitive best evidence in the ocean of medical information. What is worse, some evidence is contradictory and some defective or groundless. Moreover, expectations of patients grow high and new technologies which are immature may increase the risk in medical activities. As many factors may influence the process, it is particularly important to learn and master the steps of evidence-based decision-making.

14.2 The basic steps of evidence-based decision-making

The steps of evidence-based decision-making are the processes of EBM practice. Concretely, they can be divided in five steps: asking questions; acquiring evidence; appraising evidence; applying evidence; reevaluating evidence. How to put forward and build clinical question, how to acquire evidence and how to appraise evidence have been described in the previous chapters. We will not repeat it in this chapter. This chapter focuses on how to analyze the evidence scientifically in the process of decision-making, how to apply evidence correctly and appropriately in combination with clinical experience and patients' expectations, and how to conduct reevaluation.

14.2.1 Analyzing evidence

Evidence alone is insufficient for decision-making. Each patient has his/her own characteristics apart from the common symptoms and signs. Physicians need to analyze the evidence before making clinical decisions. They need to weigh the advantages and disadvantages of various treatments and consider the patients' values in combination with their clinical experience. Then the appropriate decision would be made after sufficient communication with the patients, let patients understand the importance of weighing the advantages and disadvantages of treatment. Therefore, evidence needs to be analyzed as follows before applying (Table 14-1).

Table 14-1 Factors to consider when appraising evidence

Points	Items
Applicability	Are your patients similar with those in the study?
	What difference between your patient and study standards would affect the applicability of the evidence?
Advantages and Disadvantages	Do the advantages exceed the disadvantages?
	Are alternatives available?
	What if you do not use the relevant therapy?
	Does the evidence affect your current management?
	What are the patient's values and opinions on the benefits and side effects?
Feasibility	Is the inspection or treatment technology carried out in your hospital? Has the technology been well developed?
	How about the compliance?
	How about the patients' financial capability?

14.2.1.1 Are your patients similar with those in the study?

Because patients are not really involved in the experimental study, it is important to first compare the PICO in the evidence with the patient's PICO before making clinical decisions, evidence can be applicable only if the PICO in evidence is similar to the PICO of your patient. Physicians need to compare the characteristics of patients before applying the evidence. The following factors should be taken into account: basic characteristics (e.g., age, sex, severity of the patient's condition, types of disease), criteria of diagnosis, inclusion and exclusion criteria, and so on. If patients in the trial are all in mild condition while your patient is a severe one, then your patient cannot benefit from the evidence even if it has high quality. Many trials exclude the older population, whereas many drugs have higher adverse effects in the aged population. Therefore, even for the same treatment, the risk among older patients may be different from patients in the evidence. The inclusion and exclusion criteria in evidence may be the starting point when analyzing the applicability. Of course, it is impossible that your patient could exactly match those in evidence. Sackett et al. have recommended framing this question in reverse: whether the difference between your patient and study standards would affect patients' results and the applicability of the evidence?

14.2.1.2 What benefits and risks will your patients take?

To make a clinical decision, physicians should evaluate not only benefits but also the risks that patients would take from the evidence. Physicians should use their clinical experience to assess the individual's risk after taking his or her characteristics into account. Some interventions could bring significant curative effects, whereas the side effects are obvious or the adverse effects increase. Your patients may prefer the therapy which is less effective but with less harm. Moreover, many patients have several complications, and the drugs they take may have interactions with each other. While weighing the advantages and disadvantages, the greater the gap is, the easier to make a clinical decision. When the gap is narrow, the decision is difficult to make and some may depend on patients' values, or even on expense.

14.2.1.3　What about the feasibility of the interventions in local areas?

How about the accessibility of the diagnostic test in the local area? Is the intervention feasible in the local area? Is it limited by some other factors (e.g., economy, technology and patients' acceptance)? Especially for trial with invasive treatments, physicians' skill is a critical factor to be concerned. If physicians' skill in the local area can't meet the requirements in the trial, the applicability of evidence should be considered carefully. Moreover, the compliance of patients needs to be taken into consideration. If taking drugs is the intervention, patient's compliance may decrease when he takes some other drugs at the same time or he needs to take drugs several times a day. Besides, the dosage and the route of administration can also affect the compliance. Overall, not all of the evidence with high-quality and great advantage could be successfully applied in clinical practice. For example, evidence with benefit and low risk has great difficult to be applied if the cost is huge.

14.2.2　The role of clinical experience in evidence-based decision-making

Clinical experience has three different levels. The first is the basic ability of the medical practice, such as interrogation, physical examination and the ability to communicate with patients. The second is the ability of making-decision after comprehensive identification of various factors. The third is about the ability of experience accumulation.

The first two are indispensable basic skills for evidence-based practice. The third is the unprocessed evidence which has not been confirmed by rigorous tests. Its quality is lower than scientific evidence. Therefore, clinical decision should be made on the basis of evidence when high quality evidence exists. Whereas, clinicians' experience should give some supplements when no high quality evidence exists. In addition, evidence is always limited while physicians' clinician experience is vast and extensive. On many occasions, clinical experience is the only and the best evidence.

Thus, clinical experience is the foundation of evidence-based practice. The research evidence and clinical experience need to complement each other and are both indispensable. Physicians need to guard against experience-oriented practice while emphasizing the importance of experience. The evidence-based medicine reminds that related scientific researches should be actively carried out when important evidence is lacking.

14.2.3　The role of values of patients and their families and the role of communication between patients and physicians in evidence-based decision-making

Evidence-based decision-making stresses and ensures that the decisions are made on the basis of values and expectations of patients and their families, for different people have different values. Patients' values may be quite different from physicians'. In order to ensure that clinical decisions meet with patients' values and expectations, it is necessary that patients participate in decision-making. This process depends on effective communications between physicians and patients.

In the communication, physicians often encounter very complicated situations. On the one hand, with the development of the society and the improvement of life quality, patients tend to have more desires and take less risk. On the other hand, due to the rapid development of the Internet, resources of medical information are more available for patients. As a result, some patients may get more related information than physicians. Sometimes patients with lower level of education or poor comprehension still can't understand their conditions despite lengthy communication, don't want to make decisions. And they may ask physicians to make decisions for them. Friends and false advertisements may have negative effects on patients, who may firmly refuse certain best evidence or blindly demand a certain technology. Sometimes it is also difficult to make a decision if patients and their family members could not reach an agreement, or when economic burden is heavy for the family.

Apart from the above reasons, it is still a huge challenge for physician to effectively deliver these complex messages to patients, and to correctly guide patients and their families to make the most appropriate decisions after fully understanding their values and expectations. Firstly, after analyzing evidence, physicians should clearly list the strategy of diagnoses and treatments, including alternatives, point out the source of evidence, and the process of evidence analyses. Secondly, physicians should provide effective, practical, and related information to the patients, including costs, benefits and risks, the complications and the consequences of each strategy, helping patients to make choices. Patients must be informed of the fact that there are possible exceptional cases in the development of diseases and each individual may acquire special body constitution. Besides, due to the limitation of medical technologies, patients should have unrealistic expectation of the outcomes of the treatment program. Thirdly, both physicians and patients need to participate in treatment decisions after full communication. Patients' knowledge on the disease differs based on their experiences and education level. Physicians should clearly deliver accurate information as much as possible and guide the patients to make correct selection by analyzing and communications. For patients' requirement which goes against the medical principles, physicians need to refuse it resolutely. It is proved that the more patients understand the evidence and participate in making a decision, the more the decision meets patients' values and wills. Full communication and patients' participation may enhance patients' trust in physicians, improve the compliance and results of treatments, and lay the foundation of building a harmonious environment for medical treatment.

14.2.4 Reevaluating evidence

The final step is to observe the result of evidence in clinical practice, and to guide the next practice. Physicians need to follow up the patients, evaluate the results, spread the evidence if there are good results, analyze reasons if there are bad results, identify the problem and carry out next evidence-based practice.

14.3 The basis for evidence-based decision-making

14.3.1 Highly qualified physicians

Physicians are the main part of the EBM. Excellent physicians are necessary to guarantee the practice of EMB. Firstly, physicians are required to strictly follow medical ethics and have excellent communication skills. Patients, not diseases, are the center in making evidence-based decisions. By understanding the expectations and values of patients, thinking it over in the viewpoint of patients and fully communicating with patients, physicians can finally make the best decision together with patients. Secondly, physicians are required to observe carefully and collect the first-hand information accurately, such as history, physical examination, diagnosis, etc. Incorrect first-hand information from patients can lead to incorrect diagnosis, and make the best decisions no sense. Besides, physicians could not accurately apply the best evidence if they are lack of practical experience. Physicians are required to constantly update their knowledge and skills, and keep learning the latest related medical progresses, instead of searching for evidence when encountering clinical questions, for in this case, the optimal time for treatment may be missed. Moreover, the most important point is that physicians are required to master the basic theories and methodologies of clinical epidemiology. Physicians should have the ability to master finding, evaluating, analyzing and applying evidence for evidence-based decision-making.

14.3.2 Best evidence

The best evidence refers to the latest and the most reliable achievements of clinical researches, which have been assessed by the principles, methodology of clinical epidemiology and the standards of quality assessment. The best evidence mainly comes from rigorously designed RCT, and high-quality meta-analysis and systematic review of these RCT studies. It can be obtained from *Annals of Internal Medicine* published by *ACJC* supplement, *Evidence-Based Medicine*, Cochrane Library, Clinical Evidence, and so on to give guidance to the clinical practice.

14.3.3 Patients' participation in decision-making

As one of the main participants in clinical practice, patients are the center of medical activities. The therapeutic effects of physicians' treatments could be improved by full analyses and communications between patients and physicians. The equal and friendly relationship between patients and physicians and their participation in decision-making are the key points of evidence-based practice.

14.4 Points need to be noticed in evidence-based practice

14.4.1 Value of expert's advice

In the past few years, expert's advice was regarded as a golden rule. It would lead to serious mistake in decision-making when the experts' advice comes from low-quality clinical studies, animal experiments, laboratory researches, or outdated textbooks. However, expert's advice based on the evidence-based medicine is trustworthy. EBM does not preclude the accumulation of scientific experiences. It just reminds physicians to pay attention to the source of experts' advice.

14.4.2 Cochrane systematic review as the evidence of highest-level in EBM

The Cochrane Library is constituted of six databases which contain high-quality evidence of different aspects and provides guidance to the clinical decisions. The editorial board of the Cochrane consists of authoritative statisticians, epidemiologists and methodologists. The researches referenced in systematic review have to meet a certain quality. Authors of Cochrane systematic reviews also use different methods to reduce the bias during the assessment of literature. Besides, Cochrane Reviews update the evidence timely. So, Cochrane systematic review not only provide evidence with high quality to medical researches and physicians, but also deliver medical information to patients.

14.4.3 Making clinical decisions when no best evidence exists

No best evidence does not mean no evidence. Physicians should treat patients based on lower-level evidence or clinical experience (rare diseases), if no high-quality evidence exists. Shortly, the best evidence which is available could be applied during clinical practice. New evidence should be used as soon as high-level evidence is published. Physicians need to take into consideration of the side effects of the treatment, patients' affordability and choice synthetically when a treatment does not have reliable evidence. At the same time, physicians should carry out high-quality clinical researches which could provide best evidence actively.

14.4.4 Contributing factors to clinical decisions beyond evidence

Evidence is one of the factors which affect evidence-based clinical decisions. Some evidence just explores the effects of treatments under ideal medical conditions, whereas the cost maybe too high to afford for patients, or the treatment is too complicated and is hardly to be implemented in local areas. Besides, physicians may make different clinical decisions in consideration of different regions or countries or applied to different patients, economic level, payment method, clinician's experience, patient's ethics and values, the size of the burden caused by the disease in question, and the patient's acceptance of the treatment measures, even for the same high-quality evidence.

14.4.5 Lack of corresponding evidence

It is estimated that a physician encounters about 60 questions per week on average, while each patient has multiple questions. It is unrealistic to answer each clinical issue with proven evidence. RCT is high-level evidence in EBM, whereas the cost of high-quality RCT is too heavy for its large sample size and long follow-up period. Besides, RCT could not be conducted in rare disease. Uncertainty is the characteristic of clinical medicine, which cannot be avoided even with fully developed EBM. Highly qualified physicians should have the ability to achieve an optimal balance between scientificity and uncertainty, which is the art of clinical medicine and is also a reflection of the overall quality of the physicians.

14.5   Evidence-based decision-making clinical examples

14.5.1   Evidence-based decision-making clinical examples 1

Case 14-1

A 67-year-old male patient was admitted to hospital for palpitation and short of breath for one year and dizzy for half a month. One year ago, the patient felt palpitation and short of breath without any obvious precipitating factors. His electrocardiogram in the local hospital showed atrial fibrillation. The coronary angiogram showed a narrow of 30% in the middle of left anterior descending coronary artery. He had taken medicine (without details) prescribed by the local physician. His symptom became more and more severe since then. Half a month ago, he felt dizzy and feeble. The patient had a history of glomerulonephritis for 5 years. He has no other positive medical history.

Physical examination: The patient was in an orthopnea position with his lips cyanosed. The lung breath sounds were not clear. A few moist rales were audible over both lung bases. Border of the heart was enlarged to the lower left side. The heart rate was 92 beats per minutes. The cardiac rhythm was irregular. The force of the first heart sounded also varied. Diastolic gallop rhythm could be heard at the 3-4th ribs of the left sternal border. Both lower extremities showed mild pitting edema.

Auxiliary examination: Electrocardiogram showed atrial fibrillation with rapid heart rate. The level of BNP was 165pg/ml. The echocardiography showed a dilated left ventricle and diffused decrease of ventricular wall motion with 35%EF. Pulmonary vein imaging showed no thrombus in the atrium.

Diagnosis: The patient was diagnosed with tachycardia induced cardiomyopathy, persistent atrial fibrillation combined with cardiac dysfunction (NYHA functional class III), coronary arteries arteriosclerosis and chronic glomerulonephritis.

14.5.1.1   Asking question

The clinical issues are mainly divided into four categories: diagnoses, treatments, etiologies and prognosis. Physicians always translate the clinical issues into searchable questions according to the PICO principle (Table 14-2). P: clinical characteristics of the patients; I: interventions or exposures of interest; C: control measures or the "diagnostic criteria" for diagnostic experiments; O: the outcomes.

Table 14-2   Clinical questions to Case 14-1 according to PICO

Categories	Clinical questions	PICO	Answerable questions
Diagnosis	The diagnostic value of pulmonary vein imaging for thrombus in atrium	P: Patients with persistent atrial fibrillation I: Pulmonary vein imaging C: Transesophageal echocardiography O: Confirm the existence of thrombus in atrium	The sensitivity and specificity of pulmonary vein imaging to diagnosis of thrombus in atrium
Treatment	Could dronedarone be applied for patients with atrial fibrillation combined with heart failure?	P: patients with atrial fibrillation combined with heart failure I: Dronedarone C: Placebo O: Mortality	Would dronedarone decrease the mortality of patients with atrial fibrillation combined heart failure?
Etiology and adverse reactions	Does glomerulonephritis increase the prevalence of cardiomyopathy induced by tachycardia?	P: Patients with tachycardia I: suffering from glomerulonephritis C: no glomerulonephritis O: prevalence of cardiomyopathy induced by tachycardia	Does glomerulonephritis increase the prevalence of cardiomyopathy induced by tachycardia?
Prognosis	Would patients with cardiomyopathy induced by tachycardia be cured after the termination of tachycardia?	P: patients with cardiomyopathy induced by tachycardia I: terminate the tachycardia C: still with tachycardia O: cure rate of cardiomyopathy	How much is the probability for patients with cardiomyopathy induced by tachycardia to be cured after the termination of tachycardia?

14.5.1.2   Acquiring evidence

The convenient way of acquiring the best evidence starts from searching databases with the highest level evidence, then turning to the next level if no relevant evidence exists. The databases physicians always use can be divided into two categories: one is the traditional databases, which contain original literature, such as PubMed, Embase etc. These databases require physicians to retrieve relevant literature, to analyze the evidence, and to draw corresponding conclusions on their own. Timeliness and free of charge are the advantages of these databases, these can access to the latest and most up-to-date clinical research evidence. But physicians are required to have robust knowledge of clinical epidemiology and have the ability of analyzing the evidence. Besides, it is time consuming. The other is the secondary analysis database, such as UpToDate, Best Evidence, EBM guidelines, MD consult, Cochrane library etc. Literature listed in these databases has been screened, appraised and analyzed by experts and could be applied by physicians directly. But these databases are not always free and can't be updated timely.

We used "Does dronedarone decrease the mortality of patients with atrial fibrillation combined with heart failure?" to retrieve relevant literature. The detailed search strategy could be referenced in relevant chapter of this book. In this chapter, we used "atrial fibrillation" and "dronedarone" as the key words to search evidence in Embase database and found 1 systematic review of Tarapués M and 2 meta-analyses published by Xia Y. and Hohnloser S. While 2 randomized control trail (RCT) studies published by Connolly SJ and Køber L were found in UpToDate database, 1 systematic review published by Dagres N and 1 meta-analysis written by Chatterjee S were obtained in Cochrane Library and 323 original literature were retrieved in PubMed.

14.5.1.3 Appraising evidence

EBM requires researchers to use studies with high quality. The quality of evidence has a great influence on their reliability. Entries listed in Table 14-3 could be referenced when physicians appraise the validity of the evidence based on their research purposes.

Table 14-3   Levels of evidence of different researches

Level	Diagnosis	Treatment	Etiology and adverse reactions	Prognosis
I	Systematic review (including meta-analysis)			
II	Cross-sectional study (randomized patients or patients at various stages of the disease)	Randomized controlled trail(RCT)	Prospective cohort study	Initial cohort study
III	Non-randomized cross-sectional study or case-control study	Non-randomized controlled trail or cohort study or case-control study	Retrospective cohort study or case-control study	Retrospective cohort study or case-control study
IV	Case report	Case report	Cross-sectional study	Case report

According to the grading of recommendation, the level of systematic review and meta-analysis can be graded as level I while two RCT studies of Connolly SJ and Køber L as level II. The paper entitled "Increased Mortality after Dronedarone Therapy for Severe Heart Failure" of Køber L was a randomized, double-blinded, placebo-controlled and parallel-group trial. The study was design strictly with proper inclusion and exclusion criteria and definite end points. Besides, the trial was terminated prematurely for safety. Another paper entitled "Dronedarone in High Risk Permanent Atrial Fibrillation" published by Connolly SJ on the journal of *New England Journal of Medicine* was also terminated prematurely for safety. This study was reasonably designed in inclusion criteria, interventions, data analyses and quality control. Besides, it was carried out rigorously. The validity and materiality of the two RCT studies are good enough to provide best evidence for clinical decisions.

As for the question proposed in this case, the result of Køber L's RCT study showed that dronedarone could deteriorate heart failure and increase the risk of early death for patients with severe heart failure and left ventricular systolic dysfunction. At the median follow-up of 2 months, mortality of the intervention group was significantly higher than the placebo group (8.1% vs 3.8%). Another RCT study conducted by Connolly SJ also showed that dronedarone could increase the risk of heart failure, stroke, and death in patients with permanent atrial fibrillation. Their results indicated that dronedarone should not be used in such patients. The meta-analysis published by Chatterjee S indicated that dronedarone could increase all-cause mortality, cardiovascular mortality and deteriorate heart failure. Another meta-analysis of 9 664 patients with atrial fibrillation conducted by Hohnloser S. demonstrated that significant heterogeneity exists in the effects of dronedarone among different subtypes of atrial fibrillation. As for patients with non-permanent AF, they could benefit from dronedarone; while there was an obvious raise in cardiovascular mortality [hazard ratio (HR) = 2.32; 95% confidence interval (CI) 1.13~4.75] and hospitalization for heart failure (HR=1.674; 95%CI 1.05~2.67) for patients with permanent AF.

14.5.1.4 Applying evidence

The inclusion criteria of the RCT conducted by Connolly SJ et al were: patients with permanent atrial fibrillation or flutter; over than 65 years old; have at least one of the following risk factors: coronary artery disease; history of stroke or transient ischemic attack; symptomatic heart failure (class II or III of New York Heart Association); EF≤40%; peripheral arterial disease; hypertension or diabetes with age over than 75 years old. The exclusion criteria were paroxysmal or persistent atrial fibrillation with an implantable cardioverter–defibrillator; heart rate is below 50 beats per minute during daytime; QTc>500ms (>530ms for patients with accelerated ventricular desynchrony). Patients enrolled in Køber L's study were over than 18 years old, hospitalized due to new or worsening heart failure with class III or IV of heart function (New York Heart Association). The clinical characteristics of patients in the evidence were basically consistent with that in the case, so the evidence was applicable for the patient.

After full communication with the patient and his families, the physicians provided anticoagulation and anti-heart failure treatments to the patient. Besides, transfusions of sinus rhythm or control of ventricular rate were applied to alleviate the atrial fibrillation. The strategies for transfusions of sinus rhythm are listed as follows:

Oral intake of amiodarone: The drug's price is cheap and does not lay much financial burden on patients. Besides, it is applied to patients with heart failure combined with atrial fibrillation. Whereas, it has various toxic side effects on different organs such as skin's allergic reaction to light, corneal micro-deposition, thyroid gland dysfunction, pulmonary interstitial fibrosis and hepatic injury.

Radiofrequency ablation: It is a rapid and radical treatment for atrial fibrillation which would alleviate patients' symptoms and improve their life quality significantly. However, only about 70% surgeries succeed and some have risk of hematoma, pneumothorax, myocardial perforation, pericardial tamponade etc. Moreover, the cost is a little expensive.

Control of ventricular rate is always carried out by oral intake of anti-arrhythmia drugs. But heart failure may be aggravated if atrial fibrillation persists.

Patient and his families decided to receive transfusions of sinus rhythm treatments to avoid the aggravation of heart failure after a comprehension of all treatment strategies. They refused to use amiodarone for its severe side effects and consulted if dronedarone which is a new anti-arrhythmia drug was suitable for the patient. After each step of evidence-based decision-making, the physician told them that dronedarone was likely to aggravate heart failure and increase all-cause and cardiovascular mortalities for patients with cardiac dysfunction although it had fewer side effects than amiodarone. So the patient and his families gave up the treatment of dronedarone. After full communication with the patients and his families about the pros and cons of radiofrequency ablation, they signed the consent form and accepted the surgery.

14.5.1.5　Reevaluating evidence

After the surgery of radiofrequency ablation, the patient's fibrillation was terminated and cardiac rhythm was converted to sinus rhythm while his symptom of palpitation and shortness of breath was alleviated a lot. After one year of follow-up, the X-ray showed a shrunk heart and the ejection fraction had escalated to 51% based on echocardiography. No severe adverse effects or major vascular events occurred during his therapy.

14.5.2　Evidence-based decision-making clinical examples 2

Case 14-2

A 35-year-old woman presented with right lower abdominal pain for 15 days, and a cyst was found in the right ovary 10 days before admission. She experienced needle-like pain in the right lower abdomen during night, lasting for 2 hours 15 days ago. Afterwards, she felt bulge pain in the right lower abdomen intermittently. 10 days ago, the ultrasound examination revealed that the right ovary had a cystic echo and the size was about 7.5cm × 8.0cm. She was diagnosed with "polycystic ovary" 3 years ago, and used clomiphene for 3 cycles to stimulate ovulation. 2 years ago, she underwent cesarean section. Menstrual history: menstruation is always irregular. The age at onset of menstruation was 14 years old. The menstrual cycle is about 30~65 days, bleeding for up to 3~5 days, with hypomenorrhea, and without dysmenorrhea. She got married at 28, got pregnant once, and delivered a baby girl through cesarean section.

Physical examination: Vital signs were stable. The heart and lung examinations were normal. Abdominal examination showed normal. Gynecological examination: both vulva and vagina were normal. The cervical columnar epithelium had moderate extracellular migration, and the uterus was normal. On the right of uterus, we could touch a regular, mobile, smooth, painless cystic and solid mass about 8cm×7cm. No masses or tenderness was found on the left side of the adnexa.

Auxiliary examination: Transvaginal ultrasound revealed that on the right side of uterine there was a cystic and solid echo about 8.0cm × 7.5cm, and the cystic area was multilocular, and the sound can pass the cystic part. The solid area showed rich blood flow signals and the blood flow resistance index (RI) was 0.4. The ultrasound diagnosis was: a cystic solid tumor in the right ovary (malignant tumor not excluded). Tumor marker series were in the normal range. Other examination results were normal.

Diagnosis: Ovarian Tumor.

14.5.2.1　Asking question

As for the case, clinical questions can be proposed as follows according to the principle of PICO (Table 14-4).

Table 14-4   Clinical questions to Case 14-2 according to PICO

Categories	Clinical questions	PICO	Answerable questions
Diagnosis	The value of MRI in the identification of benign and malignant ovarian tumor	P: the patients suspected of ovarian tumor I: MRI C: Ultrasonic examination O: pathological diagnosis	The difference of sensitivity and specificity between MRI and ultrasonic examination for benign and malignant ovarian tumor
Treatment	Should patients suffered from benign ovarian tumor with focal cancer be treated with postoperative chemotherapy?	P: patients suffered from benign ovarian tumor with focal cancer I: surgery combined with chemotherapy C: surgery O: mortality	Could postoperative chemotherapy decrease the mortality for patients suffering from benign ovarian tumor with focal cancer?
Etiology and adverse reactions	Would ovulation-promoting drugs increase the risk of ovarian cancer?	P: infertile patients I: use ovulation-promoting drugs C: not use ovulation-promoting drugs O: ovarian cancer	Would ovulation-promoting drugs increase the risk of ovarian cancer?
Prognosis	What is the recurrence rate after unilateral oophorectomy for patients with unilateral benign ovarian tumor and focal cancer	P: Patients with unilateral ovarian benign tumor and focal cancer I: unilateral oophorectomy C: bilateral oophorectomy O: the recurrence of ovarian cancer	Does unilateral oophorectomy increase the recurrence rate of ovarian cancer for patients with unilateral benign ovarian tumor and focal cancer?

14.5.2.2   Acquiring evidence

We used "whether ovulation-promoting drugs would increase the risk of ovarian cancer" to retrieve relevant literature in the example. "Ovarian cancer/ ovarian neoplasm/ ovarian carcinoma" and "ovulation induction/ stimulate/ promote/ clomiphene" in English and corresponding terms in Chinese are set as the keywords while the date was limited to June 2016. The search results are listed below (Table 14-5).

Table 14-5   Search results

Databases	The search results	Relevant Literature
PubMed	114	18
The Cochrane Library	4	1
UpToDate	14	14
Embase	75	48
Springerlink	2 537	8
Wanfang Database	22	2

14.5.2.3 Appraising evidence

Physicians need to find out papers with the highest quality after retrieving the relevant evidence. One systematic review by Ivana Rizzuto entitled "The system to evaluate the risk of ovarian cancer in women treated with ovarian stimulating drugs for infertility (Review)" and two prospective cohort studies by Modan B et al. entitled "Cancer incidence in a cohort of infertile women" and Venn a et al. entitled "Risk of cancer after use of fertility drugs with relative fertilisation" were selected after screening.

The evidence needs to be analyzed after screening. The evaluation criteria for different studies are not completely consistent and the detailed information can be referenced in relevant chapters of this textbook or Table 14-2. Three articles were selected after screening for this case. The systematic review by Ivana Rizzuto summarized 11 cases-control studies and 14 cohort studies. It had a detailed description of the inclusion criteria, intervention programs, literature retrieval and access methods, data processing and quality control. So the evidence could be graded as level one. Venn A's research was a prospective cohort study. It presented the inclusion criteria, follow-up period, indicators of outcomes, data processing and controlled the confounders. Overall, the research methods are reasonable, the statistical methods are accurate, and the evidence is reliable. Modan B's study was also designed as prospective cohort study. It gave a detailed description on the recruitment time, exposure, the source and chosen process of participants. Besides, it listed the statistical indicators and methods. Whereas, it neither stated the exclusion criteria, ways of follow-up and outcome indicators, nor used blind and quality control. So, it is not evidence with high quality.

14.5.2.4 Applying evidence

Two articles with high quality were obtained after appraising the evidence. In the systematic review, Ivana Rizzuto pointed out that no effective evidence could prove that ovulation-promoting drugs increased the risk of ovarian cancer in patients. Venn A found that primary infertility itself might increase the incidence of ovarian cancer, whereas ovulation-promoting drugs showed no effects on it. Still, more analyses needed to figure out whether the evidence are applicable to the specific patient.

We evaluated the differences between the characteristics of the patient and those in the study group. In the systematic review, one of the inclusion criteria was women aged over than 18 years old with at least one ovary. It was similar with the patient. While in Venn A' research, the inclusion criteria required women registered for infertility in Australia, and applied ovulation-promoting therapy for at least one cycle. They excluded no-residents of Australia, or women with unclear age. In this case, it should be more cautious when the evidence was applied to the patient.

According to the available evidence, it cannot yet reach the conclusion that ovulation-promoting drugs could increase the risk of ovarian cancer. It is safe to use the drugs for the infertility patients. However, as infertility itself is a risk factor for ovarian cancer, infertility patients are still recommended to take the physical examinations on time.

14.5.2.5 Reevaluating evidence

We can follow up the infertility patients taking the ovulation-inducing drugs, evaluate its effects on ovarian cancer and analyze the results statistically. Then we can compare the results with the original literature and publish the evidence after summarizing relevant data.

Summary

Although evidence-based medicine has brought about a medical revolution, it is not perfect, let alone omnipotent. It cannot be exaggerated in clinical decision-making, let alone mechanically applied. With the continuous development of medical science, evidence is also developing and changing. When applying evidence, clinicians should analyze and think more and carefully evaluate its quality. Clinicians should not regard current evidence as the supreme dogma and continue to follow the emergence of new evidence.

(Liu Guangzhi)

15

Evidence-based clinical practice guidelines

Learning objectives

1. **To master** the definition of evidence-based practice guidelines; the criteria to assess the quality of the guidelines.
2. **To be familiar with** the process and method for the development of evidence-based guidelines.
3. **To know** how to practice the guidelines.

Clinical practice guideline (CPG) has always been a part of medical practice which helps clinicians achieve better treatment outcomes and care for patients. Clinical practice guidelines can help clinicians translate the best evidence into the best clinical practice. With the development of evidence-based medicine, guidelines that reflect the essence of evidence-based medicine have become an integral part of the clinical practice of modern medicine. To develop and promote evidence-based CPGs is an important measure to standardize medical and health services. Unfortunately, published practice guidelines are not always evidence-based. A good practice guideline must be based on scientific evidence, which can reduce the inconsistency of clinical practice, reduce the variation in the level of care between providers and clinicians and avoid unnecessary diagnostic tests. A good practice guideline can also prevent the use of ineffective or harmful treatment, and help to apply the most cost-effective treatment for patients.

15.1 Basic concepts

In 1990, the Institute of Medicine (IOM) of USA defined CPG as "systematically developed statements to assist practitioner and patient decisions about appropriate health care for specific clinical circumstances". The development and application of CPGs have evolved dramatically in the 20 years since the IOM first became involved in this area. Evidence-based clinical practice guidelines have gradually become the trend of developing the guidelines. Therefore, in 2011, the new definition updated by IOM is as follows: clinical practice guidelines are statements that include recommendations intended to optimize patient care that are informed by a systematic review of evidence and an assessment of the benefits and harms of alternative care options.

Evidence-based practice guidelines are systematically developed and their content is subject to rigorous evaluation to assist healthcare practitioners in making decisions about medical activities in specific clinical settings.To be trustworthy, guidelines should: be based on a systematic review of the existing evidence; be developed by a knowledgeable, multidisciplinary panel of experts and representatives from key affected groups; consider important patient subgroups and patient preferences, as appropriate; be based on an explicit and transparent process that minimizes distortions, biases, and conflicts of interest; provide a clear explanation of the logical relationships between alternative care options and health outcomes, and provide ratings of both the quality of evidence and the strength of the recommendations; be reconsidered and revised as appropriate when important new evidence warrants modifications of recommendations.

15.2   Development of evidence-based practice guidelines

The development of high-quality clinical practice guidelines has been an effective method to standardize medical services, strengthen medical quality management and control medical costs internationally in recent years. Clinical practice guidelines are generally divided into two categories: "expert consensus guidelines" and "evidence-based practice guidelines". The development of expert consensus guidelines is relatively simple, usually by a group of experts to meet and discuss, and the consensus reached after several discussions to form a recommendation as a guideline, most of these guidelines lack evidence base, and the recommendation is vulnerable to the influence of various factors of the participating experts. Thus, the reliability and quality of these guidelines are poor.

As the evidence-based medicine has grown over the past several decades, more and more guidelines are developed after systematically searching and evaluating the relevant evidence. The development of evidence-based practice guidelines including 5 steps: composition of the guideline development group, selection of guideline topics, systematic literature review, assessing the quality of evidence and making recommendations. In addition, it includes a post-launch work plan for systematic evaluation, promotion and dissemination, and revision and updating of the guidelines so that they can keep up with the times. The methodology for developing evidence-based clinical practice guidelines is evidence-based methodology, and its conclusions or recommendations must be supported by reliable evidence, and linking recommendations clearly to the quality of relevant evidence is a distinctive feature of evidence-based clinical guidelines.

The Scottish Intercollegiate Guidelines Network was formed in 1993. The processes of evidence-based guidelines development recommended by SIGN is rather inclusive. The main steps are as follows.

15.2.1   Composition of the guideline development group

There is international agreement that guideline development groups should be multidisciplinary in their composition, with representation from all relevant professional groups, and participation of patients, careers and appropriate voluntary organizations. This facilitates both the guideline development process and the resulting recommendations.

15.2.2 Selection of guideline topics

Producing evidence-based clinical practice guidelines is a time and resource intensive process. To make best use of these resources, guidelines should address a specific healthcare need and there should be an expectation that change is possible and desirable and that, if the guidelines are followed, there is potential to improve the quality of care and/or patient outcomes. There must also be robust evidence of effective practice on which to base guideline recommendations.

15.2.3 Systematic literature review

SIGN guidelines must be based on systematic evaluation of evidence-based medicine The SIGN approach is to produce a systematic review of the evidence for each key question to be addressed in the guideline. Evidence tables are produced as supporting documents and the essential elements of systematic review are met in that the literature is: identified according to an explicit search strategy; selected according to defined inclusion and exclusion criteria; evaluated against consistent methodological standards.

15.2.4 Assessing the quality of evidence

The guideline development group has to assess the overall quality of all included literature.

15.2.4.1 Evaluating the overall quality of evidence

The guideline development group will consider the overall quality of the evidence for all critical outcomes for the key questions:

How reliable are the studies in the body of evidence?

Are the studies consistent in their findings?

Are the studies relevant to our target population?

Are we sure we have all the relevant evidence?

15.2.4.2 Interpreting the evidence

Interpretation of the evidence should be oriented to answer the following questions:

How can we balance benefits and harms?

How sure are we that any given option will work?

How can we minimize costs and maximize benefits?

15.2.5 Making recommendations

After a rigorous evaluation of the evidence to reach consensus, the strength of the recommendation can be marked with reference to the level of evidence and the strength of the recommendation comparison table. When there is sufficient evidence, recommendations are made based on the evidence; when there is no evidence or very weak evidence, recommendations are made based on the consensus (or unanimous) opinion reached in the discussion. Sometimes the recommendation level of high-quality evidence is not necessarily higher, and both the cost and acceptability to the target population need to be considered.

Evidence-based practice guidelines are generally marked recommendation level and the level of evidence, but the standards are different by different countries and academic institutions. In order to establish an international standard system for evaluating evidence and grading recommendations, the GRADE (Grading of Recommendations Assessment, Development and Evaluation) system developed the GRADE quality of evidence and grading of recommendations in 2004. The GRADE grading system breaks away from the limitations of considering evidence quality only from the perspective of study design. It classifies the quality of evidence into high, moderate, low, and very low (see Table 4-2) based on whether future studies change the investigator's confidence in the current efficacy assessment and the likelihood of change, and classifies recommendations into strong and weak. When it is clearly shown that the benefits of the intervention outweigh the harms or the harms outweigh the benefits, it should be rated as a strong recommendation; when the benefits and harms are uncertain or when the evidence of either high or low quality shows comparable benefits and harms, it is considered a weak recommendation. Evidence based on randomized controlled clinical trials was rated as high quality in the GRADE evidence quality grading system. Evidence based on randomized controlled trials begins as high-quality evidence, but our confidence in the evidence may be decreased for several reasons, including study limitations, inconsistency of results, indirectness of evidence, imprecision, reporting bias. GRADE system covers a wide range of clinical recommendations in all medical specialties and clinical areas of care, and is simple and easy to follow. the Cochrane Collaboration, the World Health Organization (WHO), and many other international organizations have made extensive use of the rating system.

Before the GRADE system, "Oxford Centre for Evidence-based Medicine - Levels of Evidence (2001)" was widely used. The level of evidence was classified into five levels based on the study design and the strength of the argument for causality. Recommendations were then classified into four levels of A (excellent), B (good), C (satisfactory), and D (poor) based on the quality, consistency, clinical significance, generalizability, and applicability of the evidence. Only the level of evidence and grades of recommendation for therapeutic studies were listed in Table 15-1.

Table 15-1   Oxford Centre for Evidence-based Medicine - Levels of Evidence (2001)

Grades of Recommendation	Evidence Level	Source of Evidence (Evidence from therapeutic studies)
A	1a	SR (with homogeneity) of RCTs
	1b	Individual RCT (with narrow Confidence Interval)
	1c	All or none
B	2a	SR (with homogeneity) of cohort studies
	2b	Individual cohort study (including low quality RCT, e.g., <80% follow-up)
	2c	"Outcomes" Research (refers to a category of studies that describe, explain, and predict the role and impact of interventions on clinical end outcomes, which are different from intermediate indicators and include primarily survival, quality of life, and burden of disease)
	3a	SR (with homogeneity) of case-control studies
	3b	Individual case-control Study
C	4	Case-series (and poor quality cohort and case-control studies)
D	5	Expert opinion without explicit critical appraisal

15.2.6 Consultation and peer review

All SIGN guidelines are reviewed in draft form by independent referees who are selected for their expertise and to reflect the multidisciplinary nature of the guideline. The guideline team further revised the draft based on the recommendations. The draft is also sent to at least two lay reviewers in order to obtain comments from the patient's perspective. Reviewers are asked to comment primarily on the comprehensiveness and accuracy of interpretation of the evidence base supporting the recommendations in the guideline.

15.2.7 Presentation and publication

Clarity of definitions, language, and format is likely to be important. Guidelines should, therefore, be written in unambiguous language and should define all terms precisely. The most appropriate format for presenting guidelines will vary depending on the target group(s), the subject matter, and the intended use of the guideline.

15.2.8 Implementation

It is important to ensure the implementation of evidence-based guideline recommendations. There are two types of barriers to the implementation of guidelines: those internal to the guideline itself, and the external barriers relating to the clinical environment and particular local circumstances. SIGN addresses the internal barriers by: developing guidelines according to a highly respected methodology; ensuring clarity of definitions, language, and format; presenting the guideline in a way appropriate to target group(s), subject matter, and the intended use. SIGN addresses the external barriers by developing guideline specific implementation strategies consisting of elements from the following four domains: improving processes, awareness raising and education, networking and implementation support resources.

15.2.9 Involving patients and their representatives

Patients may have different perspectives on healthcare processes, priorities, and outcomes from those of health professionals. The involvement of patients in guideline development is therefore important to ensure that guidelines reflect their needs and concerns. The purpose of patient involvement is to ensure that the guideline addresses issues that matter to them and that their perspectives are reflected in the guideline.

15.3 Appraisal of guidelines

High quality clinical practice guidelines can help physicians and/or other healthcare practitioners and patients to make decisions about appropriate health care for specific clinical circumstances, while low quality clinical practice guidelines will mislead the clinicians. Before using the clinical practice guidelines, we should assess the quality of clinical practice guidelines: how well a guideline is developed and reported.

15.3.1 Principles for evaluating clinical practice guidelines

The evaluation of clinical practice guidelines is mainly divided into three aspects: validity, importance and applicability.

15.3.1.1 Evaluation of validity

Guidelines of high quality must follow the principles and methods of evidence-based medicine, that is, clinical practice guidelines should be based on evidence and that recommendations should be graded according to the credibility of the evidence.

Key points of evaluation include:

Did the guideline composers do a comprehensive and reproducible literature search? Was the search conducted within one year?

Was the grade of evidence associated with each recommendation indicated and links to the original evidence or literature provided?

The evaluation focused on the collection, evaluation, and synthesis of the evidence and how closely the recommendations were integrated with the relevant evidence.

15.3.1.2 Evaluation of importance

After evaluating the validity of the guidelines, it is also important to clarify whether the guidelines answer the important questions that clinicians need to address. However, it should be noted that the problems faced by clinicians are quite complex and guidelines cannot encompass all clinical problems.

15.3.1.3 Evaluation of applicability

Evaluation of applicability should consider whether the burden of disease is low in the region and therefore there is no need to refer to guidelines. Are patients' opinions of the pros and cons of treatment consistent with the guidelines? What is the cost of implementing the guideline, that is, is there a greater benefit of using the same resources for other measures? Are there insurmountable difficulties for the patient in implementing the guideline? Thus, the successful implementation of a guideline relies on four factors, namely burden, belief, bargain and barrier, which need to be considered together when applying the guideline according to the principle of individualization.

15.3.2 Evaluation tools for clinical practice guidelines

For scientific and objective evaluation of evidence-based practice guidelines, different countries and academic groups have developed a number of specialized clinical practice guidelines evaluation tools. So far, there are more than 20 evaluation tools. At present, three evaluation tools are widely used, which are the Cluzeau scale (37 items), the United States COGS evaluation criteria (18 items) and the European AGREE evaluation criteria (23 items). We will mainly introduce the European AGREE (appraisal of guidelines research and evaluation, AGREE) evaluation criteria.

AGREE consists of 23 key items organized in 6 domains (Table 15-2). Each domain captures a unique dimension of guideline quality.

Table 15-2 Appraisal of Guidelines Research and Evaluation (AGREE Ⅱ)

Ⅰ **Scope and purpose**

    1. The overall objective(s) of the guideline is (are) specifically described

    2. The clinical question(s) covered by the guideline is (are) specifically described

    3. The patients to whom the guideline is meant to apply are specifically described, and their characteristics (age, sex, clinical type, etc.) are described

Ⅱ **Stakeholder involvement**

    4. The guideline development group includes individuals from all the relevant professional groups

    5. The patients' views and preferences have been sought

    6. The target users of the guideline are clearly defined

    7. The guideline has been piloted among target users

Ⅲ **Rigor of development**

    8. Systematic methods were used to search for evidence. A detailed strategy for retrieving evidence should be provided, including the search terms used, the sources of information, and the time period covered by the literature

    9. The criteria for selecting the evidence are clearly described

    10. The methods used for formulating the recommendations are clearly described

    11. The health benefits, side effects, and risks have been considered in formulating the recommendations

    12. There is an explicit link between recommendations and the supporting evidence

    13. The guideline has been externally reviewed by experts prior to its publication

    14. A procedure for updating the guideline is provided

Ⅳ **Clarity and presentation**

    15. The recommendations are specific and unambiguous

    16. The different options for management of the condition are clearly presented

    17. Key recommendations are easily identifiable

    18. The guideline is supported with tools for application (e.g. outlines, educational tools, leaflets for patients, etc.)

Ⅴ **Applicability**

    19. The potential organizational barriers in applying the recommendations have been discussed

    20. The potential cost implications of applying the recommendations have been considered

    21. The guideline presents key review criteria for monitoring and audit purposes

Ⅵ **Editorial independence**

    22. The guideline is editorially independent from the funding body

    23. Conflicts of interest of guideline development members have been recorded

Each of the AGREE Ⅱ items is rated on a 7-point scale (1– strongly disagree to 7–strongly agree). A score between 2 and 6 is assigned when the reporting of the AGREE Ⅱ item does not meet the full criteria or considerations. A score is assigned depending on the completeness and quality of reporting. Since evaluation is inevitably somewhat subjective, each guideline should be evaluated by two to four participants. The scores of all participants are then combined according to the formula to obtain a standardized total score for the domain. Standardized total score = (actual total score − lowest possible score) / (highest possible score − lowest possible score) (Table 15-3)

Table 15-3 An example for calculating domain scores

Appraisers	Item 1	Item 2	Item 3	Total
Appraiser 1	5	6	6	17
Appraiser 2	6	6	7	19
Appraiser 3	2	4	3	9
Appraiser 4	3	3	2	8
Total	16	19	18	53

Maximum possible score = 7 (strongly agree) × 3(items) × 4 (appraisers) = 84.

Minimum possible score = 1 (strongly disagree) × 3 (items) ×4 (appraisers) =12.

The scaled domain score = (obtained score−minimum possible score)÷(maximum possible score−minimum possible score) = (53−12)÷(84−12)= 0.57×100% =57%.

The six domain scores are independent and should not be aggregated into a single quality score. Although the domain scores are useful for comparing guidelines and will inform whether a guideline should be recommended for use, the Consortium has not set minimum domain scores or patterns of scores across domains to differentiate between high quality and poor-quality guidelines. These decisions should be made by the user and guided by the context in which AGREE II is being used.

15.4 Clinical application of evidence-based practice guidelines

Clinical practice guideline is the technical guidance to help clinicians to deal with the clinical problems. It is not a legal document. It is recommended, but not mandatory. It is noteworthy that clinicians can decide whether to use or change the recommendations according to the specific circumstances. Mandatory, blind dogmatic application of clinical practice guidelines without regard to patient specificity should be avoided. Inevitably, there is a gap between evidence-based practice guidelines and specific clinical practice. Clinicians should consider the following issues in the process of applying evidence-based practice guidelines.

15.4.1 Are the recommendations valid?

15.4.1.1 Are all important options and outcomes considered? These must be considered from the perspective of the patient as well as the physician. All reasonable physician options should be considered including comments on those options not evidence-based but in common practice.

15.4.1.2 Is a reasonable, explicit, and sensible process used to identify, select, and combine evidence? Explicit rationale for choice of studies should be done. Evidence should be presented and graded by quality indicators.

15.4.1.3 Is a reasonable, explicit, and sensible process used to consider the relative value of different outcomes? The different outcomes should be described explicitly and the reasons why each outcome was chosen should be given.

15.4.1.4 Is the guideline likely to account for recent important developments? The bibliography should include the most recent evidence regarding the topic.

15.4.1.5 Has a peer-review and testing process been applied to the guideline? Ideally, it should be tested in various settings to determine if physicians are willing to use it and to ensure that it accomplishes its stated goals.

15.4.2 What are the recommendations?

15.4.2.1 Are practical and clinically important recommendations made? The guidelines should be simple enough and make enough sense for most clinicians to use them.

15.4.2.2 How strong are the recommendations? The evidence for the guideline should be explicitly listed and graded using a commonly used grading scheme. The results of the studies should be compelling with large effect sizes to back up the use of the evidence.

15.4.2.3 How much uncertainty is associated with the evidence and values used in creating the guideline? It should be clear from the presentation of the evidence how uncertainty in the evidence has been handled. Some sort of sensitivity analysis should be included.

15.4.3 Will the recommendations help me in caring for my patients?

15.4.3.1 Is the primary objective of the guideline important clinically? The guidelines ought to meet your needs for improving the care of the patient you are seeing. They should be consistent with your patient's health objectives.

15.4.3.2 How are the recommendations applicable to your patients? The patient must meet the criteria for inclusion into the guideline.

Summary

In the clinical application of evidence-based practice, we should promote the medical decision not only based on scientific evidence, but also based on the clinical experience and patient benefits. Clinical medicine is not only scientific but also artistic. We should pay attention to the evidence-based practice, and should not neglect the importance of personal clinical skills, such as good communication with patients and other clinical skills. Scientific and flexible use of evidence-based practice guidelines will enable patients to get the best results.

(Li Yafei)

16

Systematic review and meta-analysis

Learning objectives

1. **To master** the basic steps of meta-analysis conduction, principles of literature evaluation and interpretation of results.
2. **To be familiar with** special types of meta-analysis.
3. **To know** the basic concepts of systematic review and meta-analysis.

16.1   The concept of systematic review

The core concept of evidence-based medicine is that clinical practice should be based on evidence. Therefore, the formation and quality of "evidence" is the key point to practice evidence-based medicine. All completed and ongoing medical research can become evidence. Systematic review, as well as meta-analysis, is one of the most important methods to produce high quality evidence in evidence-based medicine. Systematic reviews based on large randomized controlled trials, which evaluate the efficacy and safety of a therapy, are always considered as the best evidence, and widely cited in clinical guidelines.

Systematic review refers to a research method that extensively collects studies on a certain health question in accordance with strict inclusion criteria, conducts comprehensive quality assessment and analysis on the included studies, and conducts quantitative and statistical processing when necessary to draw comprehensive conclusions. This method aims to collate and summarize multiple research results, provide reliable evidence for clinical decision making. The systematic review is not limited to efficacy assessment, but has been expanded to etiology, diagnosis, prognosis and animal experiments etc.

Cochrane collaboration is a British international organisation formed to organise medical research findings to facilitate evidence-based choices about health interventions. Cochrane systematic review is a systematic review published in the Cochrane Library under the guidance of the uniform Cochrane handbook and with the help of the corresponding professional review groups. With strict quality control throughout the implementation process and professional software as an auxiliary, Cochrane systematic review is recognized as the most mature and highest quality method at present.

16.2 Basic steps of systematic review

Systematic review is a research method that draws comprehensive conclusions by collecting, evaluating and synthesizing the results of original clinical studies. Systematic review is not only a scientific research method, but also a system in itself, there are many research steps involved. This section outlines the general steps of systematic review based on the Cochrane systematic review handbook.

16.2.1 Defining the review questions

It is the first step in systematic review to develop a good review question. This step takes time, expertise and engagement with intended users of the review. The detailed specification of the review question(s) requires consideration of several key components which are often called as "PICO", an acronym for population, intervention, comparison(s) and outcome.

16.2.2 Defining the criteria for including studies

Eligibility criteria are based on the PICO elements of the review question plus a specification of the types of studies that have addressed these questions. The type of study design, year of publication and the published language are often set as eligibility criteria besides the PICO elements.

16.2.3 Searching for studies

The main process is developing a search strategy on the basis of PICO, which includes clarifying the retrieval database, determining the retrieval words, formulating the retrieval strategy, and implementing the retrieval and literature management. It is important to conduct a comprehensive search of all relevant clinical studies. The Cochrane Central Register of Controlled Trials (CENTRAL) and MEDLINE, together with Embase (if access to Embase is available to the review team) should be searched for all Cochrane reviews. We should also try to search thematic database, citation database, dissertation database and other grey literature sources. Trials registers should be searched for all Cochrane reviews and other sources such as regulatory agencies and clinical study reports (CSRs) are an increasingly important source of information for study results. We strongly suggest that reviewers should work closely with an experienced medical librarian or information specialist.

16.2.4 Selecting studies

A typical process for selecting studies recommended by Cochrane is as follows: merge search results from different sources and remove duplicate records of the same report; examine titles and abstracts to remove obviously irrelevant reports; retrieve the full text of the potentially relevant reports; link together multiple reports of the same study; examine full-text reports for compliance of studies with eligibility criteria; correspond with investigators, where appropriate, to clarify study eligibility (it may be appropriate to request further information, such as missing methods information or results, at the same time); make final decisions on study inclusion and proceed to data collection; tag or record any ongoing trials which have not yet been reported so that they can be added to the ongoing studies table. In the process of study selection, the reasons for exclusion should be recorded in detail and the flow chart of selecting studies could be drawn meanwhile.

16.2.5   Data extraction

Data collected for systematic reviews should be accurate, complete, and accessible for future updates of the review and for data sharing. Note to minimize biases and human error. Studies are reported in a range of sources, and it is important to link together multiple reports of the same study. It is better to extract data independently by two researchers and double check to ensure the accuracy. And, results extracted from different study reports need to be converted to a consistent, or usable, format for analysis.

16.2.6   Quality assessment of the included studies

It is necessary to evaluate the quality of individual studies to prevent or reduce bias or systematic error during design, implementation and analysis. Numerous tools have been developed for randomized controlled trials, including Jadad scale, Cochrane risk-of-bias tool and risk-of-bias tool version 2 (RoB 2). Due to the variety of non-randomized studies, there is no universal tool. Newcastle-Ottawa Scale (NOS) is one of the most commonly used tools, which is simple and easy to use. There are corresponding items for cohort study and case control study respectively.

16.2.7   Analyzing Data

Conduct meta-analysis when necessary. Meta-analysis is the statistical combination of results from two or more separate studies. We need to identify and measure the heterogeneity of multiple individual studies. If heterogeneity is identified, several solutions are available, which will be described in the following part. Forest plots are often used to present the results of meta-analysis. Funnel plots and related tests may help review authors to identify evidence of non-reporting biases.

16.2.8   Summarizing results and drawing conclusions

Reporting results of systematic review should follow the PRISMA 2020 statement.

16.3   Tools for study quality assessment

Quality assessment of the included studies is one of the core steps of systematic review. Quality assessment of the original individual studies is very important to objectively judge the authenticity and reliability of the results of a systematic review. Since the conclusions drawn in a review depend on the results of the included studies, if these results are biased, then a meta-analysis of the studies will produce a misleading conclusion.

There are many methods to assess the quality of included studies and risk of bias, such as checklist, scales, or domain-based tools. Quality evaluation tools and methods also differ significantly for different types of study designs.

The Jadad scale and Cochrane risk-of-bias assessment tool are widely used in assessing the quality of randomized controlled trials. The former emphasizes the quality of the research report, which is simple and easy to operate, but some items are not clearly defined. The latter emphasizes the quality of study design, methodology and implementation. The items are clearly defined and standardized. Therefore, the Cochrane risk-of-bias assessment tool is recommended here.

The Jadad scale was developed and published by Alejandro R. Jadad and his colleagues in 1996. The initial version included 3 items (randomization, blinding and withdrawals), scored $0 \sim 5$ points. Subsequently, a modified Jadad scale with 8 items was developed. The modified Jadad scale is listed below (Table 16-1).

Table 16-1　Modified Jadad Scale

Items	Response	Score
Was the study described as randomized?	Yes	+1
	No	0
Was the method of randomization appropriate?	Yes	+1
	No	0
	No described	−1
Was the study described as blinded?	Yes	+1
	No	0
Was the method of blinding appropriate?	Yes	+1
	No	0
	No described	−1
Was there a description of withdrawals and dropouts?	Yes	+1
	No	0
Was there a clear description of the inclusion/exclusion criteria?	Yes	+1
	No	0
Was the method used to assess adverse effects described?	Yes	+1
	No	0
Was the method of statistical analysis described?	Yes	+1
	No	0

In 2008, Cochrane released the Cochrane risk-of-bias (RoB) assessment tool, which was slightly revised in 2011, an updated version (RoB 2) was released. This tool was developed by a working group of many methodologists, editors, and reviewers. The tool focused on assessing the risk of bias. It was based on a domain-based approach, in which different types of bias were considered in turn. The tool covered six domains: Selection bias, implementation bias, information bias, follow-up bias, reporting bias, and other bias. Note that there was no scoring system in the tool. The assessment of risk of bias required judgement and should thus be completely transparent. Reviewers provided a judgement for each domain, rated as "low", "high" or "unclear" risk of bias, and provided reasons to support their judgement.

This tool has been implemented widely since being released. And a new version of the Cochrane risk-of-bias assessment tool, RoB 2, was developed in 2019. Several changes are noticed in the updated version. Signaling questions and algorithms are introduced; assessment of bias is at the level of an individual result; the names given to the bias domains describe more clearly; an explicit process for making a judgement about the overall risk of bias in the result is introduced. Detailed items of the Cochrane risk-of-bias assessment tool is listed in Table 16-2. More information on the Cochrane risk-of-bias assessment tool 2 is available via the risk of bias tool website.

Table 16-2　Version 2 of the Cochrane risk-of-bias assessment tool for randomized trials

Bias domain and signaling question*	Response options		
	Lower risk of bias	Higher risk of bias	Other
Bias arising from the randomization process			
1.1　Was the allocation sequence random?	Y/PY	N/PN	NI
1.2　Was the allocation sequence concealed until participants were enrolled and assigned to interventions?	Y/PY	N/PN	NI
1.3　Did baseline differences between intervention groups suggest a problem with the randomization process?	N/PN	Y/PY	NI
Risk-of-bias judgment (low/high/some concerns)			
Optional: What was the predicted direction of bias arising from the randomization process?			
Bias due to deviations from intended interventions			
2.1　Were participants aware of their assigned intervention during the trial?	N/PN	Y/PY	NI
2.2　Were clinicians delivering the interventions aware of participants' assigned intervention during the trial?	N/PN	Y/PY	NI
2.3　If Y/PY/NI to 2.1 or 2.2: Were there deviations from the intended intervention that arose because of the trial context?	N/PN	Y/PY	NA/NI
2.4　If Y/PY/NI to 2.3: Were these deviations likely to have affected the outcome?	N/PN	Y/PY	NA/NI
2.5　If Y/PY to 2.4: Were these deviations from intended intervention balanced between groups?	Y/PY	N/PN	NA/NI
2.6　Was an appropriate analysis used to estimate the effect of assignment to intervention?	Y/PY	N/PN	NI
2.7　If N/PN/NI to 2.6: Was there potential for a substantial impact (on the result) of the failure to analyze participants in the group to which they were randomized?	N/PN	Y/PY	NA/NI
Risk-of-bias judgment (low/high/some concerns)			
Optional: What was the predicted direction of bias due to deviations from intended interventions?			

continue

Bias domain and signaling question*	Response options		
	Lower risk of bias	Higher risk of bias	Other
Bias due to missing outcome data			
3.1 Were data for this outcome available for all, or nearly all, participants randomized?	Y/PY	N/PN	NI
3.2 If N/PN/NI to 3.1: Was there evidence that the result was not biased by missing outcome data?	Y/PY	N/PN	NA
3.3 If N/PN to 3.2: Could missingness in the outcome depend on its true value?	N/PN	Y/PY	NA/NI
3.4 If Y/PY/NI to 3.3: Was it likely that missingness in the outcome depended on its true value?	N/PN	Y/PY	NA/NI
Risk-of-bias judgment (low/high/some concerns)			
Optional: What was the predicted direction of bias due to missing outcome data?			
Bias in measurement of the outcome			
4.1 Was the method of measuring the outcome inappropriate?	N/PN	Y/PY	NI
4.2 Could measurement or ascertainment of the outcome have differed between intervention groups?	N/PN	Y/PY	NI
4.3 If N/PN/NI to 4.1 and 4.2: Were outcome assessors aware of the intervention received by study participants?	N/PN	Y/PY	NI
4.4 If Y/PY/NI to 4.3: Could assessment of the outcome have been influenced by knowledge of intervention received?	N/PN	Y/PY	NA/NI
4.5 If Y/PY/NI to 4.4: Was it likely that assessment of the outcome was influenced by knowledge of intervention received?	N/PN	Y/PY	NA/NI
Risk-of-bias judgment (low/high/some concerns)			
Optional: What was the predicted direction of bias in measurement of the outcome?			
Bias in selection of the reported result			
5.1 Were the data that produced this result analyzed in accordance with a prespecified analysis plan that was finalized before unblinded outcome data were available for analysis?	Y/PY	N/PN	NI
Was the numerical result being assessed likely to have been selected, on the basis of the following results, from:			
5.2 Were multiple eligible outcome measurements (e.g., scales, definitions, time points) within the outcome domain?	N/PN	Y/PY	NI
5.3 Were multiple eligible analyses of the data?	N/PN	Y/PY	NI
Risk-of-bias judgment (low/high/some concerns)			
Optional: What was the predicted direction bias due to selection of the reported results?			
Overall bias			
Risk-of-bias judgment (low/high/some concerns)			
Optional: What was the overall predicted direction of bias for this outcome?			

Y=yes; PY=probably yes; PN=probably no; N=no; NA=not applicable; NI=no information.

* Signaling questions for bias due to deviations from intended interventions relate to the effect of assignment to intervention.

Non-randomized controlled studies are more susceptible to the risk of bias than randomized controlled studies. Non-randomized studies, including non-randomized controlled trials, case-control and cohort studies, can be challenging to implement and conduct. There is no universal assessment tool for these studies at present. The Newcastle-Ottawa Scale (NOS) is one of the most commonly used tools. The scale developed a 'star system', in which a study is judged on three broad perspectives: the selection of the study groups; the comparability of the groups; and the ascertainment of either the exposure or outcome of interest for case-control or cohort studies respectively, total 8 entries. A maximum of 13 stars can be given for cohort study and 9 stars for case-control study (Table 16-3, Table 16-4).

Table 16-3   Newcastle-Ottawa quality assessment scale for cohort studies

Domains	Items	Evaluation criterion
Selection	Representativeness of the exposed cohort	a) truly representative of the average (describe) in the community * b) somewhat representative of the average in the community * c) selected group of users e.g., nurses, volunteers d) no description of the derivation of the cohort
	Selection of the non-exposed cohort	a) drawn from the same community as the exposed cohort * b) drawn from a different source c) no description of the derivation of the non-exposed cohort
	Ascertainment of exposure	a) secure record (e.g. surgical records) * b) structured interview * c) written self-report d) no description
	Demonstration that outcome of interest was not present at start of study	a) yes * b) no
Comparability	Comparability of cohorts on the basis of the design or analysis	a) study controls for the most important factor * b) study controls for any additional factor * (These criteria could be modified to indicate specific control for a second important factor.)
Outcome	Assessment of outcome	a) independent blind assessment * b) record linkage * c) self-report d) no description
	Was follow-up long enough for outcomes to occur	a) yes (select an adequate follow up period for outcome of interest) * b) no
	Adequacy of follow up of cohorts	a) complete follow up - all subjects accounted for * b) subjects lost to follow up unlikely to introduce bias - (prescribed lost to follow up rate, or description provided of those lost) * c) prescribed lost to follow up rate and no description of those lost d) no description

Note: A study can be awarded a maximum of one star for each numbered item within the selection and exposure categories. A maximum of two stars can be given for comparability.

Table 16-4   Newcastle-Ottawa quality assessment scale for case-control studies

Domains	Items	Evaluation criterion
Selection	Is the case definition adequate?	a) yes, with independent validation * b) yes, e.g. record linkage or based on self-reports c) no description
	Representativeness of the cases	a) consecutive or obviously representative series of cases * b) potential for selection biases or not stated
	Selection of Controls	a) community controls * b) hospital controls c) no description
	Definition of Controls	a) no history of disease (endpoint) * b) no description of source
Comparability	Comparability of cases and controls on the basis of the design or analysis	a) study controls for the most important factor* b) study controls for any additional factor * (This criterion could be modified to indicate specific control for a second important factor.)
Exposure	Ascertainment of exposure	a) secure record (e.g. surgical records) * b) structured interview where blind to case/control status* c) interview not blinded to case/control status d) written self-report or medical record only e) no description
	Same method of ascertainment for cases and controls	a) yes * b) no
	Non-Response rate	a) same rate for both groups * b) non respondents described c) rate different and no description

Note: A study can be awarded a maximum of one star for each numbered item within the selection and outcome categories. A maximum of two stars can be given for comparability.

16.4   Meta-analysis

In 1976, Gene Glass first proposed the method of integrating statistics from several similar studies, which he called a meta-analysis. A meta-analysis is a statistical analysis of a series of individual studies. Subsequently, the method was widely used in the field of health care. In the late 1980s, meta-analysis was introduced into China.

In the *Cochrane Handbook*, the meta-analysis was defined as the statistical combination of results from two or more separate studies. Meta-analysis is an important statistical technology and tool to provide clinical evidences for evidence-based medicine. Potential advantages of meta-analyses include an improvement in precision, the ability to answer questions not posed by individual studies, and the opportunity to settle controversies arising from conflicting claims. However, they also have the potential to mislead seriously, particularly if specific study designs, within-study biases, variation across studies are not carefully considered.

Therefore, we recommend meta-analysis only when the data included in the systematic evaluation are suitable for meta-analysis, which can greatly improve the reliability and accuracy of the analysis results. However, when the data are not suitable for meta-analysis, it is recommended to summarize and describe all studies and be cautious about the analysis conclusions.

16.4.1 Heterogeneity test

The variation between studies in systematic review is called heterogeneity. The core of meta-analysis is to combine results of multiple studies. According to the statistical principle, only homogeneous data can be combined, and vice versa. If the confidence intervals of individual study results overlap poorly, this usually indicates statistical heterogeneity. More formally, a statistical test of heterogeneity indicates whether observed differences are caused by chance. Generally, P values < 0.1 indicates heterogeneity. The heterogeneity can also be evaluated by I^2, which is calculated by the following formula:

$$I^2 = \left(\frac{Q - df}{Q} \right) \times 100\%$$

Where, Q is the Chi-square statistic of heterogeneity test, and df is the degree of freedom. The formula describes the percentage of variation (heterogeneity) in the intervention estimates rather than sampling error (chance). It is generally considered that heterogeneity is acceptable when $I^2 < 50\%$. Substantial heterogeneity may exist when $I^2 \geqslant 50\%$.

If the P-value of heterogeneity test is more than 0.10, the fixed effect model can be used. When the heterogeneity test P-value < 0.10 or $I^2 > 50\%$, we should first explore the causes of heterogeneity by conducting subgroup analysis or meta-regression. It is an option to fit a random effects model to summary estimates of studies. The random effects model and the fixed-effects model will give identical results when there is no heterogeneity among the studies. When heterogeneity is present, a confidence interval around the random effects summary estimate is wider than a confidence interval around a fixed effects summary estimate. It should be noted that the random effects model is a statistical method for unexplained heterogeneity, but it cannot replace analyzing the causes of heterogeneity.

16.4.2 Meta-analysis of outcomes

The core component of meta-analysis is to combine the results of multiple similar studies into some single effect size. For different types of indicators, results are combined in different ways, so meta-analysis begins by determining the combined statistic and calculating the results for each study. The summary statistics commonly used for meta-analysis of dichotomous data are odds ratio (OR), risk ratio (RR) or risk difference (RD). Summary statistics commonly used for meta-analysis of continuous data are the mean difference (MD) and the standardized mean difference (SMD).

There are four widely used methods of meta-analysis for dichotomous outcomes, three fixed-effects methods (Mantel-Haenszel, Peto and inverse variance) and one random-effects method (DerSimonian and Laird inverse variance). The Peto method can only combine odds ratios, whilst the other three methods can combine odds ratios, risk ratios or risk differences. For continuous data, fixed-effects model with inverse variance is widely used.

The inverse variance method is so named because the weight given to each study is chosen to be the inverse of the variance of the effect estimate (e.g., 1 over the square of its standard error). Thus, larger studies, which have smaller standard errors, are given more weight than smaller studies, which have larger standard errors. When data are sparse, either in terms of event risks being low or study size being small, the estimates of the standard errors of the effect estimates that are used in the inverse-variance methods may be poor. The Mantel-Haenszel methods are fixed-effects meta-analysis methods using a different weighting scheme that depends on which effect measure (e.g., risk ratios, odds ratios, risk differences) is being used. The Mantel-Haenszel methods show better statistical properties when there are few events. The simplest and most commonly used method of random-effects model is the DerSimonian and Laird inverse variance method. More detailed statistical formulas are not shown here. Readers can refer to relevant literature for further study.

16.4.3　Forest plot

Forest plot is commonly used in meta-analysis to display the results. An example appears in Figure 16-1. A forest plot displays effect estimates and confidence intervals for both individual studies and meta-analyses. The vertical line in the middle with a value of 0 or 1 is invalid line. When the effect size is the mean difference between groups, the invalid vertical line values 0; when the effect size is the risk ratios, odds ratios, risk differences, it values 1. Each study is represented by a block at the point estimate of intervention effect with a horizontal line extending either side of the block. The area of the block indicates the weight assigned to that study in the meta-analysis while the horizontal line depicts the confidence interval (usually with a 95% level of confidence). When the horizontal line touches or crosses the midline, it indicates that the difference in the outcome effect between the test group and the control group is not statistically significant. Conversely, if the horizontal line falls completely to the left or right of the invalid line and does not intersect the invalid line, it indicates that the difference is statistically significant. The location of the center of the bottom diamond indicates the estimate of the combined effect value, and the width of this diamond indicates the confidence interval range of the combined effect.

16.4.4　Funnel plot

The funnel plot is a common method to assess the potential impact of publication bias. The funnel plot is a graphical representation of the size of trials (or the standard error of the effect size or the inverse of the standard error) plotted against the effect size they report. It assumes small studies are more likely to be susceptible to publication bias than large ones. If researchers complete a large randomized trial, they are likely to want to see it published even if the result is negative because of the effort involved. For small trials, however, the situation may be different. If publication bias does exist, it is most likely to be due to small negative trials not being published. As the size of the trial increases, trials are likely to converge around the true underlying effect size.

Because there are usually more small than large samples, the points that represent each mean value are widely spread at the base and narrow as they move to the top, thus resembling an inverted funnel. When publication bias has occurred, one expects an asymmetry in the scatter of small studies, with more studies showing a positive result than those showing a negative result. So there will be an asymmetric funnel plot, and the more pronounced the asymmetry, the greater the degree of bias.

The funnel plot is a qualitative method, mainly through the observation of the scatter plot to make a judgment of subjectivity. At present, there are several quantitative methods to evaluate publication bias. Egger's test and Begg's test are commonly used quantitative methods. The Egger's test is a regression analysis of the precision (inverse of the standard error) of the effect estimates using standardized effect sizes, and the intercept size to indicate the degree of asymmetry of the funnel plot; if there is publication bias, the intercept of the regression line will deviate from the starting point. Begg's test examines the relationship between the standardized treatment effect and the variance of the treatment effect using rank correlation test. Egger's test has a slightly higher power than Begg's test. However, when the number of included studies is small (less than 10), both methods are lack of power.

16.4.5 Subgroup analysis

Subgroup analysis refers to splitting all the participant data into subgroups based on certain factors, often in order to make comparisons between them. For example, subgroup analyses may be done according to different subject characteristics (e.g., sex, age, or disease severity) or different studies (e.g., conducted at different locations). Subgroup analysis can also be used as an important method to explore heterogeneous outcomes, or to answer questions about specific patients, types of interventions, or types of studies, which has important implications for guiding clinical individualization.

Findings from multiple subgroup analyses may be misleading. The sample size of each subgroup may be too small to detect effects between groups with enough statistical power. The more subgroup analyses, the higher likelihood of false-negative and false-positive significance tests. Therefore, the results of the subgroup analysis should be interpreted with caution. The Cochrane recommends that authors should clarify whether subgroup analysis is pre-specified or undertaken after the results of the studies had been compiled (post-hoc). Performing extensive post-hoc subgroup analysis to explore heterogeneity is data fishing, its reliability is low.

16.4.6 Sensitivity analysis

A sensitivity analysis is a repeat of the primary analysis or meta-analysis by changing ranges of values or criteria which were arbitrary or uncertain. The arbitrariness or uncertainty will influence the robustness of results and conclusion of the meta-analysis. With the help of a large amount of sensitivity analysis, review authors could fully assess the robustness and reliability of the results, and to discover or determine the influence of the arbitrariness or uncertainty. When doing the sensitivity analysis, you can always ask the question, "Are the findings robust to the decisions made in the process of obtaining them?"

In practice, review authors could analyze a specific subgroup by changing the arbitrary or uncertain criteria. For example, exploring the treatment effect of randomized controlled trials or non-randomized controlled trials to assess the impact of study design; excluding some studies with low quality or high bias to assess the influence of research quality on the integrate effect. Be careful not to confuse the sensitivity analysis with the subgroup analysis. Although some sensitivity analyses involve restricting the analysis to a subset of the totality of studies, it does not attempt to estimate the treatment effect in the group of studies removed from the analysis. And in sensitivity analysis, informal comparisons are made between different ways of estimating the same thing.

Sensitivity analysis can usually be considered from the following perspectives. ① study design: characteristics of participants, characteristics of intervention, characteristics of comparator, characteristics of endpoints, and type of study; ② data: analysis dataset, sample size of studies, and imputation methods of missing values; ③ Analysis methods: the choice of statistical models, for example, fixed-effects model or random-effects model. Sensitivity analysis is not limited to these perspectives mentioned above.

Some sensitivity analyses should be pre-specified in the study protocol, but many issues suitable for sensitivity analysis are only identified during the review process where the individual peculiarities of the studies under investigation are identified. Where sensitivity analyses identify particular factors or missing information that greatly influence the findings of the review, greater resources can be deployed to try and resolve uncertainties and obtain extra information, possibly through contacting trial authors and obtaining individual participant data. If this cannot be achieved, the results must be interpreted with an appropriate degree of caution. The Cochrane recommends that review authors should produce a summary table to report the summary of sensitivity analysis.

16.4.7 Example

The efficacy difference between metformin and rosiglitazone in the treatment of type 2 diabetes is controversial. Therefore, some researchers conducted a systematic review and meta-analysis to evaluate the efficacy and safety of metformin and rosiglitazone in the treatment of type 2 diabetes. The search keywords were metformin, rosiglitazone, diabetes and HbA1c. A total of 12 articles met the inclusion criteria and was extracted. The data of HbA1c after 6 months of treatment were listed as follows (Table 16-5).

Table 16-5 HbA1c outcomes after 6 months of treatment of 12 studies

Included studies	Publish year	Metformin group			Rosiglitazone group			Mean difference	S.E.
		n1	mean1	s1	n2	mean2	s2		
Viljanen AP et al.	2005	12	−0.60	0.82	14	−0.30	0.90	−0.30	0.337 5
Stocker DJ et al.	2007	38	−1.19	0.13	37	−1.08	0.14	−0.11	0.031 2
Bilezikian JP et al.	2013	84	−0.49	0.75	73	−0.49	0.70	0.00	0.115 8
Yoon KH et al.	2011	114	−0.92	0.96	117	−0.82	0.79	−0.1	0.115 8
Natali A et al.	2004	28	−0.33	1.10	24	0.09	12.00	−0.42	2.458 3
Yener S et al.	2008	16	−1.00	1.11	23	−1.10	1.57	0.10	0.429 2
Iliadis F et al.	2007	15	−1.70	1.10	14	−1.00	0.70	−0.70	0.340 1
Kiyici S et al.	2009	16	−0.30	0.79	19	−0.70	0.79	0.40	0.268 1
Jung HS et al.	2005	13	−1.00	0.98	14	−1.50	1.01	0.50	0.383 1
Skov V et al.	2014	90	−1.31	0.15	93	−1.26	0.19	−0.05	0.025 3
Fidan E et al.	2011	20	−1.20	0.95	20	−1.00	0.92	−0.20	0.295 7
Rosenstock J et al.	2006	150	−1.80	1.00	155	−1.60	1.00	−0.20	0.114 5

The primary endpoint of this study was continuous (HbA1c), and the aggregate effect size was weighted mean difference (WMD). Based on the result of heterogeneity test, we could select the fixed-effects model with the inverse-variance method or the random-effects model with D-L method. We used Stata software to complete the meta-analysis and draw related figures. The operation steps and codes of meta-analysis are as follows.

16.4.7.1 The extracted data was sorted in the following format and imported into the Stata software (Table 16-6).

Table 16-6 Extracted data in Stata

name	year	studylabel	n1	m1	s1	n2	m2	s2
Viljanen AP	2005	ViljanenAP(2005)	12	−0.60	0.82	14	−0.30	0.90
Stocker DJ	2007	StockerDJ(2007)	38	−1.19	0.13	37	−1.08	0.14
Bilezikian JP	2013	BilezikianJP(2013)	84	−0.49	0.75	73	−0.49	0.70
Yoon KH	2011	YoonKH(2011)	114	−0.92	0.96	117	−0.82	0.79
Natali A	2004	NataliA(2004)	28	−0.33	1.10	24	0.09	12.00
Yener S	2008	YenerS(2008)	16	−1.00	1.11	23	−1.10	1.57
Iliadis F	2007	IliadisF(2007)	15	−1.70	1.10	14	−1.00	0.70
Kiyici S	2009	KiyiciS(2009)	16	−0.30	0.79	19	−0.70	0.79
Jung HS	2005	JungHS(2005)	13	−1.00	0.98	14	−1.50	1.01
Skov V	2014	SkovV(2014)	90	−1.31	0.15	93	−1.26	0.19
Fidan E	2011	FidanE(2011)	20	−1.20	0.95	20	−1.00	0.92
Rosenstock J	2006	RosenstockJ(2006)	150	−1.80	1.00	155	−1.60	1.00

16.4.7.2 Entered the following code in Stata (Version 16 or above).

Meta esize n1 m1 s1 n2 m2 s2, esize(mdiff, unequal) fixed studylabel(studylabel)

Meta-analysis setting information
  Study information
    No. of studies: 12
      Study label: studylabel
      Study size: _Meta_studysize
    Summary data: n1 m1 s1 n2 m2 s2
    Effect size
        Type: mdiff
        Label: Mean Diff.
        Variable: _Meta_es
        Precision
        Std. Err.:   _Meta_se
  Std. Err. adj.:   Unequal
        CI: [_Meta_cil, _Meta_ciu]
        CI level: 95%
Model and method
        Model: Fixed-effects
        Method: Inverse-variance

16.4.7.3   Entered the command "Meta summarize", the results of the Meta-analysis were printed as below.

  Effect-size label: Mean Diff.
  Effect size: _Meta_es
  Std. Err.:   _Meta_se
  Study label: studylabel
Meta-analysis summary   Number of studies = 12
Fixed-effects model   Heterogeneity:
Method: Inverse-variance   I2 (%) = 18.36
                                          H2 = 1.22

Study |	Mean Diff.	[95% Conf. Interval]		% Weight
Viljanen AP(2005) |	−0.300	−0.961	0.361	0.31
Stocker DJ(2007) |	−0.110	−0.171	−0.049	35.71
Bilezikian JP(2013) |	0.000	−0.227	0.227	2.60
Yoon KH(2011) |	−0.100	−0.327	0.127	2.59
Natali A(2004) |	−0.420	−5.238	4.398	0.01
Yener S(2008) |	0.100	−0.741	0.941	0.19
Iliadis F(2007) |	−0.700	−1.367	−0.033	0.30
Kiyici S(2009) |	0.400	−0.125	0.925	0.48
Jung HS(2005) |	0.500	−0.251	1.251	0.24

Skov V(2014) |	−0.050	−0.100	−0.000	54.53
Fidan E(2011) |	−0.200	−0.780	0.380	0.40
Rosenstock J(2006) |	−0.200	−0.424	0.024	2.65
------------------+--				
theta |	−0.075	−0.112	−0.038	
--				

Test of theta = 0: $z = -4.02$ Prob > |z| = 0.000 1

Test of homogeneity: Q = chi2(11) = 13.47   Prob > Q = 0.263 5

In the Stata output, the Chi-squared statistic Q of the heterogeneity test was 13.47 (degree of freedom =11), and the P-value of the heterogeneity test was 0.264. Therefore, it cannot be considered that the heterogeneity of the 12 studies exist (0.10 is generally used for alpha level of heterogeneity test). In this example, another heterogeneity statistic [I-squared (variation in WMD attributablel to heterogeneity)] was $I^2=18.4$, which means insignificant heterogeneous variation (<50%), which indicated low heterogeneity. So the fixed-effects model with inverse-variance method was appropriate.

The pooled mean difference of the fixed-effects model was −0.075, with statistically considerable differences (P-value=0.000 1). The 95% confidence interval of the mean difference was (−0.112, −0.038). Since the upper limit of the 95% confidence interval (−0.038) is less than 0, it can be inferred that the average level of HbA1c in diabetic patients taking metformin was lower than that in those taking rosiglitazone. In other words, it can be inferred that metformin had better hypoglycemic effect than rosiglitazone.

16.4.7.4 Entered the command "meta forestplot, nullref", the software outputted the forest plot (Figure 16-1).

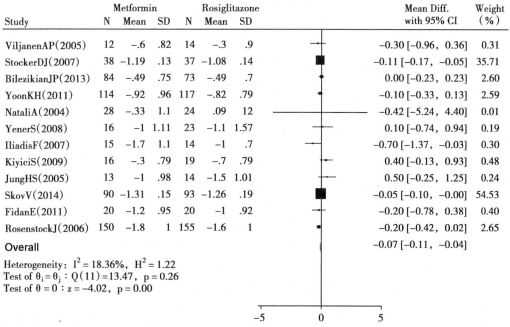

Figure 16-1　Forest plot

The forest plot output in this case showed that the distribution of the effects across studies was on both sides of the invalid line, with the combined effect values falling to the left of the invalid line 0 and the upper limit of the confidence interval <0, suggesting that the differences between the two groups were statistically different and that the mean glycosylated hemoglobin levels were lower in the diabetic population taking metformin than in the diabetic population taking rosiglitazone.

16.4.7.5 Typed the command "Meta funnel plot" to output a funnel plot to explore the reporting bias. Entered the command "meta bias, begg" or "meta bias, egger" to conduct the Begg's test or Egger's test. The funnel plot of this data (Figure 16-2) showed that the scattered points of the effect estimations of all individual studies fell within the funnel reference line, indicating that there was no obvious sign of publication bias.

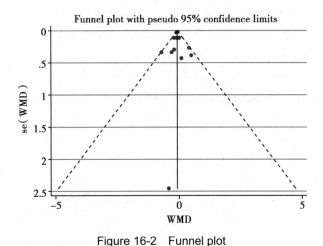

Figure 16-2   Funnel plot

16.5   Special topics of systematic evaluation and meta-analysis

16.5.1   Network meta-analysis

Systematic review and Meta-analysis are commonly used to assess the effectiveness and safety of interventions, which can provide reliable medical information for clinicians, policymakers and patients. The reality is that there are multiple interventions for the specific disease, but traditional meta-analysis only compares two interventions at a time. Lack of "head-to-head" trials acts as a block to obtain the direct evidence of comparing two interventions. To address this issue, methods have emerged that compare multiple interventions simultaneously, known as network meta-analyses (NMA), or mixed treatment comparisons and multiple treatments meta-analysis.

Network meta-analysis is a technique for comparing three or more interventions simultaneously in a single analysis by combining both direct and indirect evidence across a network of studies. With all available direct and indirect evidence, the network meta-analysis produces estimate of the relative effects between any pair of interventions in the network, and usually yields more precise estimates than a single direct or indirect estimate. It also allows the estimation of their relative ranking for a given outcome.

Any set of studies that links three or more interventions via direct comparisons forms a network of interventions. The network diagram is a graphical depiction of the structure of a network of interventions. It consists of nodes representing the interventions in the network and lines showing the available direct comparisons between pairs of interventions. The area of nodes represents the sample size of patients included in the intervention, and the thickness of lines represents the number of available studies that contribute to direct comparisons.

An example of a network diagram with four interventions is given in Figure 16-3. In this example, intervention A was directly compared with intervention B, intervention C and intervention D, and more studies involving direct comparison between A and B were included. No lines between node C and D indicated no direct comparisons between intervention C and D. However, we can compare interventions C and D via intervention A, which is called indirect treatment comparison (ITC). Indirect comparisons allow us to estimate the relative effects of two interventions that have not

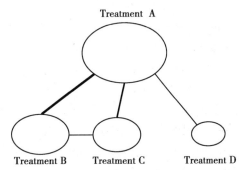

Figure 16-3 Network diagram

been compared directly within a trial. The underlying assumption of indirect comparisons is that we can learn about the true relative effect of C versus D via treatment A by combining the true relative effects A versus C and A versus D. Indirect comparisons provide observational evidence across randomized trials and may suffer the biases of observational studies, such as confounding bias.

Network meta-analysis can be performed using several approaches. The main technical requirement for all approaches is that all interventions included in the analysis form a "connected" network. A straightforward approach that be used for many networks is to use meta-regression. Another popular approach to conducting network meta-analysis is using hierarchical models, commonly implemented within a Bayesian framework.

16.5.2 Individual patient data reviews

Individual participant data (IPD) review is a specific type of systematic review. Unlike common systematic reviews, it does not directly extract data from published reports. IPD review authors may obtain data either from study investigators or via data-sharing repositories or platforms, and check and reanalyze the original data for each participant in each study. The IPD will usually contain de-identified demographic information for each participant such as age, sex, nature of their health condition, as well as information about treatments or tests received and outcomes observed. The process always requires more time, resources and expertise than other types of systems reviews, but is of higher quality. IPD reviews are carried out by a collaborative group, comprising a project management team, the researchers who contribute their study data, and an advisory group.

The IPD reviews have advantages that traditional approach cannot surpass. The IPD approach can bring substantial improvements to the quality of data available and offset inadequate reporting of individual studies. IPD reviews always include studies that are unpublished or not reported in full. If such unreported data is available and analyzed, publication bias will be greatly avoided. With original data of every subject and necessary extra data, risk of bias can be assessed more thoroughly and IPD enables more detailed and flexible analysis than is possible in systematic reviews of aggregate data. Review authors can deal with missing data at the patient level, analyze all interesting and important outcomes, check analytical assumptions, conduct subgroup analysis conveniently, and conduct more detailed and complex analysis. For example, the characteristics of patients can be analyzed in depth to develop complex prediction or prognostic models. Review authors can also update follow-up of survival or other outcomes beyond that reported. When interpreting findings of IPD, review authors can discuss implications for clinical practice and research with a multidisciplinary group of collaborators including study investigators who supplied data.

An IPD review usually takes longer and costs more than a conventional systematic review of the same question, and requires a range of skills to obtain, manage and analyze data. Generally, IPD reviews should be considered in circumstances where the available published or other aggregate data do not permit a good quality review. Another important consideration is whether sufficient IPD is likely to be available to permit credible analysis. Before embarking on an IPD review, review authors need to think carefully about which skills and resources will be required for the project to succeed.

It is important to note that while the IPD approach helps avoid bias associated with analysis and reporting, it generally does not avoid bias associated with study design or implementation. Such studies should be considered to be excluded from the meta-analysis. It is not always possible to obtain all the desired data for an IPD review. Review authors should be wary of bias related to the unavailable data. If investigators do not respond or refuse to participate, it might be to suppress unfavorable results, and therefore not including such trials could bias the meta-analysis. Therefore, the reasons for the failure to obtain data and the possibility of resultant bias should be explained, and conclusions should be drawn cautiously.

16.5.3 Prospective meta-analysis

Prospective meta-analysis (PMA) is a planned and active meta-analysis method, which refers to combining single-site randomized trials with a concurrent meta-analysis. This is different from the traditional approach of researchers designing, conducting, and publishing a clinical trial without any further plans. They often passively wait for other researchers to combine the results of the study with other similar randomized trials in a traditional retrospective meta-analysis as part of a systematic review. Alternatively, they may plan to conduct a traditional meta-analysis that includes the study. However, in prospective meta-analysis, researchers can design a meta-analysis while planning and implementing a component trial.

Prospective meta-analysis (PMA) avoids some problems and challenges existing in the traditional retrospective meta-analysis. In a PMA, results of randomized trials are recognized and determined to be included in meta-analysis before they are known. Investigators specify hypotheses without prior knowledge of the results of individual trials and establish selection criteria to be applied to trials prospectively. Moreover, PMAs allow a prior declaration of planned analyses, including subgroup analysis, prior to the findings of any component trial. Therefore, PMA avoids the potential difficulties in interpretation arising from data-dependent decisions in traditional meta-analysis.

In addition, all centers in a PMA must have uniform interventions and outcomes. This avoids differences between interventions and differences in different outcome measures in retrospective meta-analysis. Without common provisions by PMA investigators, certain individual centers may produce conflicting data that cannot be combined in a scientific meta-analysis.

If initiated early enough, PMA provides an opportunity for trial design, data collection and other trial processes to be standardized across the eligible ongoing trials. All sites in a PMA may agree to use the same instrument to measure a particular outcome, and to measure the outcome at the same time-points in each trial. Therefore, some of the issues raised by lack of standardization in a traditional retrospective meta-analysis could be addressed. Without PMA researchers' collective decision and common regulations, some single sites may produce conflicting data that cannot be combined in a scientifically acceptable meta-analysis.

PMAs based on IPD are similar to multicenter clinical trials and have similar advantages, including increased sample size, increased diversity of treatment settings and populations, and the ability to examine heterogeneity of intervention effects across multiple settings. However, whereas traditional multicenter trials implement a single protocol across all sites to reduce variability in trial conduct among centers, PMAs allow investigators greater flexibility in how their trial is conducted. Sites can follow a local protocol appropriate to local circumstances, with the local protocol being aligned with elements of a PMA protocol that are common to all included trials.

Therefore, PMAs are often carried out by a collaborative group that usually collects and analyzes individual patient data. Unlike traditional multicenter trials, they allow variation in the protocols of the included studies, while maximizing power in the pre-designed meta-analyses. For culture researchers, a PMA often requires fewer resources than a multicenter randomized trial. PMA projects can increase research capacity through collaboration.

16.6 The registration and reporting of systematic review

To address the suboptimal reporting of meta-analyses, QUOROM (Quality Of Reporting Of Meta-analyses) guideline was developed by an international group and published in 1999. In 2009, the guideline was updated to address several conceptual and practical advances in the science of systematic reviews, and was renamed PRISMA (preferred reporting items of systematic reviews and meta-analyses). With the widespread use of these statements, the quality of systematic review reports has been improved. In recent years, the PRISMA statement has derived many different versions to accommodate different types of systematic reviews. Over the past decade, there have been many innovations in methodology and terminology. In 2017, an international group set out to update the PRISMA 2009 statement to ensure its currency and relevance. The PRISMA 2020 statement was published online in several top medical journals, including *BMJ*, *PLOS Medicine* and so on.

The PRISMA 2020 statement provides updated reporting guidance for systematic reviews that reflects advances in methods to identify, select, appraise, and synthesize studies. It incorporates advances in systematic review methodology and terminology occurring in the last decade. The PRISMA 2020 statement consists of a 27-item checklist, an expanded checklist that details reporting recommendations for each item, the PRISMA 2020 abstract checklist, and revised flow diagrams for original and updated reviews.

In order to guarantee the reviews' authenticity and transparency, systems reviews are required to register as other types of research. PROSPERO is an international database of prospectively registered systematic reviews, which is the most popular registered platform. Key features from the review protocol are required to fill in the platform and maintained as a permanent record. A PROSPERO registration number will be awarded upon approval.

Summary

The core concept of evidence-based medicine is that clinical practice should be based on evidence. Therefore, the formation and quality of "evidence" are the key point to practice evidence-based medicine. All completed and ongoing medical research can become evidence. Systematic review, as well as meta-analysis, is one of the most important methods to produce high quality evidence in evidence-based medicine.

(Lü Minzhi, Li Chunbo)

17

Health-related quality of life

Learning objectives

1. **To master** the definition and evaluation of health-related quality of life.
2. **To be familiar with** the establishment and evaluation of health-related quality of life scale; the application of patient reported outcomes in evaluation of health-related quality of life.
3. **To know** the clinical practice of health-related quality of life assessment.

The harm caused by chronic diseases on patients is not only the complaint of physical symptoms and physiological functions, but also the influence of emotion, social activities, interpersonal relationship, family roles, etc. In 1948, World Health Organization (WHO) pointed out that health "is a state of complete physical, mental and social well-being and not merely the absence of disease or infirmity." However, the conventional assessment methods of chronic diseases mainly focus on patients' biological changes. Apparently, the results of these assessment can only answer whether the patients are sick or not, rather than the entire health condition. For example, two patients had been diagnosed with a malignant tumor. One accepted surgery with better prognosis. However, he frequently visited doctors because of panic, depression and insomnia throughout the whole day. Another patient with advanced cancer was very optimistic, trying his best to take part in family and social activities. How should we evaluate the health status of those two patients?

17.1 Definition of health-related quality of life

17.1.1 Definition of quality of life

In 1993, according to the statement by WHO quality of life assessment team, quality of life (QOL) was defined as "individual's perceptions of their position in life in the context of the culture and value systems in which they live and in relation to their goals, expectations, standards and concerns". This definition emphasized the unique life experiences of persons and respected their individual and social values. Thus, QOL shows its obviously subjective characteristics.

17.1.2 Definition of health-related quality of life

Application of the principles and assessment methods of QOL in health care produces health-related quality of life (HRQOL) which is the self-perception of satisfaction in relation to economic and cultural background and value orientation under the influence of disease, medical intervention, individual economic incomes, aging and social environment. HRQOL can reflect health condition comprehensively, which conforms to the bio-psycho-social pattern, and established the domains and dimensions needed to evaluate HRQOL. Every domain in the evaluation of HRQOL not only is related to the disease, but constitutes causal relationship with each other, and has complex connection with social, economic and other factors. Although disease brings damage and disability, which results in worse HRQOL, the relationship between disease and HRQOL is not always linear or one-way. For example, a patient has left hemiparesis after a stroke. With deepened understanding of the disease, improved compensatory ability of the healthy side, family support and the reattendance of social activities, his HRQOL can be obviously improved even without the function recovery of the affected side.

17.1.3 Content of health-related quality of life assessment

Established HRQOL systems, including the *International Classification of Functioning, Disability and Health* and WHO Quality of Life (WHOQOL), combine the objective criteria with disease related parameters and patient reported symptoms and feelings. Usually, five major domains are chosen in the assessment of HRQOL as follows.

Physical symptoms: disease symptoms, etc.

Physiological function: organic function, cognition, role state, sexual function, etc.

Psychological function: good emotion, depression, anxiety, etc.

Social function: social relationship, job role, hobby, financial condition, etc.

Mental status: religion, individual values, etc.

The above domains fully demonstrate that the assessment of HRQOL is patient-centered and subjective. However, whether the current HRQOL assessment should include some objective items such as incomes and ecological environment has sparked great controversy.

17.1.4 The evaluation methods of health-related quality of life

As the majority of contents in HRQOL assessment is the subjective experience of subjects, the most common methods at present are scales and patient reported outcomes.

17.2 Establishment and evaluation of scales

17.2.1 Classification of scales

According to the users, the HRQOL scales have been divided into two types, generic QOL instrument and disease-specific QOL instrument.

The generic QOL instrument includes routine activities and psychological status. It can be applied to an extensive range of diseases and patients with different races and languages. The advantage of generic QOL instrument is that it is not affected by disease diagnosis and it is able to compare directly the severity of different diseases and the benefit-risk balance of various inventions. For example, after comparing the disease adverse outcomes and therapeutic effects between systemic lupus erythematosus (SLE) and gastrointestinal ulcer, the administrators will make a better decision on the rational use of medical resources. Nevertheless, such scales usually exclude the items in relation to the specific characteristics of the diseases and neglect some important functional assessment. Therefore, for evaluating the HRQOL of a specific disease, the reliability of this kind of instrument is not high and for some questions may have low response rate. For instance, the European Health-Related Quality of Life 5 Dimensions (EQ-5D) questionnaire includes mobility, self-care, daily activities, pain/discomfort, anxiety/depression, etc. Choosing no pain often represents better HRQOL, but for a patient losing algesia, the reality is opposite.

The disease-specific QOL instrument is created for a disease or a subtype of disease, which can reflect the patient's HRQOL specifically and mainly be applied to compare different inventions. But the specific QOL instrument has some limitations. It may be affected by regional features, cultural tradition, religion, custom and lifestyle, etc. Sometimes it needs to establish different scales for the subtypes of a disease. The disease-specific QOL instrument is unable to compare HRQOL of different diseases. Now there are some specific QOL instrument that are utilized widely, such as health assessment questionnaire (HAQ) for rheumatoid arthritis, European Organization for Research and Treatment of Cancer scale (EORTC) for cancers, etc.

17.2.2   The contents of a scale

The general frame of a scale includes several domains (or subscales) such as physiological function, social function, overall condition and role function, etc. Every domain also contains various facets, for instance, physiological function can be divided into daily physiological function, cognitive level and role function. Every facet is composed of quantitative items.

17.2.3   The establishment of a scale

There are some factors needed to be considered in the design of a scale, such as clinical background, research purpose, users, conceptual framework, items' pool and selection, responding options, data collection methods, monitoring models, response time windows, scoring standards, items' or subscales' weights, format, filling burden, translation and cultural adaptation, etc.

The establishment of a scale must experience a series of rigorous and standardized steps. Firstly, form conceptual framework of the scale and make clear the study population and content according to the disease background and research purpose. Secondly, establish research group and its core team. Thirdly, form items pool by summarizing disease characteristics, searching literature, organizing medical staffs and patient interview. Furthermore, the items are selected into the scale by discussion of the research group. Fourthly, pretest the validity, rationality, completion and response of the scale. Correct or delete items that are ambiguous, incomprehensible and recurring. Then, deeply analyze and select items by traditional methods as comprehensive scoring from physicians and patients, variation coefficient, principal component analysis and new models like grade response model and division scoring model. Fifthly, enlarge samples to test reliability, validity and feasibility of the scale and adjust content and structure of the scale on the basis of results. Sixthly, evaluate the quality of the scale again.

17.2.4　The evaluation of a scale

When a scale is established or when its applicable subjects or languages change, it is vital to re-evaluate the reliability, validity, feasibility and reactivity of the scale (see Table 17-1) in order to ensure the survey results are true and reliable.

Table 17-1　Evaluation of HRQOL scale

Aspects	Index	Test parameter or examples
Reliability	Test-retest reliability	Intra-class correlation coefficients (ICC)
	Inter-reviewer reliability	Intra-class correlation coefficients (ICC)
	Internal consistency reliability	Cronbach's alpha
Validity	Content validity	Applicability of all items to the composition of the scale
		Relevance of all items to study population characteristics
		Relevance of all items to the scale
		Patient's ability to understand the contents of the scale
	Construct validity	Discriminant and convergent validity
	Criteria-related validity	ROC curve (Continuity variable)
		Sensitivity and specificity (binary variable)
	Cross-cultural validity	Conceptual equivalence
		Item equivalence
		Semantic equivalence
		Operational equivalence
		Measurement equivalence
Reactivity		Minimal important difference, MID
		Patient changes over time
Feasibility		Completion rate
		Completion time
		Items response rate

17.2.4.1 Reliability

Reliability is the stability of the same question answers and the consistency of all items results in the same field. There are three factors affecting reliability of a scale, namely content, time of measurement and rater. The common test methods include test-retest reliability, inter-reviewer reliability, internal consistency reliability, and half-fold reliability.

Test-retest reliability is an important indicator for the scale stability. It means the degree of consistency that such a scale can be achieved twice in the same patient under the same condition during a certain interval. The length of interval has a great impact on test-retest reliability. The subjective experience of the patient is influenced by his/her memory when the interval is too short. In contrast, the HRQOL of the patient will change if the interval is too long. In principle, the test-retest reliability should be carried out during the period of no change in HRQOL. The Kappa value is often used to test the consistency of two measurements. For continuous variables, intra-class correlation coefficients (ICC) is used for statistics. Generally, a Kappa value of $0.40\sim$ 0.75 or ICC>0.6 indicates that the test-retest reliability is good; if Kappa or ICC > 0.75, it is excellent.

Inter-reviewer reliability can reflect the consistency among different reviewers. The standardization of managing measurement instruments and the training of reviewers on this standard are the premises to improve inter-reviewer reliability. The Kappa value or intra-class correlation coefficients is often used for testing.

Internal consistency reliability

For example, Cronbach's alpha measures the level of consistency between items within the subscale. Ideally, Cronbach's alpha of each subscale is $\geqslant 0.70$, which indicates that the contents of each item are homogeneous. But in clinical trials, it should be noted that internal consistency reliability will be doubted in the absence of test-retest reliability.

17.2.4.2 Validity

Validity is the agreement between the contents of the testing scale and those of the real world, which means the authenticity and accuracy of the test. But it is difficult to confirm the truth of patients' subjective experience, which makes it necessary to evaluate multi-faceted validity including content validity, construct validity, criteria-related validity and cross-cultural validity.

Content validity is one of the primary characteristics of a scale, which indicates whether the content of the measurement can truly reflect or represent the phenomenon measured. However, content validity is so extensive that it cannot apply the quantitative method for testing. Therefore, it faces with the huge difficulties to evaluate the validity of content. We can only observe the description of content validity in the literature to estimate whether it is accurate, comprehensive and detailed. Content validity includes item generation (such as generation method, item source, selection, editing and deletion, quantitative tools for item evaluation, research objects, etc.), data collection methods and tool supervision modes, recall cycles, response options, measurement tool standardization and training, patients' comprehension, scoring system for items and subscales, responsibility of respondents and managers etc.

Construct validity is the degree of the measurement of an instrument on the basis of the theoretical structure and characteristics. It indicates the consistency between research results and hypotheses, which means whether the instrument can meet the requirements of the measurement to the hypothesis test. Construct validity also can be divided into discriminant validity and convergent validity. Discriminant validity is applied to clarify whether the measuring tool can identify a detected object with a certain characteristic. Convergent validity refers to the similarity degree of different measurements when they are used to test the same feature.

Criteria-related validity refers to the degree of consistency between an established scale and the existing standard measurement (gold standard). The standard measurement could be wide-accepted scales, clinical indicators or long-term clinical follow-up results. Criteria-related validity is divided into two types: one is concurrent validity, which means that measuring a group of subjects with the assessed scale and standard measurement tools simultaneously, and evaluating the consistency between the results; the other is predictive validity which can predict future events (such as disease recurrence, treatment response, etc.) However, it is hard to find "gold standard" in most of the quality of life research. If a standard measurement tool is used in the study, information such as its rationale, sensitivity, specificity, and predictive value will be required.

Cross-cultural validity

A scale needs to be translated and adjusted culturally when the same scale is applied to people of different countries, races and languages due to discrepancies in social, economic, religious, cultural backgrounds, etc. This kind of literature reports should provide information concerning the development of the source language version, the translation process of the target language version, the experts participating in the translation and back-translation, the independence of the translators, the adjustment of cultural differences, and the pretest for testing the level of patients' understanding, etc.

17.2.4.3   Reactivity

With the lapse of time or intervention, patients' conditions change, so does their corresponding quality of life. The ability of a scale to reflect this change is called reactivity. Clinical studies often use "statistically significant" to determine the difference in efficacy, but significant differences in values do not always mean clinical significance. The threshold called minimal important difference (MID) is the degree of improvement on the features of patients that make health care professionals believe it important or meaningful. MID is a quantitative reactivity indicator that is often used in therapeutic efficacy assessments and comparative studies.

17.2.4.4   Feasibility

The implementation of a scale should not be time-consuming, difficult to operate, burdensome, or risky for the patients. It should be finished within 20 minutes to obtain complete, effective and authentic information. The completion rate of the scale and the response rate of the item are commonly used as indicators for the feasibility evaluation of a scale.

17.3   Application of patient report outcomes in HRQOL evaluation

The core content of HRQOL is the patient's level of satisfaction in terms of health. It is often necessary for patients to provide information about their self-perception, activities they are doing, and their own health and life satisfaction through self-reporting. This assessment is also called patient reported outcomes (PROs), which has been proven to be effective and practicable. The effective PROs usually require to be wide-ranged and irrelevant to age, gender or diagnosis. It is sensitive enough to detect tiny but important clinical differences. PROs are more and more popular in clinicians partly because they supplement the important symptom information from the patient's point of view that cannot be obtained by objective examinations. PROs have become a necessary evaluation index for clinical research. For example, in the evaluation of the efficacy of new drugs for rheumatoid arthritis(RA), the patient's overall self-assessment of disease status, feeling of joint pain, HAQ (specific QOL instrument) and SF-36 (generic QOL instrument) are usually included to detect the effect of new drugs on HRQOL of RA patients.

PROs include all reports from the patients. It can be a single indicator measurement, an event record, a symptom complaint or a health-related quality of life questionnaire, which provide important information of patient's response to a disease or treatment via hospital records, the patients' diaries or any other possible sources. PROs view patients' conditions and overall physical health from the patients' own perspective, which is conductive to patients' participation in the treatment decisions and understanding of the disease burden. What's more, it can also provide guidance for decisions on health resource allocation.

17.4   The clinical application of HRQOL evaluation

The clinical application of HRQOL evaluation has been more and more widespread in the past decade, and continues to receive attention. The health care sector and its guidelines need to take the impact of HRQOL results into considerations.

Numerous HRQOL scales provide important information for clinicians and researchers, which helps to evaluate the overall influence of the disease on patient survival. The study of QOL has opened up a new field of clinical medical research. Establishing and evaluating QOL with the scientific methods in this field could help clinicians further access the patient's condition comprehensively and guide them to choose drugs correctly and rationally. At the same time, it also helps the medical management department compare medical costs of different disease, conduct cost-utility, cost-benefit analysis, optimize the allocation of medical resources and medical policies.

Summary

Health-related quality of life emphasizes the evaluation of health through concepts and methods of quality of life, focusing on the individual and social values of patients. HRQOL scales provide valuable support and reference for making clinical decision and conducting clinical researches.

(Ma Lili)

18

Cost-effectiveness analysis

Learning objectives

1. **To master** basic elements and types of clinical economic evaluation.
2. **To know** literature evaluation standards for cost-effectiveness analysis.

18.1 Basic concepts

In clinical practice, doctors and patients not only consider the clinical outcome of different diagnosis and treatment methods, but also pay attention to the medical treatment and related costs. Our country is a developing country with insufficient investment in health, and the total health expenditure only accounts for about 5% of the gross domestic product (GDP). At the same time, our country is currently facing a serious population aging problem, as well as factors such as increased service access and technological advancement, and our country's health expenditure and demand are rising rapidly. Therefore, applying the principles and methods of economics to research in the field of medicine and health has very important theoretical and practical significance. The government needs to consider the allocation of health resources when formulating health policies. Clinicians play the role of gatekeepers in the utilization of health care resources. Clinicians are faced with how to use the money well. For every examination and every treatment plan, it needs to consider whether it is worthwhile and whether it is cost-effective. Therefore, the medical practice of clinicians must have an economic perspective. It is necessary to comprehensively conduct medical services in terms of clinical results and resource consumption, carry out relevant research and clinical practice, and provide evidence-based medicine for the government to formulate relevant policies.

Clinical economics is the application of the principles and methods of economics by clinicians and other stakeholders to evaluate the economic effects of clinical diagnosis, prevention and treatment technologies and measures, and to find out the factors that affect the rational use of limited resources so as to provide scientific basis for decision-making in clinical practice.

The purpose of clinical economics research is to scientifically evaluate the emerging diagnostic and therapeutic measures in clinical practice, make an economic analysis from the perspective of their benefits to the society, and put forward an economic basis to allocate and utilize limited health resources in a reasonable and effective way. Clinicians should be familiar with the basic concepts in clinical economic evaluation, master clinical economic evaluation methods, and apply them in clinical practice.

18.1.1　Basic elements in clinical economic evaluation

18.1.1.1　Costs refer to the input or resource consumption in the process of clinical medical treatment or health services. Generally speaking, in clinical economics, costs include direct medical costs, direct non-medical costs, indirect costs and hidden costs.

Direct medical costs are the costs for treatment, prevention, and health care in the process of health services, including hospitalization, medicine, diagnosis and treatment, laboratory examination fees, imaging examination fees, surgery fees, and ward fees, rehabilitation fees and other expenses.

Direct non-medical costs refer to resources other than medical resources directly consumed by patients in seeking medical services, such as transportation expenses, food and lodging expenses, and nutritious food expenses. Under normal circumstances, direct non-medical costs vary greatly due to varying conditions and are difficult to accurately calculate. Therefore, if the proportion is small, it can be ignored in the study.

Indirect costs, also known as social costs, refer to resources lost due to disease, including costs related to morbidity and mortality. There are some difficulties in calculating indirect costs. Commonly used methods include human capital method and willingness to pay method. Human capital method uses wage rates, unemployment rates, life expectancy, retirement age, etc. to calculate the reduction in income caused by sickness or death. But the disadvantage is that different groups of people have different incomes, and it is difficult to measure the elderly, children, and unemployed who have no income. Willingness to pay method is to directly measure the voluntary payment of the individual due to the reduction of sickness, disability and death. The disadvantage is that the poor and the rich have different willingness to pay, and the size of the individual's subjective expected results affects the willingness to pay.

Hidden costs refer to the physical and mental pain and discomfort caused by diseases or the implementation of medical services such as prevention and diagnosis. Hidden costs are also called intangible costs. They are usually not measured separately for two reasons. First, it is difficult to accurately measure hidden costs with currency, and measuring hidden costs itself usually requires more costs; second, in measuring utility, the hidden costs have been included in the measurement of output, which makes it unnecessary to repeat the calculation.

18.1.1.2　Effectiveness is the output measurement, which refers to the output in the process of clinical medical treatment or health service, that is, the medical result. Broadly speaking, the effects refer to the results obtained after the implementation of the medical or health service program. It may be a good result or a bad result. In a narrow sense, effects refer to good and useful results, that is, results that can meet the needs of the population, bring benefits or satisfaction to people, such as a decrease in morbidity, complications, and mortality. Commonly used effects include efficacy, survival or mortality. More broadly used effects include utility and benefit. For the sake of comparison, in evaluating the input and output of different health measures, the effects are converted into benefits, which are often measured in monetary units. In assessing the outcome of survival or death, if the quality of life is corrected, the effects is converted to utilities.

18.1.2 The basic types of clinical economic evaluation

18.1.2.1 Cost minimization analysis (CMA), also called cost identification analysis, measures the costs of different medical measures and compares the costs. CMA assumes that the effects of these measures are the same in order to choose the most economical and effective measure. For example, to prevent stress ulcers during the perioperative period, the preventive measures are the application of acid-suppressing drugs, which can be proton pump inhibitor (PPI) administered intravenously or orally. In patients who can take the drug orally, the efficacy of the two regimens is the same. However, the cost of the former is much higher. Therefore, the oral program has the least cost but the same effect, and oral medication should be selected for prevention. However, this method has certain limitations. It can only compare the costs of interventions for the same disease with the same effect, so the scope of application is narrow.

18.1.2.2 Cost-effectiveness analysis (CEA) is to analyze the effect obtained after cost consumption. It is expressed as the cost of each effect unit (cost-effectiveness ratio) or the incremental cost (incremental cost-effectiveness ratio) required for each additional effect. This allows two different medical measures to be compared and selected with the same evaluation unit, thereby providing a scientific basis for clinical decision-making.

Cost/effectiveness (C/E) is a way of expressing CEA, that is, the cost of each additional life-year, 1 death saved, 1 new case diagnosed, or 1 result unit increased. Generally, the smaller the C/E value, the more economic efficiency. A single C/E value is meaningless. It is mainly used to compare two or more items and compare two items with the same result unit. Clinically, when comparing the two measures, we often pay attention to the changes in costs as the new measures increase their efficacy. If the new measures not only increase the efficacy, but also reduce the cost, we will definitely choose the new measures if other conditions are the same (such as indications). If the cost of the new measures increases while the effectiveness of the new measures also increases, we compare the cost-effectiveness ratio of the two measures, that is, the cost per unit effect, and choose the solution with a lower cost-effectiveness ratio. If the new measures increase their effectiveness, but at the same time, the cost also increases, and the cost-effectiveness ratio is higher than that of the traditional measures, how do we choose? Whether from the perspective of groups or individuals, clinical efficacy is our first consideration, and the cost-effectiveness ratio is only applicable in case of limited resources for infinitely magnified groups. If we want to increase input to obtain higher output, how to judge the results of cost-effectiveness analysis? Incremental analysis can help us weigh.

Incremental cost-effectiveness analysis is often used to express the relationship between any two measures, which usually cannot be fully demonstrated by cost-effectiveness analysis for it involves the comparison of two or more measures. By calculating the ratio of the difference in cost between the study group and the control group to the difference in health output, called the incremental cost-effectiveness ratio (ICER), we can judge the economic advantages and disadvantages of the study versus the control. ICER can fully explain what the corresponding effect of the additional measures is and whether they are worth recommending. It is the most commonly used analytical index in the economic evaluation of health intervention programs. In economic theory, marginal analysis is usually used to guide economic decision-making. In clinical economic evaluation, the results of marginal analysis, or incremental cost-effectiveness analysis, must be reported.

$$\frac{\text{new cost} - \text{old cost}}{\text{new effect} - \text{old effect}} = \frac{\text{increased cost}}{\text{each additional effect unit}}$$

$$\frac{\Delta C}{\Delta E} = \frac{C_N - C_0}{E_N - E_0}$$

ΔC represents the difference between the costs of the two programs, ΔE is the difference between the effects of the two programs, and $\Delta C/\Delta E$ is the incremental ratio.

C_N means the new cost, C_0 means the old cost, E_N means the new effect, and E_0 means the old effect.

ICER is a comparison of the two dimensions of cost and output between the two groups. It represents the increase in cost that the study group needs to pay to obtain a unit increase in health output compared to the control group. The current World Trade Organization (WTO) recommendation on cost-effectiveness threshold analysis is that when ICER < per capita GDP, the increased cost can be considered completely worthwhile and has cost-effectiveness advantages; When per capita GDP < ICER < 3 times per capita GDP, the increased cost is considered acceptable and has a cost-effective advantage; when ICER > 3 times per capita GDP, the increased cost is considered not worthwhile, and there is no cost-effective advantage. The ICER indicator also reflects the consideration of the net benefits of health intervention programs. The decision-making method of comparing ICER and threshold is equivalent to monetizing health output through the threshold, and then comparing the net benefits of different options.

18.1.2.3   Cost-utility analysis (CUA) is a special form of cost-effectiveness analysis. The measurement of the results is to convert the different results of different programs into utility indicators. The utility value is a numerical value obtained by quantifying each disease or different health level according to the physiological or psychological function, ranging from 0 to 1, with complete health as 1, and death as 0. It is usually measured by quality-adjusted life year (QALY) and disability-adjusted life year (DALY). QALY can be measured directly or indirectly. Standard gamble (SG), time trade-off (TTO), visual analogue scale (VAS) are direct measurement methods; European Qualify of Life Five Dimensions scale (Euro-Qol-5 Dimensions, EQ-5D), Short-Form Six-Dimensions (SF-6D), health utilities index (HUI) and health quality scale are all indirect measurement methods.

18.1.2.4   Cost-benefit analysis (CBA)

When comparing different medical measures, in addition to the above-mentioned QALY as the unit, we can also use currency as the unit for all costs and effects of a certain item and medical service. This is cost-benefit analysis (CBA). As an economic decision-making method, cost-benefit analysis is used in government planning and decision-making to find out how to obtain the maximum benefit with the smallest cost in investment. It is often used to evaluate the value of public health projects that need to quantify social benefits.

18.2　Literature evaluation criteria for cost-effectiveness analysis

18.2.1　Clinical economic evaluation methods

Clinical economic evaluation methods include four types: minimum cost analysis, cost-effectiveness analysis, cost-utility analysis, and cost-benefit analysis. Table 18-1 answers two questions: Have you compared two or more programs? Have you checked the costs and effects of each program at the same time?

Table 18-1　Evaluation methods of clinical economics

Dimension		Have you checked the costs and effects of various programs at the same time?		
		No		Yes
		Only checked the effects	Only checked the costs	
Have you compared two or more programs?	No	1A Partial evaluation Effect description	1B Partial evaluation Cost description	2 Partial evaluation Cost-effectiveness description
	Yes	3A Partial evaluation Effectiveness or effect analysis	3B Partial evaluation Cost analysis	4 complete economic evaluation Minimal cost analysis Cost-effectiveness analysis Cost-utility analysis Cost-benefit analysis

18.2.2　The literature evaluation criteria of cost-effectiveness analysis

The literature evaluation criteria of cost-effectiveness analysis include three aspects, namely, whether the results of economic analysis are correct, what are the results, and whether the results are applicable to my patients.

18.2.2.1　Is the result correct?

Is a complete economic analysis provided? From whose perspective to evaluate? Have all relevant clinical measures been compared? Is the measurement of cost and effect correct? Are the cost and effect data incrementally analyzed? Whether a sensitivity analysis was performed? Does the estimated cost and effect come from the intervention population?

18.2.2.2　What is the result?

What are the incremental cost and effect? Are there differences in incremental costs and effects in each subgroup? What is the uncertain result of the allowable change?

18.2.2.3 Does the result apply to my patient?

Do the benefits or advantages of the treatment outweigh the costs or harms? Does my patient have similar clinical results? Does my patients have similar costs?

18.3 Evidence-based practice of cost-effectiveness analysis

18.3.1 Clinical case

A 12-year-old male patient was admitted to the hospital with the main complaint of "dry mouth, polydipsia, polyuria for 3 years with nausea and vomiting for 2 days". After the patient was hospitalized, relevant examinations were performed, and the diagnosis was type 1 diabetes and diabetic ketoacidosis. The patient's condition improved after the use of insulin, fluid and potassium supplementation and other treatments. The follow-up plan is to take further measures to control blood sugar. Between multiple daily injections (MDI) insulin and continuous subcutaneous insulin infusion (CSII) the two intensive insulin treatment programs recommended by the International Juvenile Diabetes Federation to effectively control blood sugar and improve microvascular disease, which one should we choose? Compared with MDI, CSII can better control blood sugar and reduce the incidence of acute complications of diabetes. However, the cost of treatment for CSII is higher. When medical resources are limited and there are multiple effective treatment options, which method is used to control blood sugar?

18.3.2 Clinical problems

To control the blood sugar of patients with type 1 diabetes, should I choose to inject insulin multiple times a day or use continuous subcutaneous insulin infusion?

18.3.3 Literature search

By entering keywords, you can retrieve the corresponding literature.

18.3.4 Literature evaluation

18.3.4.1 Is the result correct?

This question emphasizes whether clinical economic analysis truly reflects that one of the clinical measures may provide better cost-effectiveness. As with other types of research, the authenticity of clinical economic evaluation depends on whether the methods used are correct.

The literature provides a complete economic evaluation, and compares the clinical results and costs of multiple daily insulin injections with those of continuous subcutaneous insulin infusion.

From the perspective of saving resources for the society.

Describe in detail the plans to be compared.

Adopt appropriate measurement and evaluation methods for costs and clinical effects. The clinical results are derived from literature analysis, including a single randomized controlled clinical trial, a systematic summary of a series of clinical trials, and synthetic data of clinical trials (meta-analysis). The results include the credibility interval and could fit real clinical practice.

The research conducts incremental cost-effectiveness analysis.

Adopt single factor and probability sensitivity analysis.

Estimate the baseline cost-effectiveness of the treatment population.

18.3.4.2 What is the result?

The results should include the incremental cost and effect of each measure. Has the study analyzed the incremental costs and effects in different subgroups of people? According to the results of single factor sensitivity analysis and probability sensitivity analysis, judge the impact of uncertainty factors have on the results. From the above research, we can know that for 60 years of simulation, for children and adolescents suffering from T1DM in Qingdao, the direct medical cost of the CSII group was 67 137 yuan higher than that of the MDI group; the life expectancy and quality-adjusted life year of the CSII group were both higher than those of the MDI group by 0.41 years; the incremental cost-effectiveness ratio of the CSII group was 163 749 yuan/QALY, which was 1.5 times (186 423 yuan) lower than that of Qingdao's per capita gross domestic product (GDP) in 2019; CSII treatment was cost-effective. Sensitivity analysis showed that under the circumstance of the price of the insulin pump as 60 000 yuan and simulated for 60 years, the greater the price drop of the insulin pump, the lower the ICER. When the upgrade price of insulin pumps dropped by 10%, 20%, 30%,40%, and 50%, the ICER of the CSII group was lower than 1.5 times the per capita GDP of Qingdao in 2019. Therefore, CSII was cost-effective. When the threshold is 1.5 times and 3.0 times of Qingdao's per capita GDP in 2019, the probability that the CSII group has cost-effectiveness is 62.8% and 93.7%, respectively.

18.3.4.3 Whether the results can be used in clinical practice?

After obtaining the economic analysis results of the two measures and the accuracy evaluation of the economic analysis, we need to answer whether this result is suitable for our patients, and which treatment is more reasonable for our patients. There are two points that can help you make a choice: one is the incremental ratio of the cost-effectiveness analysis, and the other is the degree to which your patients are similar to the case population in the economic analysis. In clinical practice, it is also necessary to consider factors other than the evidence-based decision-making evidence such as the patient's willingness and the convenience of operation.

In conclusion, the findings of clinical economics analysis can provide health care payers and decision makers with important reference information that can help optimize the allocation of health care resources, as well as motivate clinicians to make more rational clinical decisions in the course of clinical treatment.

Summary

The purpose of clinical economic analysis is to scientifically evaluate new diagnostic and therapeutic measures that constantly emerge in clinical practice, make economic analysis from the perspective of whether they are beneficial to society, and present the economic rationale to achieve the purpose of allocating and utilizing limited health resources in the most rational and effective way. Clinicians should be familiar with the basic concepts in clinical economics evaluation, master the methods of clinical economics evaluation, and apply them to clinical practice.

(Chen Shiyao)

Evidence-based decision analysis

Learning objectives

1. **To be familiar with** concepts and models of clinical decision analyses.
2. **To know** how to read and evaluate literature on evidence-based decision analysis.

19.1　Overview of clinical decision analysis

In clinical practice, the issues to be decided are often complicated. For example, although a certain diagnostic method is highly accurate and reliable, it is also expensive or may cause new trauma; although surgical treatment can control the disease progression and prolong the life of the patient, but at the same time it will cause new and serious damage to health and affect the quality of life of patients. Doctors may weigh the pros and cons to make treatment decisions based on clinical experience, but this is a simple, even perfunctory decision-making method. Sometimes the decision is left to the patient or family member. Even if the doctor informs the benefits and risks of various diagnosis and treatment methods and the related data, and the patient and family member comprehensively consider the treatment effect and their own financial ability to make the decision, it is still non-quantitative, non-scientific clinical decision-making. These two commonly used clinical decision-making methods are difficult to comprehensively consider and accurately measure the impact of various factors on the outcome, and it is difficult to give convincing answers. What I want to discuss here is the decision-making based on quantitative analysis, which can help doctors analyze and solve decision-making problems more comprehensively, systematically, and scientifically. So, in clinical economics, how should we judge disease diagnosis more accurately and choose diagnostic tests reasonably? How to evaluate the pros and cons of treatment more comprehensively and objectively?

Decision-making is the process of selecting the best course of action from a number of alternative courses of action for solving the current problems. Clinicians need to make clinical decisions for the diagnosis and treatment of patients at any time. Scientific decision-making emphasizes establishing models based on the thoroughly collected scientific evidence from relevant research results and using appropriate methods of quantitative analysis to fully evaluate the risks and benefits of the diagnosis and treatments plans available and to weigh the pros and cons of each alternative. This process helps to reduce clinical uncertainty and achieve maximum benefit with limited resources. This approach of using evidence-based medicine to make clinical decisions is decision analysis in evidence-based decision-making.

19.2 Implementation of decision analysis

19.2.1 Basic steps of decision analysis

The evidence-based decision-making process includes the following five basic steps: propose clinical problems to be solved; search literature; build models, analyze and compare the expected results; select and implement plans; evaluate the effect. Decision-making can be aimed at a specific patient, through decision analysis to select the best treatment for the patient, or for groups with the same attributes, through decision analysis to determine the first-line or preferred treatment measures, alternative treatment measures.

19.2.2 Building a decision analysis model

The decision tree and Markov model are the two most commonly used clinical decision analysis models. The decision tree model is the most commonly used, especially in the decision analysis of acute diseases or short-term projects, and the Markov model is mainly chosen for chronic diseases. For complex clinical problems, the decision tree and Markov model can be combined.

19.2.2.1 Decision tree model

The steps of decision tree model analysis include: clarify the purpose of the analysis based on clinical problems; determine alternatives based on clinical experience and literature reading and evaluation; and list all possible important clinical outcomes of each plan; establish a decision tree model; determine the analysis timeframe and decision evaluation criteria based on literature data; determine the probability of various clinical outcomes of each plan; clarify outcome indicators and profit and loss values of various clinical outcomes; comprehensively analyze and evaluate the plan; and conduct a sensitivity analysis of the possible uncertainties of the parameters used in the analysis.

The following figure (Figure 19-1) shows the analysis principle of the decision tree model.

The triangle at the far right represents the final outcome. The utility value of recovery and healthy survival is 1.0, and death is 0. Because total gastrectomy has a serious impact on the patient's quality of life, the utility value is 0.6. However, for non-gastric cancer, its' degree of influence on the quality of life after surgery is slightly lighter, with a utility value of 0.8. Draw a tree structure from left to right in chronological order. Each branch represents a clinical result or decision within a period of time. Use different nodes to represent decision-making, clinical outcome or final outcome. Usually, small squares are used to indicate the decision points where the decision maker wants to compare different options. The branches extending from the decision point represent the different options being compared. The nodes shown in circles are often called probability nodes, and the branches connected to the probability nodes represent possible occurrences, event or clinical outcome.

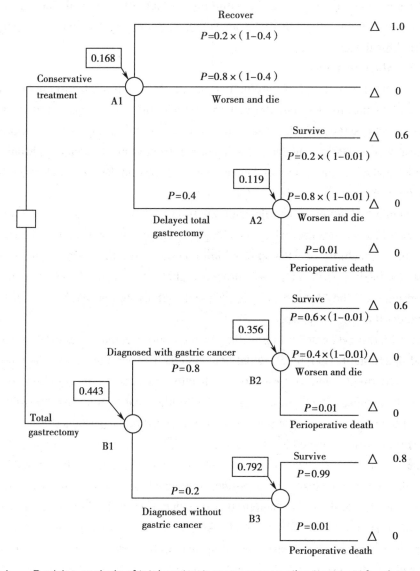

Figure 19-1   Decision analysis of total gastrectomy or conservative treatment for giant gastric ulcer

In decision tree analysis, first, determine the timeframe according to the specific disease, and the analysis period is usually a disease cycle. Next, determine the profit and loss value of various clinical outcomes, that is, quantify the various results. After the decision tree is established, calculate the expected utility value. It is calculated by multiplying the probability and utility values starting from the rightmost end of the decision tree branches, and then add the values of each branch on a node, step by step from right to left. Finally, calculate the expected utility of each scheme.

In addition, sensitivity analysis and threshold analysis are required for the model. The lack of relevant research to provide the required parameters for analysis is the main cause of uncertainty in decision analysis, and it is also an important factor affecting the reliability of clinical decision-making results. Sensitivity analysis can analyze only one factor at a time (single-factor sensitivity analysis), or simultaneously analyze the combined effects of two or all factors (two-factor sensitivity analysis, probability sensitivity analysis). The scope of the analysis depends on the source of the clinical data.

19.2.2.2　Markov model

In the natural development of chronic diseases, there is a process of conversion between different states of the disease, but the general trend is that the disease gradually worsens, complications occur, and eventually lead to death. Decision tree analysis is not appropriate for chronic diseases. The Markov model can analyze recurrent clinical events in chronic diseases. Markov model analysis requires a lot of calculations, and relevant decision analysis software such as TreeAge Pro can be used.

The principle of Markov model decision analysis is to divide the researched disease into several different health states according to the degree of its impact on health, and then according to the transition probability of each state within a certain period of time, estimate the health outcome or cost of disease development through multiple loop calculations by combining the resource consumption and health results of each state. Applying the Markov model to decision analysis includes the following steps.

Establish Markov state according to the research purpose and the natural outcome of the disease, and determine the possible mutual conversions between the states. The whole disease process is usually divided into several different health states according to the research purpose and the natural outcome of the disease, the so-called Markov state. Simulate all possible events as the process of transitioning from one state to another, and divide the period to be analyzed into the same time period, which is called Markov cycle period. In each cycle, the patient may transition from one state to another. Figure 19-2 shows the principal diagram of Markov model decision analysis. In the decision analysis of preventing esophageal varices bleeding from cirrhosis, the six Markov states in the figure are: comprehensive state after rebleeding (comprehensive state, re-endoscopic treatment or re-TIPS comprehensive treatment status), no rebleeding and stable state of hepatic encephalopathy (well), rebleeding state (RB), hepatic encephalopathy state (HE), rebleeding and hepatic encephalopathy simultaneous state (RB+HE) and death state (death). The arrow between the states in the figure indicates that the patient can transition from one state to another in a cycle.

Determine the cycle period and the transition probability between the states in each cycle. The length of the Markov cycle is usually set according to clinical significance. For esophageal varices bleeding from cirrhosis, a cycle usually lasts for 1 year. After determining the Markov state and cycle period, estimate the patient's stay in each state or the possibility of transitioning to another state based on relevant clinical research or epidemiological results. The transition probability between states in each subsequent cycle can be fixed, or different transition probabilities can be determined according to the actual condition of the disease.

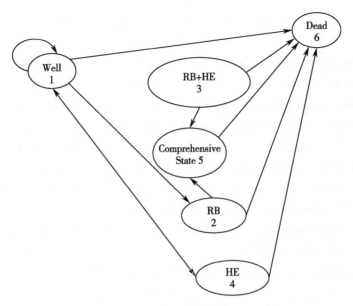

Figure 19-2   Six-state Markov model

Determine the utility value of each health state. It can also be formulated in terms of time, efficacy, safety, quality of life, and economic indicators according to the impact of specific diseases on patients and specific conditions.

Estimate the utility of the entire analysis period by calculation. First, calculate the distribution probability of each state in each cycle. Then, calculate the utility value and cumulative utility value of each cycle according to the probability and utility value of different states.

Perform sensitivity analysis. Like the decision tree analysis, the Markov model analysis should also be based on baseline analysis to perform sensitivity analysis to determine the stability of the analysis results and the main uncertain factors that affect the analysis results.

19.3   How to read and evaluate the literature on decision analysis

The evaluation of decision analysis literature is similar to other studies, and the following aspects should be considered comprehensively.

19.3.1   Is the research design reasonable and are the analysis results true and reliable?

19.3.1.1   Does the evaluated plan include all important strategies and clinical outcomes?

First of all, we should clarify how many different options are in the decision tree, what kind of disease state transitions are in the Markov model, and whether all important strategies and clinical outcomes are included.

19.3.1.2 Is the clinical plan for comparison a commonly used clinical plan?

In the decision analysis, the researcher should not only point out which clinical strategies to compare, but also give a detailed description of the various clinical strategies to be compared. Explain the respective advantages and disadvantages of the schemes, as well as the reasons for the comparison and the difficulties in clinical selection.

19.3.1.3 Have all relevant clinical results been considered?

Clinical decision analysis and research should be based on the patient or the whole society, that is, it should include all important clinical benefits and risks. It should be ensured that the trade-offs reflected in the model are the current patients and society's concerns, such as treatment effects, adverse reactions, quality of life, cost-effectiveness, compliance, etc.

19.3.1.4 Are clear and reasonable methods used to obtain and determine the parameters required for analysis?

Decision analysis needs to synthesize a large amount of information. Researchers need to search literature, consult experts and visit patients. First, it is necessary to search the literature comprehensively, evaluate the authenticity, validity and consistency of these studies, and further use quantitative analysis methods (such as meta-analysis) to estimate the possibility or probability of clinical events, and assign these probabilities to the branches of each node in the analysis model. The paper should report the literature retrieval, source and calculation method of the probability used, and list the relevant literature.

19.3.1.5 Is the setting of the utility value reasonable, and is the source reliable?

The utility value represents the quantitative measurement value of various outcomes in the decision analysis. The author should explain the method of assignment in the text. The clearer the understanding of the possible outcomes and the setting of utility values, the more reliable the utility value assignment method.

19.3.1.6 Are there any uncertain factors that may affect the results in the choice of data? Has a sensitivity analysis been performed? Is the sensitivity analysis reasonable?

Most of the parameters used in decision analysis come from published research results. These results often have the problem of inaccurate estimation, which is usually manifested by a wide confidence interval. It is necessary to carefully understand which factors and in what scopes the author makes sensitivity analysis, and make clear whether these analyses are reasonable.

19.3.2 Evaluate the results of decision-making analysis

On the basis of determining that the decision-making analysis method is reasonable and the results are reliable, we should further clarify how much benefit the proposed scheme of the research may bring to patients, and how credible the benefit is.

19.3.2.1 What is the evaluation result obtained in the baseline analysis?

Baseline analysis means that the probability or other parameters set in the analysis is the best estimate according to the analyst, that is, the estimate that is closest to the overall level. Decision analysis is to compare the total "expected utility" that may be obtained by each plan, and choose the most effective plan as the recommended best plan.

19.3.2.2　How strong is the evidence used in the analysis? Will the uncertainty of the evidence affect the results of the decision analysis?

The research results with relatively strong research design, reliable method and high quality are selected as the estimated value. At the same time, the sensitivity analysis of the important parameters of the model is carried out.

19.3.3　Application of research results

If all aspects of the research are performed well and the clinical patient situation is consistent with the research subjects in the literature analysis, then the research conclusions can be used to help us make clinical decisions.

19.4　Cases of evidence-based clinical decision analysis

19.4.1　Clinical case

A 52-year-old male patient with hepatitis B cirrhosis had bleeding from esophageal gastric varices, with liver function Child-Pugh grade B. After active blood volume supplementation, reduction of portal pressure, inhibition of gastric acid, hemostasis and other medications, the bleeding stopped. In order to prevent rebleeding, what kind of treatment should I choose?

By consulting related literature, we can find that after rupture of esophageal and gastric varices in patients with liver cirrhosis and portal hypertension, the rate of rebleeding in 1 year is as high as 50%, and the risk of bleeding to death is also high. The efficacy of drug therapy is not good, and surgical treatment has many limitations and drawbacks. Endoscopic variceal ligation + beta-blocker (EVL + β-B) and interventional therapy (transjugular intrahepatic portosystemic stent-shunt, TIPSS) are choices made by clinicians for most patients. How do clinicians recommend treatment measures for patients in terms of efficacy, adverse reactions, and treatment costs?

19.4.2　Clinical problems

For patients with hepatitis B liver cirrhosis and portal hypertension, esophageal and gastric varices bleeding, should I choose combined endoscopic and drug therapy or interventional therapy?

19.4.3　Literature search

By searching related databases, the corresponding literature can be retrieved.

19.4.4　Research process and research results

Refer to the third section of this chapter for literature evaluation (Table 19-1). The literature concludes: The results of a 7-year baseline simulation study (Figure 19-3) showed that the expected cost of EVL+β-blocker is \$7 444.25/person, and 1.98 quality-adjusted life years can be obtained. The expected cost of the TIPSS stent graft was 13 151.69$/person, and 2.34 quality-adjusted life years can be obtained. In the 7th year, ICER=$16 001.74/QALY. Based on China's willingness to pay threshold (WTP=3GDP, $19 887), it can be concluded that the covered stent TIPSS has a cost-effective advantage over endoscopic band ligation combined with β-blocker therapy. It was cost-effective if the stent graft is introduced into China for no more than $5 401.52 (¥33 627.04).

Table 19-1   1-year, 3-year, 5-year, 7-year baseline analysis results

Treatment plan	Time	Cost /$	LYs	QALYs	ICER LY/Per LY per QALY
EVL+β-B	1 year	4 492.47	0.95	0.64	
TIPSS		10 175.96	0.94	0.64	—
EVL+β-B	3 year	6 188.65	2.12	1.41	
TIPSS		11 560.49	2.25	1.51	42 655.63 55 963.19
EVL+β-B	5 year	7 026.18	2.71	1.79	
TIPSS		12 513.84	3.04	2.03	16 841.08 23 469.50
EVL+β-B	7 year	7 444.25	3.00	1.98	
TIPSS		13 151.69	3.51	2.34	11 274.48 16 001.74

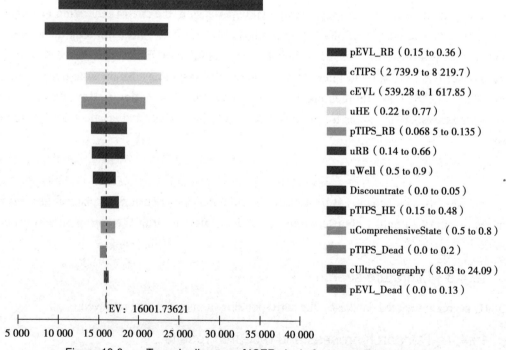

Figure 19-3   Tornado diagram of ICER single factor sensitivity analysis

The results of univariate sensitivity analysis (Figure 19-4) show that the rebleeding rate of endoscopic band ligation combined with β-blocker therapy was the factor that has the greatest impact on ICER, followed by the cost of TIPSS treatment and hepatic encephalopathy utility value, etc. Therefore, when choosing endoscopic treatment, clinicians need to continuously improve its effect; when choosing interventional treatment, the cost of stent is an important factor influencing the choice. Centralized procurement by the state to control and reduce stents and other consumables is an effective measure.

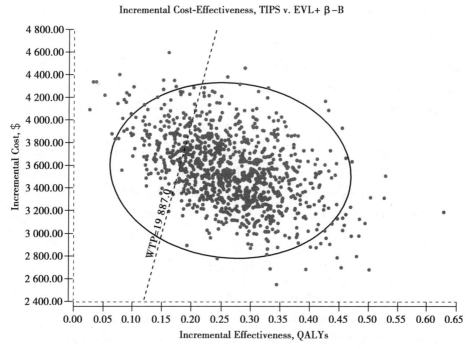

Figure 19-4   ICER scatter plot for probabilistic sensitivity analysis

The study conducted a two-factor sensitivity analysis (Figure 19-5) and a threshold analysis (Table 19-2). The results shown that when the price of the stent graft was not higher than $5 401.52, TIPSS was cost-effective.

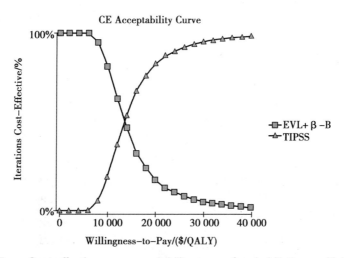

Figure 19-5   Cost-effectiveness acceptability curve of probabilistic sensitivity analysis

Table 19-2　Threshold analysis results

Variable	Baseline value	threshold
Risk of **rebleeding** in the endoscopic treatment group	0.25	0.21
Risk of **rebleeding** in the TIPSS group	0.10	0.13
Stent graft price	$4 015.74	$5 401.52
TIPS treatment cost	$5 479.80	$6 865.58
Endoscopic band ligation treatment cost	$1 078.57	$658.63
Hepatic encephalopathy utility value	0.55	0.35

In addition, the study conducted a probability sensitivity analysis. Through Monte Carlo simulation calculations, the incremental cost-effect chart (Figure 19-4) shown that when the willingness to pay threshold in China was $19 887, 83% of the simulations show that TIPSS was cost-effective.

From the acceptability curve in the probabilistic sensitivity analysis (Figure 19-5), it can be seen that if WTP>$13 920.9/QALY, greater than 50% simulations shown that TIPS was cost-effective. When WTP was greater than $39 774/QALY, more than 98% of the simulations shown that TIPSS was cost-effective, that is, almost all patients undergo TIPSS treatment were cost-effective.

Summary

In short, decision analysis exists in every process of clinical treatment of diseases. Evidence-based clinical decision-making not only allows us to reasonably choose diagnostic measures, but also allows us to avoid vague and empirical treatment methods when dealing with patients, make clinical decision-making more scientific and maximize the interests of patients and society.

(Chen Shiyao, Li Ying)

20

Evidence-based medicine for social advancement

Learning objective

To be familiar with evidence-based practice on social advancement including field investigation, questionnaire survey, simulation test, decision and promotion on social perception and regulation.

China's current car ownership is growing rapidly year by year, accompanied by rapidly increasing car accidents. Some child passengers die from accidents and child road trauma is becoming a significant public health problem in China.

Evidence-based medicine practice is not limited to the formulation and implementation of medical decisions, but also enhances the understanding of social subjects as well as recent regulations and serves as reference for legislation promotion based on the updating of evidence and the collection of data, contributing to the health of patients and the harmony of society. Evidence-based medicine practice for the population needs to identify real public problems, conduct researches, and generate evidence to help alteration of social perception and regulation for social advancement.

20.1　Background

World Health Organization (WHO) estimates that global burden of road traffic injuries will increase from the ninth in 2004 to the third by 2030. In 2000, 10 642 children aged 0~4 years and 16 034 children aged 5~14 years respectively died of road traffic injuries in China.

Data show that the number of motor vehicle drivers in China had exceeded 199.77 million by the end of 2009. With the increase in car ownership in China, it becomes increasingly urgent to take actions to prevent child passenger injury. Research on child passenger safety should focus on child passenger safety standards, requirements, design, injury prevention and formulation of regulations.

20.2　Formulate questions

It is a problem of relationship between child passengers' seating position or restraint practices and child road traffic injuries.

First, we need to ask the following questions.

How is the use of child safety seats and restraint practice in China?

What are the factors influencing child passengers' use of restraint practices in China?

What is the relationship between child passengers' different seating position or restraint practices and child road traffic injuries?

20.3　Current situation investigation

20.3.1　Child passenger seating and restraint practices in China

Direct observational studies of child passenger safety practice were still lacking in China. To have an idea of actual seating and restraint practice, the researcher conducted a cross-sectional observational study to describe child passenger safety practices in Shanghai in 2009. Observations of restraint practices were made at toll-gates of the G2 highway in Shanghai, to understand the actual seating position of child passengers, the use of restraint practices and the factors influencing. Pilot observations over 3 consecutive mornings (between 9:00 a.m. and 11:00 a.m.) identified that cars and other passenger vehicles accounted for 93% and 7% of total traffic respectively, of which 10% of cars transported child passengers. We used multivariate binomial regression to estimate the adjusted risk ratio (RR) for the two outcome measures, proper rear seating compared with other suboptimal seating position and any restraint use compared with no restraint use, respectively (Table 20-1).

Table 20-1　Risk ratios for children being restrained or properly rear seated when traveling in cars, Shanghai 2009

Variables	Risk ratios (95% confidence interval)			
	Properly rear seated		Traveling restrained	
	Unadjusted	Adjusted	Unadjusted	Adjusted
Age group				
≤4 years	**0.36 (0.28 ~ 0.45)** *P*<0.000 1)	**0.35 (0.28 ~ 0.44)** *P* <0.000 1	0.73 (0.39~1.36)	0.91 (0.43~1.93)
>4 years(referent)				
Gender				
Male	0.92 (0.82~1.03)	0.96 (0.87~1.06)	1.05 (0.82~1.35)	1.07 (0.65~1.75)
Female (referent)				

continue

Variables	Risk ratios (95% confidence interval)			
	Properly rear seated		Traveling restrained	
	Unadjusted	Adjusted	Unadjusted	Adjusted
Driver belt use				
No	1.04 (0.90~1.21)	0.99 (0.87~1.12)	**0.09 (0.01 ~ 0.64)** *P*= 0.016 2	**0.09 (0.01 ~ 0.60)** *P*= 0.013 7
Yes (referent)				
Number of children in a car				
Single	**0.74 (0.64 ~ 0.85)** *P*<0.000 1	**0.84 (0.74 ~ 0.96)** *P*= 0.012 4	3.52 (0.50~24.94)	3.33 (0.55~20.01)
Multiple(referent)	0.94 (0.72~1.22)	1.00 (0.87~1.15)	0.94 (0.49~1.81)	1.03 (0.57~1.86)
Rear seated alone				
No	n/a	n/a	1.11 (0.67~1.84)	0.89 (0.49~1.61)
Yes (referent)				
Traveling restrained				
No	1.05 (0.82~1.35)	1.07 (0.82~1.39)	n/a	n/a
Yes (referent)				
Accompanying adult passengers				
No	**0.77 (0.57 ~ 1.04)** *P*= 0.083 4	**0.66 (0.49 ~ 0.89)** *P*= 0.006 6	**5.09 (2.94 ~ 8.82)** *P*<0.000 1	**5.28 (2.86 ~ 9.76)** *P*<0.000 1
Yes (referent)				

Note: Children sitting on adult laps in the rear was not counted in the rear-seated alone category.

This study demonstrated that in Shanghai, China children commonly used suboptimal seating positions such as sitting in the front or on an adult's lap (in the front or rear). Restraint use was relatively rare among child car passengers in Shanghai, China. Child car passengers traveling with unrestrained drivers were less likely to use any type of restraint than those traveling with restrained drivers (RR 0.09, 95%CI 0.01~0.60). Compared with children accompanied by other adult passengers, those traveling without adult passengers were more likely to be restrained (RR 5.28, 95%CI 2.86~9.76). Compared with children aged over 4 years, younger children were less likely to be seated properly in the rear seat of cars (RR 0.35, 95%CI 0.28~0.44). Compared with children accompanied by other adult passengers, those traveling without adult passengers were less likely to be properly rear-seated (RR 0.66, 95%CI 0.49~0.89). Children traveling in cars where there were no other children were less likely to be rear seated than those traveling with other children in the car (RR 0.84, 95%CI 0.74~0.96). Given that rear seating and correct use of size-appropriate restraints are well known to reduce injury risk among child passengers, the identified gap in good practice indicates an urgent need for action.

20.3.2 Factors influencing child passengers' use of restraint in China

To clarify the factors influencing child seating position and the use of restraint, the researcher conducted parental surveys in five randomly selected kindergartens in the Songjiang and Pudong districts of Shanghai from October 2008 to October 2009 to investigated the parents on child passenger safety knowledge by questionnaires and to further explore the factors related to child seating and child passenger safety.

A total of 1010 parents participated in the survey, with a participation rate of 100%. The final study population comprised information for 970 children aged 3~7 years enrolled at kindergartens during the study, whose characteristics were similar to those of 40 children (5%) excluded from the study due to missing information on seating position, parent's education level and family income: the proportion of no restraint use in the study population was 60.8% (vs 65.0% in those excluded), the proportion of children aged ≤4 years was 44.0% (vs 42.5%) and the proportion of boys was 56.0% (vs 54.4%). In this study, 78.0% of parents reported having heard of child restraints (including booster seats) but very few owned them (about 5.9%, $n=57$) or used them (about 1.2%, $n=12$), whereas 29.4% ($n=285$) of parents reported that their children traveled in cars almost every day. Among all children, 83.1% ($n=806$) of parents reported that their child always sat separately in the rear seat (i.e., not on an adult's lap), and 39.2% ($n=380$) of parents reported that their children used some form of restraint.

Younger children (aged≤4 years) were less likely to be seated in the rear compared with children aged>4 years (RR 0.82, 95%CI 0.77~0.87). Compared with parents who were unlicensed, parents holding a driver's license were slightly less likely to report that their child occupied an optimal seating position (RR 0.95, 95%CI 0.91~0.99), but they were more likely to report restraint use by their children (RR 1.44, 95%CI 1.18~1.75). Parents with a tertiary education were slightly more likely to report that their child occupied an optimal seating position compared with those who did not have tertiary education (RR 1.08, 95%CI 1.03~1.13) (Table 20-2). It was found that misunderstanding existed among parents on child's sitting on an adult's lap and airbag impact and child passenger rear seating rate was high while restraints utilization rate was low. It suggested that parents were lack of child passenger safety knowledge.

Table 20-2 RRs for children being restrained or seated in the rear when traveling in cars, Shanghai 2008—2009

Variables	RR (95% CI)			
	Always rear seated		Traveling restrained	
	Unadjusted	Adjusted	Unadjusted	Adjusted
Age group				
≤4 years	0.83 (0.78 ~ 0.88)	0.82 (0.77 ~ 0.87)	1.05 (0.90~1.23)	1.04 (0.89~1.21)
>4 years(referent)				

continue

Variables	RR (95% CI)			
	Always rear seated		Traveling restrained	
	Unadjusted	Adjusted	Unadjusted	Adjusted
Child's gender				
Male	1.03 (0.97~1.09)	1.04 (0.99~1.09)	1.06 (0.91~1.25)	1.04 (0.89~1.22)
Female(referent)				
Parental license status				
Yes	0.96 (0.90~1.01)	**0.95 (0.91 ~ 0.99)**	**1.48 (1.22 ~ 1.79)**	**1.44 (1.18 ~ 1.75)**
No(referent)				
Family income				
High	1.05 (0.99~1.11)	1.00 (0.96~1.05)	1.17 (0.99~1.37)	1.06 (0.89~1.26)
Unknown	0.94 (0.72~1.22)	1.00 (0.87~1.15)	0.94 (0.49~1.81)	1.03 (0.57~1.86)
Low(referent)				
Parents' tertiary education				
Yes	1.03 (0.97~1.09)	**1.08 (1.03 ~ 1.13)**	1.16 (0.99~1.36)	1.08 (0.91~1.28)
No(referent)				

20.3.3 Verification of relationship between children's seating position and traffic safety

Is there any relevance between different children seating position or restraint use and road traffic accident occurrence? Studies from foreign countries found that child passengers sitting in the front without any restraint were at the highest traffic accident risk, while rear seating with appropriate restraint got the minimum. The risk of injury is more than three times higher for children who do not use restraint than for those who do use them. Among the rear seats, position behind the driver had the death risk 8.1% lower than the right one. The rear middle position had the lowest death risk of 0.27% only, 65%~71% lower than that of the driver. The rear middle position had the lowest RR of 0.29 and the highest one of 0.35 was right back, especially when tumbling. Although the rear seating can reduce the risk of injury to children passengers, the use of restraint has better effects. A child's sitting in the rear middle together with restraint device use lower the injury risk by 43% than the right side. A survey of 17 980 children in 11 506 car accidents found that the safety of rear seating was less than that of the restraint use, and the front seating increased the risk of injury by 40% compared to rear seating (OR 1.4, 95% CI 1.2~1.7).

Using MADYMO software to simulate the vehicle crash test, we verified the injury risk of different children seating based on the data we obtained from spot observation and parents' surveys. We found that rear seated child passengers in the correct use of appropriate safety seats got the best protection effect, while the most unsafe way was the child seating in the front on an adult's lap.

20.4   Promote alteration of perception and formulation of regulation

20.4.1   Relevant evidences on the children seating and use of restraint in foreign countries

There are some differences in the prevalence of child passengers using the restraint and there are relevant laws and regulations on children's restraint system used in car in Europe, the United States and other developed countries though their regulations on children's age limits vary. At the same time, the United States, Europe, Japan and other developed countries and regions have established a complete system of laws and regulations on the installation and fixation of the child restraint, such as the United States FMVSS 213, the European ECE regulation R44. Japan, Republic of Korea, Singapore and other Asian countries and regions also have the relevant legislation. The legislation is a powerful tool for the prevention of child passenger injury, and it can be seen as a test to ensure the child passenger safety.

In 1997, the U.S. Transportation Safety Board recommended that each state amend child safety laws to mandate children rear seating. There had been 7 states that passed the child's rear seating bill by 2004. The deaths rate and serious injuries rate of child passengers aged 4~15 years decreased by 42% after the *Front Passenger Seat Belt Legislation* passed in North Carolina in 1985. Child passenger injury hospitalization rate and the head injury incidence decreased by 36% and 25% respectively, and the proportion of injured child passengers aged ≤4 years old declined by 25% after the promulgation of *Child Safety Seat Law* in Michigan. The mortality rate and non-fatal injury rate of child passengers under the age of 5 decreased by 33% and 12.5% respectively after *Safety Seat Legislation* promulgated in New Mexico. All the experience has fully demonstrated that appropriate interventions can significantly reduce mortality rate and disability rate of children and adolescents in road traffic trauma. The practice has also showed that child passenger restraint systems such as child safety seats, booster seats, improved safety belt or rear seating can effectively reduce the risk of child passengers' fatal and nonfatal injury.

20.4.2   Evidence-based medicine's promotion on attention to child passengers' safety law

China has been the world's largest consumer of new cars, so it's necessary to be more attention to the safety of children passengers. Results from evidence-based practice could help clarify social issues, change the perception and raise awareness. Appropriate interventions can significantly reduce mortality of children and adolescents in road traffic injury and disability. China should continue their efforts to develop and improve the child passenger safety legislation, strengthen the education of the community and parents to promote child passenger safety.

Finally, with direct child passenger safety observation data, Shanghai parents' safety surveys and simulation of vehicle crash test, study results illustrated social issues to promote change of perception, contributing to formulation and revision of regulations. The first mandatory national standards on motor vehicle child restraints in China—*The Standards on Motor Vehicle Child Restraint System* (GB 27887—2011) was formally implemented on July 1st 2012. It helped improve the public attention to the child passenger safety; in addition, it was also a strong constraint to the child safety seat production enterprises and automobile manufacturing enterprises. *Modified Decisions on Regulations of Shanghai Municipality on the Protection for juveniles* was implemented on March 1, 2014. It is legislated that any car taken by child ≤4 years should be equipped with child safety seat and children under 12 years old shall be not arranged to the copilot seat.

Summary

The evidence-based medicine pushes forward the social development. As to the evidence-based medicine, medical decision-making including health policy formulation should be made on the basis of the best available clinical researches, it emphasizes the evidences advanced with the times, constantly updated, the collection of sufficient and reliable information, forms the assessment, and then formulates policies and regulations which are put forward according to the result of evaluation, thus ultimately ensure the patients benefits, achieve best cost-effectiveness. The practice object of public health is the crowd, which is different from clinical practice focusing on individual patient. In the field of public health, constructing the appropriate questions in order to find out the real reasons to some events and related factors is more important. Medical behavior or some decisions of the intervention would cause our attention and require critical appraisal as no matter doctors or our patients doubt on it. It requires our evidence-based medicine to clarify what kind of impact it will bring on our patients step by step.

This chapter proposed the important public health problem of road traffic injuries among children from the perspective of evidence-based medicine. It investigated the factors that influenced the child passenger safety by observation on child passenger seating, restraint practices in Shanghai and parental surveys, evaluated child passenger safety with different seating positions by vehicle collision test practice. It illustrated the relationship between child safety seating or restraint use and children's road traffic injury risk, combined with the international improvement of children's road traffic injury after the legislation of restraint use, aimed to promote the legislation on child passenger safety in our society, promote the safety of child passengers.

Evidence-based medicine has great significance for conducting social work and promoting social development. Evidence-based medicine also attaches great importance to the accumulation of research evidence and shortens the distance between research and practice.

Evidence-based practice is a possible strategy to promote social development, transform our daily experienced practice to the scientific theory guided practice, and ultimately realize social advancement.

(Pan Shuming)

循证医学基础模拟卷 A

一、单选题

1. 循证医学的核心思想,下列不恰当的是(D)
   A. 遵循证据的临床医学
   B. 临床决策的科学化
   C. 任何医疗干预都应建立在当前研究的最佳证据之上
   D. 只能根据文献上的证据进行相关治疗
   E. 使患者获得最大利益

2. 下列研究证据的结论强度最弱的是(A)
   A. 大样本病例分析结果
   B. 有阳性结果的单中心随机对照临床试验
   C. 队列研究结果
   D. Meta 分析结果
   E. 病例对照研究

3. 在治疗性研究中下列描述错误的是(E)
   A. 随机化分组是评价治疗性试验时最重要的标准
   B. 没有随机化隐藏得出的治疗效果往往小于随机化隐藏的结果
   C. 随机化使研究对象有同等的机会被分配到治疗组或对照组
   D. 一般要求失访率不小于 20%
   E. 进行双盲试验研究中,不存在随机化隐藏的问题

4. 在对有关预后的文章进行评价时,以下最重要的是(A)
   A. 观察疾病的预后是否都有一致的起点
   B. 是否介绍了研究对象的情况和病例的来源
   C. 是否有客观的预后指标
   D. 预后估计是否采用盲法
   E. 随访时间是否足够长

5. 若要进行白血病病因和危险因素研究,最适宜选用以下哪种设计方法(C)
   A. 横断面研究
   B. 大样本病例分析
   C. 病例对照研究
   D. 队列研究
   E. 临床试验

6. 若您拟设计一份类风湿关节炎生命质量量表，一般不纳入以下哪个方面（A）

    A. 药物不良反应   B. 日常生活能力

    C. 关节疼痛程度   D. 关节活动度

    E. 社会角色能力

7. 关于系统综述的说法，下列错误的是（C）

    A. 采用临床流行病学方法严格评价文献

    B. 选择高质量的文章进行综合

    C. 一定是定量综合分析

    D. 结论可靠可信

    E. 收集的文献中包括未发表的文章

8. 在应用一项临床指南之前，必须考虑的原则是（E）

    A. 同时考虑研究结果和具体指导的原则

    B. 只考虑研究结果的原则

    C. 只考虑具体指导的原则

    D. 只考虑其真实性的原则

    E. 同时考虑其真实性、研究结果和具体指导的原则

9. 一项前瞻性研究结果发现，饮酒者比不饮酒者患肺癌可能性更大，但分层研究发现吸烟者中饮酒者与不饮酒者患肺癌的危险性相同，非吸烟者中饮酒者与不饮酒者患肺癌的危险性也相同，这是下述哪项原因造成的（D）

    A. 选择偏移，选择的患者既有吸烟也有非吸烟患者

    B. 易感性偏移，饮酒的人更容易吸烟

    C. 失访偏移，该前瞻性研究可能有大量失访

    D. 混杂偏移，吸烟是混杂因子

    E. 混杂偏移，饮酒是混杂因子

二、案例题

1. 男性，67 岁。患者因"间歇性上腹部不适伴体重下降 1 年"入院。胃镜检查显示胃窦存在巨大溃疡，病理活检明确为胃窦中分化腺癌，免疫组化示 IIER2（+++，即 *HER2* 基因扩增），腹部增强 CT 示腹膜后多发淋巴结转移及肝多发转移。

问题：

（1）患者的临床特征是什么？（B）

（2）最佳的干预措施是什么？（D）

（3）最佳的干预措施是选择什么作为对照措施的？（E）

（4）希望达到什么样的预期结果？（F）

    A. 晚期胃癌

    B. HER2 阳性的晚期胃癌

    C. 手术

    D. 姑息性化疗联合分子靶向治疗（曲妥珠单抗）

    E. 姑息性化疗

    F. 长期生存

2. 女性，21 岁。某重点大学大三学生，于 2016 年 4 月 19 日以下腹痛为主诉到妇产科就诊，B 超检查提示：盆腔两处占位性病变，宫底偏右性质待定，考虑来源于双侧卵巢、盆腹腔大量积液。血常规提示白细胞总数 14.51×10⁹/L，中性粒细胞比例 74.5%，C 反应蛋白 10mg/L（正常低于 0.5mg/L），提示存在感染或炎症。

问题：

（1）对该患者的疾病进行个体描述属于（A）

（2）要了解卵巢变化在人群中的总体发生率应采用那种描述方法（B）

（3）要了解发生卵巢变化的原因可以采用的设计类型是（C）

（4）可以明确与卵巢变化有关病因的设计类型是（D、E）

（5）论证强度最高的设计类型是（E）

    A. 病例报告

    B. 横断面调查

    C. 病例对照研究

    D. 队列研究

    E. 临床试验

三、判断题

1. 病例对照研究不适于研究发病率比较低的疾病。（×）

2. 随机分配可以使治疗组和对照组均衡可比，因此随机化是评价治疗性研究的重要标准之一。（√）

3. 诊断试验评价本质上是横断面研究设计。（√）

4. 系统评价是一种二次研究方法，每篇系统评价均要进行定量分析，即 meta 分析。（×）

5. 存在混杂因素一定会导致混杂偏倚的产生。（×）

四、简答题

1. 循证决策包括的 5 个步骤分别是哪些？

【参考答案】 循证决策的 5 个步骤分别是：①针对具体患者提出并构建临床问题（asking question）；②全面收集有关证据（acquiring evidence）；③严格评价证据（appraising evidence）；④临床应用证据（applying evidence）；⑤后效评价（after assessment）。

2. 证据分析时应该从哪些方面来考虑？

【参考答案】 证据分析应从证据的适用性、可行性以及权衡利弊等方便着手，重点分析"患者与研究证据中纳入的患者特征是否相似""患者可以得到的利益和风险是什么""证据中的干预措施在当地可行性如何"。

Single-choice questions

1. As to the core of evidence-based medicine, which of the following **is inappropriate** (D)
   A. Clinical medicine following evidence
   B. Scientific decision-making
   C. Any medical intervention should be based on the best evidence from current research
   D. Relevant treatment can only be carried out based on literature evidence
   E. Maximize the benefit of patients

2. Which of the following research evidence has the weakest conclusion (A)
   A. Analysis results of large-sample cases
   B. Single-center randomized controlled clinical trials with positive results
   C. Results of cohort studies
   D. Results of meta-analysis
   E. Case-control studies

3. Which of the following is **wrong** in the therapeutic research (E)
   A. Randomization is the most important criterion when evaluating therapeutic trials
   B. The treatment effect obtained without randomization concealment is often less than the result of randomization concealment
   C. Randomization gives the research subjects the same chance to be assigned to the treatment group or the control group
   D. It is generally required that the loss to follow-up rate is not less than 20%
   E. Randomization concealment doesn't matter in the double-blind trial study

4. When evaluating prognosis studies, which of the following is the most important (A)
   A. Whether the prognosis of the disease has the same start point?
   B. Whether the characteristics of the research subjects and the source of the cases are introduced?
   C. Whether there are objective prognostic indicators?
   D. Whether blind method is conducted to estimate the prognosis?
   E. Whether the follow-up time is long enough?

5. To study the etiology and risk factors of leukemia, which of the following design methods

is most appropriate (C)

    A. Cross-sectional study

    B. Analysis of large-sample cases

    C. Case-control study

    D. Cohort study

    E. Clinical trial

6. If you plan to design a rheumatoid arthritis quality of life scale, which of the following is generally **not included** (A)

    A. Adverse reaction of drugs

    B. Ability of daily life

    C. Joint pain

    D. Motion range of joint

    E. Social skill

7. As to the system review, which of the following is **wrong** (C)

    A. It strictly evaluates the literature with clinical epidemiological methods

    B. It selects high-quality literature for synthesis

    C. It must be a quantitative comprehensive analysis

    D. Its conclusion is reliable

    E. The collected literature includes unpublished articles

8. Before applying a clinical guideline, which of the following must be considered (E)

    A. Consider the research results and specific guidelines at the same time

    B. Only consider research results

    C. Only consider specific guidelines

    D. Only consider validity

    E. Consider validity, research results and specific guidelines at the same time

9. A prospective study found that drinking alcohol is more likely to develop lung cancer than non-drinking. However, a stratified study found that drinkers have the same risk of developing lung cancer as non-drinkers among smokers; the situation is the same among non-smokers. Which of the following can explain the result (D)

    A. Selection bias: the selected patients consist of both smokers and non-smokers

    B. Susceptibility bias: drinkers are more likely to smoke

    C. Follow-up bias: the study may have a large number of lost to follow-up

    D. Confounding bias: smoking is the confounding factor

    E. Confounding bias: drinking is the confounding factor

Case question

1. A 67-year-old man was admitted to our hospital because of "intermittent epigastric discomfort with weight loss for 1 year". He underwent gastroscopy which revealed a large ulcer at the gastric antrum-body. Biopsy specimen led to the diagnosis of a moderately differentiated adenocarcinoma and immunohistochemistry (IHC) showed HER2 (3+) (means *HER2* gene amplification). Computed tomography (CT) showed two swollen para-aortic lymph nodes and multiple liver metastases.

Questions:

(1) What is the clinical characteristic of the patient? (B)

(2) What is the best intervention? (D)

(3) What is the control to the best intervention measure? (E)

(4) What is the expected result? (F)

    A. Advanced gastric cancer

    B. HER2 positive advanced gastric cancer

    C. Surgery

    D. Palliative chemotherapy combined with molecular targeted therapy (trastuzumab)

    E. Palliative chemotherapy

    F. Long-term survival

2. Miss Ma, 21, was a junior student at a key university. On April 19th, 2016, she attended the obstetrics and gynecology department due to abdominal pain. B-scan ultrasonography showed: there were two pelvic space-occupying lesions, the property of the one on the right side of the uterine fundus remained to be determined, possibly affected by the large amount of effusion in both the ovary and the pelvic cavity. Blood routine indicated that the total number of leukocytes was 14.51×10^9 /L, Neutrophil ratio was 74.5%, and C-reactive protein was 10mg/L (normally less than 0.5mg/L), indicating the presence of infection or inflammation.

Questions:

(1) Individual description of the patient's disease belongs to (A)

(2) To get an overview of the overall incidence of ovarian changes in the population, which design should be used (B)

(3) To investigate the causes of ovarian changes, which design should be used (C)

(4) To clarify the etiology related to ovarian changes, which design should be used (D, E)

(5) The design type with the highest demonstration intensity is (E)

    A. Case report

    B. Cross-sectional study

    C. Case-control study

    D. Cohort study

    E. Clinical trial

True or false

1. Case-control studies are not suitable for studying diseases with relatively low incidence. (×)

2. Random allocation can make the treatment group and the control group balanced and comparable, so randomization is one of the important criteria for evaluating therapeutic research. (√)

3. Evaluation of diagnostic test is essentially a cross-sectional study. (√)

4. Systematic review is a secondary research, and each systematic review needs to be quantitatively analyzed, that is, meta-analysis. (×)

5. The existence of confounding factors will definitely lead to the production of confounding bias. (×)

Short-answer questions

1. What are the 5 steps for evidence-based decision-making?

[Reference answer] 5 steps for evidence-based decision-making: asking and building clinical questions for specific patients (asking question); comprehensive collection of relevant evidence (acquiring evidence); strict evaluation of evidence (appraising evidence); clinical application of evidence (applying evidence); after assessment.

2. What should be considered when analyzing evidence?

[Reference answer] Evidence analysis should consider the applicability, feasibility of the evidence, the advantages and disadvantages. The following points need to be emphasized: Whether the characteristics of your patient are similar to those included in the research evidence? What are the benefits and risks of patients? How feasible is the intervention in the local area?

循证医学基础模拟卷B

一、单选题

1. 关于循证医学检索资源的来源，下列描述错误的是（B）
   A. 应包含所有已发表的文献
   B. 不应包含灰色文献
   C. 需要跟踪相关论文的参考文献
   D. 非电子版资源需要手工检索
   E. 有时需要与专家互通信息

2. PubMed 是哪种类型的数据库（C）
   A. 引文数据库
   B. 事实数据库
   C. 文摘数据库
   D. 全文数据库
   E. 以上都不正确

3. 产生选择偏倚的根本原因可以认为是（B）
   A. 不选对照
   B. 样本缺乏代表性
   C. 调查方法不统一
   D. 回忆不准确
   E. 没有进行配比

4. 用脱落细胞巴氏染色法检查宫颈癌确诊患者，患者中有 85% 的人检查结果为阳性，说明下列哪项指标为 85%（A）
   A. 敏感度
   B. 特异度
   C. 阳性预测值
   D. 阴性预测值
   E. 约登指数

5. 在一个精心设计的卵巢癌治疗的临床试验中，提供某种新药的患者 1 年的缓解率为 30%，提供安慰剂的患者为 20%。P 值为 0.4。以下最能说明对这个结果的解释的是（E）
   A. 两种治疗方法都有效
   B. 两种治疗方法都无效
   C. 本研究的统计力为 60%。
   D. 治疗效果的最佳估计是 0.4
   E. 没有足够的信息确定一种治疗方法是否比另一种更好

6. 随机对照临床试验及观察性研究 meta 分析均适用的规范为（A）
   A. PRISMA 声明
   B. QUOROM 声明

  C. MOOSE 声明　　　　　　　　　　D. STROBE 声明

  E. STARD 声明

7. 循证临床指南中常采用 GRADE 证据评估和推荐意见分级系统,如果推荐意见是 1A,说明(C)

  A. 1 类证据,A 级推荐等级　　　　　B. A 级证据质量,1 类推荐

  C. 高质量证据,强推荐　　　　　　　D. A 级证据等级,弱推荐

  E. 低质量证据,弱推荐

8. 关于药物治疗罕见的慢性副作用,应首先检索的原始研究通常是(D)

  A. 随机对照试验　　　　　　　　　　B. 横断面研究

  C. 病例系列研究　　　　　　　　　　D. 病例对照研究

  E. 队列研究

9. 生命质量评价主要的应用领域不包括(E)

  A. 慢性病干预的疗效评价　　　　　　B. 新药临床试验

  C. 人群和患者的健康状况评价　　　　D. 资源分配、计划和决策制定

  E. 基础病理研究

10. 一位研究者对新生儿黄疸的病因感兴趣,为进行研究,他选择了 100 名患此病的患儿,并同时选择在同一所医院内选择了 100 名未患此病的新生婴儿,然后查阅了婴儿母亲的妇科和分娩记录,以确定产前和分娩中的各种暴露因素,该研究属于何种类型的研究(C)

  A. 现况研究　　　　　　　　　　　　B. 队列研究

  C. 病例对照研究　　　　　　　　　　D. 临床试验研究

  E. 生态学研究

11. 系统综述有关文献的收集过程,下列说法欠妥当的是(E)

  A. 收集检索文献的范围清楚明确

  B. 对所收集到文献质量评价的标准具体客观

  C. 对使用的原始文献研究结论的分析科学有效

  D. 应采用多种渠道和系统的检索方法

  E. 不能使用未发表的文献

12. 循证医学核心思想不包括(D)

  A. 最佳的研究证据　　　　　　　　　B. 医师的临床技能和经验

  C. 患者意愿　　　　　　　　　　　　D. 最先进的实验室

  E. 临床决策个体化

13. 各项筛检试验的正常参考值都有一个范围,普查时希望诊断试验具有(A)

  A. 灵敏度高,假阳性率相对低的标准

  B. 特异度高,假阳性率相对低的标准

  C. 灵敏度高,真阳性率相对低的标准

  D. 特异度高,真阳性率相对低的标准

  E. 特异度高,真阴性率相对高的标准

14. 非小细胞肺癌患者随机分为 2 组,一组用常规化疗,一组用吉非替尼治疗,随访 3 年,比较生存率,化疗组失访率为 25%,吉非替尼组失访率 15%,可以用什么方法来考察失访对结果的影响大小(B)

A. COX 回归模型多因素分析　　　　B. 敏感性分析

C. 剔除失访人群进行分析　　　　　D. ITT 分析

E. PP 分析

15. 健康相关生命质量评价包括哪些方面（E）

A. 生理功能　　　　　　　　　　B. 心理功能

C. 社会角色　　　　　　　　　　D. 财政状况

E. 生理功能，心理功能，社会角色，财政状况

16. 量表的可行性评价不包括下列哪项（C）

A. 完成时间　　　　　　　　　　B. 难易程度

C. 文化调适　　　　　　　　　　D. 条目的可应答性

E. 对患者的风险性

二、案例题

1. 急性脑梗死患者，治疗 90 天后。

问题：

（1）评价预后的主要结局指标是（H）

（2）评价预后的次要结局指标是（G）

A. 血压　　　　　　　　　　　　B. 肝肾功

C. 心电图　　　　　　　　　　　D. 血常规

E. 颅脑 CT　　　　　　　　　　F. 颅脑 MRI

G. Barthel 指数　　　　　　　　H. Rankin 量表评分

2. 两名医师先后分别对 100 名脂肪肝患者进行 B 超检查和肝功检测。

问题：

（1）评价两人 B 超检查结果一致性的指标是（H）

（2）评价两人肝功检测结果一致性的指标是（G）

A. 灵敏度　　　　　　　　　　　B. 特异度

C. 预告值　　　　　　　　　　　D. 似然比

E. X^2 值　　　　　　　　　　　F. t 值

G. 组内相关系数　　　　　　　　H. Kappa 值

三、多选题

1. 循证医学对临床医学的作用与价值，主要体现在（ABCE）

A. 促进临床医学实践，提高医疗水平

B. 可服务于医学教育，培养高质量的人才

C. 可为临床科研的选题立题提供指导

D. 与部分临床学科相关，但和某些临床学科无关

E. 为疾病病因、诊断、治疗及预后研究证据提供一系列评价标准与方法

2. 诊断试验的对照组应包括（ADE）

A. 健康志愿者

B. 具有典型临床表现的患者

  C. 临床表现不典型的患者

  D. 易与所研究疾病相混淆的其他病例

  E. 患有与所研究疾病不同系统的其他疾病的患者

3. 以下哪些途径可以帮助对循证医学检索的检出结果进行选择和评价（ABC）

  A. 阅读文摘   B. 浏览全文

  C. 联系作者   D. 使用主题词检索

  E. 使用逻辑运算符

四、简答题

1. 简述循证医学的"三个基本要素"和"五个实施步骤"。

【参考答案】 循证医学是遵循证据的临床医学，核心思想是医务人员应该认真地、明智地、深思熟虑地运用在临床研究得到的最新、最有力的科学研究信息诊治患者。其是最佳证据与医师临床经验及患者需求和价值观三者的结合。

五个实施步骤包括①提出临床问题：将临床信息转化为可回答的问题；②寻找证据：检索与问题有关的最佳证据；③评价证据：评价证据的真实性、有效性和实用性；④应用证据：将证据评价与临床经验和患者意向结合起来；⑤后效评价：评价实施效果，并进行改进。

2. 验证病因假设的主要研究设计方法有什么？并说明各研究设计方法因果论证的强度。

【参考答案】 （1）病例报告，横断面研究，病例对照研究，队列研究，随机对照试验。（2）就因果论证强度上，试验性研究大于观察性研究，有对照的研究大于无对照的研究。

3. 为评价某减肥药的疗效，某医生设计了一个临床研究。选择 200 例肥胖症妇女，使用该减肥药物治疗 1 个疗程后减肥的有效率为 60%，而同期观察的另 200 名肥胖妇女不服该药，体重无明显变化，该医生认为该减肥药有效。请回答以下问题：

（1）该研究的临床问题是什么？请用 PICO 模式列出。

（2）该研究的设计类型是什么？

（3）根据该研究设计方案，能否得到"减肥药有效"的结论？并说明理由。

【参考答案】 （1）肥胖症妇女（P），使用减肥药（I）与不服药（C）比较，体重（O）是否有变化？（2）非随机对照试验；（3）虽然有对照，却不是随机分组，治疗前的基线情况不明。需进一步采用随机对照的临床试验。

Quiz B

Single-choice questions

1. Which one of the following descriptions about the source of evidence-based medicine retrieval resources is **wrong** (B)

    A. It should include all published literature

    B. It should not include grey literature

    C. It should track references of related literature

    D. Non-electronic resources need to be retrieved manually

    E. Sometimes researchers need to exchange information with experts

2. What type of database is PubMed (C)

    A. Citation database   B. Fact database

    C. Abstract database   D. Full-text database

    E. None of the above

3. The essential cause of selection bias could be (B)

    A. No selected control

    B. The sample is not representative

    C. The investigation method is not uniform

    D. Inaccurate recall

    E. No matching

4. Examining patients with confirmed cervical cancer by Pap staining of exfoliated cells, 85% of the patients showed positive results. Which of the following indicators is 85%? (A)

    A. Sensitivity   B. Specificity

    C. Positive predictive value   D. Negative predictive value

    E. Youden index

5. In a well-designed clinical trial of treatment for ovarian cancer, remission rate at 1 year is 30% in patients offered a new drug and 20% in those offered a placebo. The P value is 0.4. Which of the following best describes the interpretation of this result? (E)

    A. Both treatments are effective

    B. Neither treatment is effective

    C. The statistical power of this study is 60%

D. The best estimate of treatment effect size is 0.4

E. There is insufficient information to decide whether on treatment is better than the other

6. Which of the following is applicable to both randomized controlled clinical trial and observational research meta-analysis (A)

A. PRISMA statement   B. QUOROM statement

C. MOOSE statement   D. STROBE statement

E. STARD statement

7. GRADE is often used in evidence-based clinical guidelines. If the recommendation is 1A, what does it mean? (C)

A. Type 1 evidence, grade A recommendation

B. Grade A evidence quality, type 1 recommendation

C. High-quality evidence, strong recommendation

D. Grade A evidence, weak recommendation

E. Low-quality evidence, weak recommendation

8. As to the rare chronic side effects of drug treatment, the original study that should be searched first is usually (D)

A. Randomized controlled trial   B. Cross-sectional study

C. Case series   D. Case-control study

E. Cohort study

9. The main application of life quality assessment does **not include** (E)

A. Evaluation of curative effect of chronic disease intervention

B. Clinical trials of new drugs

C. Evaluation of the health status of the population and patients

D. Resource allocation, planning and decision-making

E. Basic pathology research

10. A researcher was interested in the cause of neonatal jaundice. He selected 100 children suffering from the disease, and selected 100 newborn babies who did not in the same hospital. He then reviewed the gynecological and childbirth records of the mothers to determine various exposure factors before and during childbirth. What kind of research is this study? (C)

A. Current situation study   B. Cohort study

C. Case-control study   D. Clinical trial

E. Ecological research

11. As to the collection process of relevant literature for systematic review, which of the following is **inappropriate**? (E)

A. The scope of collecting literature is clear

B. Specific and objective criteria for evaluating the quality of the collected literature

C. The analysis of the original literature used is scientific and effective

D. Multiple channels and systematic retrieval methods should be used

E. Unpublished literature cannot be used

12. Which of the following is **not** the core of evidence-based medicine? (D)

A. Best research evidence

B. Physician's clinical skills and experience

C. Patient wishes

D. Best laboratory

E. Individualization of clinical decision

13. Each screening test has a normal reference range, and during census, the diagnostic test is expected with (A)

A. High sensitivity and relatively low false positive rate

B. High specificity and relatively low false positive rate

C. High sensitivity and relatively low true positive rate

D. High specificity and relatively low true positive rate

E. High specificity, relatively high of true negative rate

14. Patients with non-small cell lung cancer were randomly divided into 2 groups: one group was treated with conventional chemotherapy and the other group was treated with gefitinib. They were followed up for 3 years, and the survival rate was compared. The rate of loss to follow-up in the chemotherapy group was 25%, and that in the gefitinib group was 15%. What method can be used to investigate the impact of loss to follow-up on the results? (B)

A. Multi-factor COX regression

B. Sensitivity analysis

C. Exclude people who are lost to follow-up and analyze

D. ITT analysis

E. PP analysis

15. Assessment of health-related quality of life includes (E)

A. Physiological function

B. Mental function

C. Social role

D. Financial situation

E. Physiological function, mental function, social role and financial situation

16. Which of the following is **not included** in the feasibility evaluation of the scale? (C)

A. Complete time

B. Degree of difficulty

C. Cultural adaptation

D. Responsibility of items

E. Risk to patients

Case question

1. After 90 days of treatment for patients with acute cerebral infarction.

Questions:

(1) The main outcome indicator among the prognostic indicators is (H)

(2) The secondary outcome indicator among the prognostic indicators is (G)

A. Blood pressure

B. Liver and kidney function

C. Electrocardiogram

D. Blood routine

E. Head CT

F. Head MRI

G. Barthel Index

H. Rankin scale score

2. Two doctors performed B-scan ultrasonography and liver function tests on 100 people with fatty liver.

Questions:

(1) The index to evaluate the consistency of the B-scan ultrasonography results of two patients is (H)

(2) The index to evaluate the consistency of the liver function test of the two is (G)

A. Sensitivity	B. Specificity
C. Forecast value	D. Likelihood ratio
E. Chi-square value	F. t value
G. Intra-group correlation coefficient	H. Kappa value

Multiple choice questions

1. The role and value of evidence-based medicine in clinical medicine are mainly reflected in (ABCE)

A. Promoting clinical practice and improving medical care

B. Serving for medical education and cultivating high-quality talents

C. Providing guidance for the topic selection of clinical scientific research

D. Related to some clinical disciplines rather than others

E. Providing a series of evaluation standards and methods for the research evidence of disease etiology, diagnosis, treatment and prognosis

2. The control group of the diagnostic test should include (ADE)

A. Healthy volunteers

B. Patients with typical clinical manifestations

C. Patients with atypical clinical manifestations

D. Other cases easily confused with the target disease

E. Patients with other diseases in different systems

3. Which of the following approaches can help us select and evaluate the results of evidence-based medicine retrieval? (ABC)

A. Read the abstract	B. Browse full text
C. Contact the author	D. Search by subject terms
E. Use logical grouping characters	

Short-answer questions

1. Briefly describe the "three basic elements " and "five implementation steps" of evidence-based medicine.

[Reference answer] Evidence-based medicine is clinical medicine that follows evidence. The core is that clinicians should seriously, wisely and deliberately use the latest and best scientific research obtained in clinical studies to diagnose and treat patients. It is a combination of the best evidence and the clinical experience of physicians and the needs and values of patients.

The five implementation steps include: asking clinical questions, transforming clinical information into answerable questions; searching for evidence, searching for the best evidence related to the problem; evaluating evidence, evaluating the validity, applicability and effectiveness of the evidence; applying evidence, combining evidence evaluation with clinical experience and patient intentions; after evaluation, evaluating implementation effects and making improvements.

2. What are the main research designs to verify the etiology hypothesis? And explain the strength of the causal argumentation of each research design.

[Reference answer] Case reports, cross-sectional studies, case-control studies, cohort studies, randomized controlled trials. In terms of the strength of causal argumentation, experimental studies are greater than observational studies, and studies with controls are greater than studies without controls.

3. To evaluate the efficacy of a weight-loss drug, a doctor designed a clinical study and selected 200 women with obesity. The effective rate of weight loss after using the drug for one course of treatment was 60%, while another 200 women observed during the same period who did not take the drug showed no significant change in weight. The doctor believed that the weight-loss drug was effective.

Questions:

(1) What is the clinical problem of the study? Please use PICO mode to list.

(2) What is the design type of the study?

(3) According to the design plan, can we get the conclusion that the weight-loss drug is effective? And explain the reason.

[Reference answer] For women with obesity (P) taking weight-loss drug (I) compared with not taking drug (C), is there any change in body weight (O)? Non-randomized controlled trial; Although there are controls, they are not randomized, and the baseline condition before treatment is unknown. The doctor needs to further adopt randomized controlled clinical trials.

推荐阅读 References

[1] Evidence-based medicine. A new approach to teaching the practice of medicine [J]. Jama, 1992, 268(17): 2420-2425.

[2] 李国荣, 乔友林, 马莉, 等. 疾病筛查方法和策略的计量评价研究 [J]. 中国卫生统计, 2011, 28(03): 261-263.

[3] BASSLER D, BUSSE J W, KARANICOLAS P J, et al. Evidence-based medicine targets the individual patient, part 1: how clinicians can use study results to determine optimal individual care [J]. Evid Based Med, 2008, 13(4): 101-102.

[4] BASSLER D, BUSSE J W, KARANICOLAS P J, et al. Evidence-based medicine targets the individual patient, part 2: guides and tools for individual decision-making [J]. Evid Based Med, 2008, 13(5): 130-131.

[5] BROUWERS M C, KHO M E, BROWMAN G P, et al. AGREE II: advancing guideline development, reporting and evaluation in health care [J]. Cmaj, 2010, 182(18): E839-842.

[6] BURNS P B, ROHRICH R J, CHUNG K C. The levels of evidence and their role in evidence-based medicine [J]. Plast Reconstr Surg, 2011, 128(1): 305-310.

[7] CITROME L, KETTER T A. Teaching the philosophy and tools of evidence-based medicine: misunderstandings and solutions [J]. J Evid Based Med, 2009, 2(4): 220-225.

[8] GRIMES D A, SCHULZ K F. An overview of clinical research: the lay of the land [J]. Lancet, 2002, 359(9300): 57-61.

[9] GUYATT G H, OXMAN A D, VIST G E, et al. GRADE: an emerging consensus on rating quality of evidence and strength of recommendations [J]. Bmj, 2008, 336(7650): 924-926.

[10] GUYATT G. Five Directions for Evidence-based Medicine [J]. 中国循证医学杂志, 2006,(03): 157-159.

[11] HAYDEN J A, CôTé P, BOMBARDIER C. Evaluation of the quality of prognosis studies in systematic reviews [J]. Ann Intern Med, 2006, 144(6): 427-437.

[12] INSTITUTE OF MEDICINE COMMITTEE ON STANDARDS FOR DEVELOPING TRUSTWORTHY CLINICAL PRACTICE G. //GRAHAM R, MANCHER M, MILLER WOLMAN D, et al. Clinical Practice Guidelines We Can Trust. Washington (DC):National Academies Press (US),2011.

[13] LAUPACIS A, WELLS G, RICHARDSON W S, et al. Users' Guides to the Medical Literature: V. How to Use an Article About Prognosis [J]. JAMA: The Journal of the American Medical Association, 1994, 272(3): 234-237.

[14] PAGE M J, MOHER D, BOSSUYT P M, et al. PRISMA 2020 explanation and elaboration: updated guidance and exemplars for reporting systematic reviews [J]. Bmj, 2021, 372(n160).

[15] POCOCK S J, STONE G W. The Primary Outcome Is Positive - Is That Good Enough? [J]. N Engl J Med, 2016, 375(10): 971-979.

[16] POCOCK S J, STONE G W. The Primary Outcome Fails - What Next? [J]. N Engl J Med, 2016, 375(9): 861-870.

[17] WOLFGANG AHRENS, IRIS PIGEOT. Handbook of Epidemiology [M]. Berlin, Heidelberg : Springer, 2013.

[18] YOUNG J M, SOLOMON M J. How to critically appraise an article [J]. Nat Clin Pract Gastroenterol Hepatol, 2009, 6(2): 82-91.

中英文名词对照索引 Index